ATLAS OF

DIABETES

Second Edition

ATLAS OF
DIABETES
Second Edition

Editor

Jay S. Skyler, MD

Director, Division of Endocrinology, Diabetes, and Metabolism
Chairman, NIDDK Type 1 Diabetes TrialNet
University of Miami
Miami, Florida

With 23 contributors

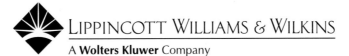

LIPPINCOTT WILLIAMS & WILKINS
A **Wolters Kluwer** Company

Philadelphia • Baltimore • New York • London
Buenos Aires • Hong Kong • Sydney • Tokyo

Current Medicine

400 Market Street
Suite 700
Philadelphia, PA 19106

Developmental Editor:	*Teresa M. Giuliana*
Commissioning Supervisor, Books:	*Annmarie D'Ortona*
Cover Design:	*John McCullough*
Design and Layout:	*Jennifer Knight, John McCullough*
Illustrators:	*William C. Whitman, Jr., Jacob C. Shoemaker, Maureen Looney, Wieslawa Langenfeld, Kay Elwood*
Assistant Production Manager:	*Margaret LaMare*
Indexer:	*Alexandra Nickerson*

Atlas of diabetes / editor, Jay Skyler.-- 2nd ed.
       p.; cm.
      Rev. ed. of: Diabetes / volume editor, C. Ronald Kahn. c2000.
      Includes bibliographical references and index.
      ISBN 0-781-74240-4 (alk. paper)
        1. Diabetes--Atlases. I. Skyler, Jay S. II. Diabetes.
      [DNLM: 1.Diabetes Mellitus--Atlases. WK 17 A8808 2002]
    RC660 .A87 2002
    616.4'62--dc21

                                      2002023752

Printed in Hong Kong

10 9 8 7 6 5 4 3 2 1

Distributed worldwide by Lippincott Williams & Wilkins

Contributors

LLOYD PAUL AIELLO, MD, PHD

Associate Professor
Department of Ophthalmology
Harvard University School of Medicine
Assistant Director, Beetham Eye Institute
Joslin Diabetes Center
Boston, Massachusetts

MARK A. ATKINSON, PHD

Professor
Department of Pathology
University of Florida
Gainesville, Florida

MICHAEL BROWNLEE, MD

Professor
Departments of Medicine and Pathology
Albert Einstein College of Medicine
New York, New York

VERONICA M. CATANESE, MD

Associate Professor
Departments of Medicine and Cell Biology
Senior Associate Dean for Education
New York University School of Medicine
New York, New York

ELE FERRANNINI, MD

Professor
Department of Internal Medicine
University of Pisa
Staff Physician
Santa Chiara Hospital
Pisa, Italy

TRACEY L. FISHER, BA

Graduate Student
Joslin Diabetes Center
Boston, Massachusetts

JOHN E. GERICH, MD

Professor
Department of Medicine
University of Rochester
Rochester, New York

NIYAZ GOSMANOV, MD

Fellow
Department of Medicine
University of Rochester School of Medicine
Rochester, New York

ROBERT R. HENRY, MD

Professor
Department of Medicine
University of California San Diego
Chief, Diabetes/Metabolism Section
VA San Diego Healthcare System
San Diego, California

LOIS JOVANOVIC, MD

Clinical Professor
Department of Medicine
Division of Endocrinology
University of Southern California
Los Angeles, California
Director and Chief Scientific Officer
Sansum Medical Research Center
Santa Barbara, California

FRANCINE RATNER KAUFMAN, MD

Professor
Department of Pediatrics
University of Southern California Keck School of
   Medicine
Head, Division of Endocrinology
Children's Hospital of Los Angeles
Los Angeles, California

ABBAS E. KITABCHI, PHD, MD

Professor
Departments of Medicine and Biological Sciences
Director of Training Program
Division of Endocrinology, Diabetes, and Metabolism
The University of Tennessee Health Sciences Center
Attending Physician
William Bowld Hospital and Regional Medical Center
Consultant
Baptist Memorial Hospital and Methodist
   Healthcare System
Memphis, Tennessee

ELEFTHERIA MARATOS-FLIER, MD

Assistant Professor
Department of Medicine
Harvard University School of Medicine
Head, Section of Obesity
Joslin Diabetes Center
Boston, MA

SUNDER R. MUDALIAR, MD, MRCP(UK), FACE

Assistant Clinical Professor
Department of Medicine
University of California San Diego
Staff Physician
Veterans Affairs San Diego HealthCare System
San Diego, California

MARY BETH MURPHY, RN, MS, CDE, MBA

Research Nurse Director
Division of Endocrinology, Diabetes, and Metabolic
   Diseases
University of Tennessee Health Sciences Center
Memphis, Tennessee

DAVID M. NATHAN, MD

Professor
Department of Medicine
Harvard University School of Medicine
Director, Diabetes Center and General Clinical
   Research Center
Massachusetts General Hospital
Boston, Massachusetts

F. JOHN SERVICE, MDCM, PHD

Professor
Department of Endocrinology
Mayo Medical School
McDonough Professor of Medicine
Mayo Clinic
Rochester, Minnesota

ARUN J. SHARMA, PHD

Instructor
Department of Medicine
Harvard University School of Medicine
Assistant Investigator
Section of Islet Transplantation and Cell Biology
Joslin Diabetes Center
Boston, Massachusetts

ROBERT C. STANTON, MD

Assistant Professor
Department of Medicine
Harvard University School of Medicine
Chief, Renal Section
Joslin Diabetes Center
Boston, Massachusetts

AARON I. VINIK, MD, PHD

Professor
Diabetes Institute
Eastern Virginia Medical School
Director, The Leonard Strelitz Diabetes Research
   Institutes
Norfolk, Virginia

GORDON C. WEIR, MD

Professor
Department of Medicine
Harvard University School of Medicine
Head, Section of Islet Transplantation and Cell Biology
Joslin Diabetes Center
Boston, Massachusetts

SUSAN BONNER-WEIR, PHD

Associate Professor
Department of Medicine
Harvard University School of Medicine
Senior Investigator
Section of Islet Transplantation and Cell Biology
Joslin Diabetes Center
Boston, Massachusetts

MORRIS F. WHITE, PHD

Associate Professor
Department of Medicine
Harvard University School of Medicine
Associate Investigator
Joslin Diabetes Center
Boston, Massachusetts

Preface

Diabetes mellitus is increasing in incidence, prevalence, and importance as a chronic disease throughout the world. In the United States, the burden of diabetes is enormous, whether one considers the magnitude of the population afflicted, the impact on the lives of people affected by diabetes, the morbidity rendered by diabetes, or the economic toll it takes. Over 17 million Americans, 6.2% of the population, have diabetes. Over 1 million Americans develop diabetes each year, or over 2800 people each day. Among those under 20 years of age, the disease pattern is changing rapidly. One out of every 400 to 500 children and adolescents has type 1 diabetes. The striking thing, however, is that the incidence of type 2 diabetes among adolescents has increased 15-fold since 1982. In some pediatric diabetes clinics, the number of patients with type 2 diabetes now equals the number with type 1 diabetes. Indeed, the average age of onset of type 2 diabetes is dropping. With more people developing the disease in their teens, 20s, and 30s, their lifetime potential for complications increases.

Strikingly, although type 2 diabetes is increasing among the young, its burden on older patients is growing as well. The prevalence among people 65 years of age or older now exceeds 20%, with diabetes afflicting 7 million Americans in this age group. Thus, 20% of the Medicare population has diabetes, but 30% of the Medicare budget is spent on diabetes, an indication of the disproportionate share of the health care budget that diabetes consumes. Diabetes accounts for 14% of total health care costs.

There are a number of paradoxes in terms of complications. Diabetic retinopathy is the leading cause of blindness in adults of working age, yet the National Eye Institute estimates that 90% of vision loss caused by diabetic retinopathy is preventable. Diabetic nephropathy is far and away the leading cause of end-stage renal disease, accounting for 43% of all new cases, yet the National Institute of Diabetes, Digestive, and Kidney Diseases estimates that most future end-stage renal disease from diabetes is probably preventable. Diabetes accounts for 60% of all nontraumatic lower extremity amputations, with diabetes imposing a 15- to 40-fold increased risk of amputation compared to the nondiabetic population, yet the American Diabetes Association and the Centers for Disease Control estimate that more than 85% of limb loss is preventable. The presence of type 2 diabetes imposes a risk of coronary events equal to that of a previous myocardial infarction in the nondiabetic population, yet people with diabetes are not as likely to be prescribed cardioprotective medication. Although in the United States the incidence and mortality rates from heart disease and stroke are decreasing in the nondiabetic population, patients with diabetes are two- to sixfold more likely to develop heart disease and two- to fourfold more likely to suffer a stroke. Optimal glycemic control is critical for reducing the risk of long-term complications associated with diabetes. The Diabetes Control and Complications Trial provided strong evidence of the importance of achieving near-normal blood glucose levels in type 1 diabetic patients by means of intensive insulin therapy programs. The United Kingdom Prospective Diabetes Study suggested similar beneficial effects of improved glycemic control in type 2 diabetes. Yet diabetes patients are still not achieving recommended target blood glucose values. Data from the Third National Health and Nutrition Examination Survey of 1988–1994 showed that approximately 60% of patients with type 2 diabetes had HbA_{1c} values greater than 7% and that 25% had HbA_{1c} values greater than 9%.

The bottom line is that neither physicians nor patients are paying enough attention to diabetes. Diabetes is underrepresented in medical school curricula compared to the burden of the disease. This is particularly the case when it is appreciated that this disease impacts virtually all medical specialties. Our health care system fails to adequately meet the needs of patients with chronic diseases in general, diabetes in particular. Referrals of patients with diabetes to diabetes specialist teams (which include medical nutrition therapists and certified diabetes educators, as well as diabetologists/endocrinologists) are infrequent, and there are not enough of these teams or the specialists who constitute them.

Meanwhile, treatment options are expanding dramatically. As recently as 1995, the only classes of medications available in the United States to lower glycemia were sulfonylureas and insulins. Now we have added biguanides, α-glucosidase inhibitors, glitazones (PPARγ activators), glinides (rapid-acting insulin secretagogues), rapid-acting insulin analogues, and long-acting basal insulin analogues. Several new classes of agents are in development. The use of insulin pumps has increased more than six-fold since 1985. Pancreatic transplantation has become a routine procedure in the company of kidney transplantation.

There has been an exciting explosion of knowledge about fundamental mechanisms related to diabetes. We have gained insights into the pathogenesis both of type 1 and type 2 diabetes, and with that, the prospect of implementing prevention strategies to delay or interdict the disease processes. Great progress has been made in islet transplantation, which offers the potential of reversing diabetes. The major challenge has become finding sources of islets sufficient to meet potential needs, given that there are annually only about 4000 organ donors nationwide. Whether diabetes prevention will come from advances in understanding the processes of islet neogenesis and proliferation, from genetic engineering, or from protecting xenoislets from attack remains unclear. All are potential avenues of pursuit.

It is with this background that we have asked leading authorities to contribute their thoughts and images concerning various aspects of diabetes. Their input makes this *Atlas* possible.

Jay S. Skyler, MD

Contents

Contents, *continued*

Color Plates

REGULATION OF INSULIN SECRETION AND ISLET CELL FUNCTION

Gordon C. Weir, Susan Bonner-Weir, and Arun J. Sharma

The β cells of the islets of Langerhans are the only cells in the body that make a meaningful quantity of insulin, a hormone that has evolved to be essential for life, exerting critical control over carbohydrate, fat, and protein metabolism. Islets are scattered throughout the pancreas; they vary in size but typically contain about 1000 cells of which about 80% are β cells located in a central core surrounded by a mantle of non–β cells. A human pancreas contains about one million islets, which comprise only about 1% of the mass of the pancreas. Insulin is released into the portal vein, which means the liver is exposed to particularly high concentrations of insulin.

Insulin secretion from β cells responds very precisely to small changes in glucose concentration in the physiologic range, thereby keeping glucose levels within the range of 70–150 mg/dL in normal individuals. β cells have a unique differentiation that permits linkage of physiologic levels of glucose to the metabolic signals that control the release of insulin. Thus, there is a close correlation between the rate of glucose metabolism and insulin secretion. This is dependent upon the oxidation of glucose-derived acetyl-CoA and also NADH generated by glycolysis, which is shuttled to mitochondria to contribute to ATP production. Insulin secretion is also regulated by various other physiologic signals. During eating, insulin secretion is enhanced by not only glucose, but amino acids and the gut hormones GLP-1 and gastric inhibitory peptide. Free fatty acids can also modulate insulin secretion, particularly to help maintain insulin secretion during prolonged fasting. The parasympathetic nervous system has a stimulatory effect exerted by acetylcholine and probably the peptidergic mediator VIP, which may also contribute to enhanced insulin secretion during eating. The sympathetic nervous system with epinephrine from the adrenal medulla and norepinephrine from nerve terminals acts upon α-adrenergic receptors to inhibit insulin secretion. This suppression of insulin is particularly useful during exercise. Important drugs include sulfonylureas, which have a stimulatory influence useful for the treatment of diabetes, and diazoxide, with an inhibitory effect used for treatment of hypoglycemia caused by insulin-producing tumors.

Type 1 diabetes is caused by reduced β-cell mass resulting from autoimmune destruction of β cells, which leads to profound insulin deficiency that can progress to fatal hyperglycemia and ketoacidosis. The non–β-cells of the islet are spared, with glucagon secretion actually being excessive, which accounts for some of the hyperglycemia of the diabetic state. The situation is more complicated in type 2 diabetes, which has a strong genetic basis predisposing individuals to obesity and insulin resistance, a problem greatly magnified by our Western lifestyle with its plentiful food and lack of physical activity. Diabetes, however, only develops when β cells are no longer able to compensate for this insulin resistance. Indeed, most people with insulin resistance never develop diabetes, but as our population ages, more β-cell decompensation occurs and the prevalence of diabetes rises. Pathology studies indicate that β-cell mass in type 2 diabetes is about 50% of normal and that islets often are infiltrated with amyloid deposits that may have a toxic effect upon β cells.

In all forms of diabetes, whether type 2 diabetes, early type 1 diabetes, or failing pancreas or islet transplants, insulin secretory abnormalities are found that seem largely secondary to exposure of β cells to the diabetic milieu and that are reversible if normoglycemia can be restored. The most prominent abnormality is an impairment of glucose-induced insulin secretion, which is more severe for early release (first phase) than the longer second phase of secretion. In contrast, β-cell responses to such nonglucose secretagogues as arginine, GLP-1, isoproterenol, or sulfonylureas are more intact. The etiology of these β-cell secretory abnormalities is not fully understood, but β cells exposed to abnormally high glucose concentrations lose the differentiation that normally equips them with the unique metabolic machinery needed for glucose-induced insulin secretion. Marked abnormalities are found at the level of gene expression that appear to have a crippling effect upon the metabolic integrity of the β cell. Abnormalities of glucagon secretion are also found in both forms of diabetes, with secretion not being appropriately suppressed by hyperglycemia or stimulated by hypoglycemia, which is problematic because glucagon is an important counterregulatory hormone for protection against hypoglycemia. This failure of glucagon to respond makes people with type 1 diabetes more vulnerable to the dangers of insulin-induced hypoglycemia.

Anatomy, Embryology, and Physiology

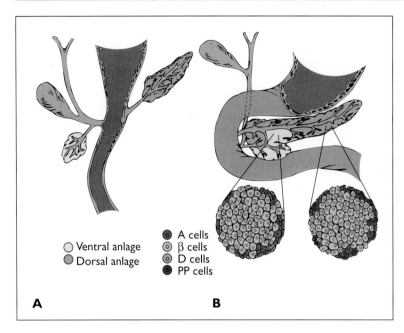

FIGURE 1-1. Embryologic origin of pancreas and islets. A dorsal anlage and one or two ventral anlagen form from the primitive gut (**A**) and later fuse (**B**) [1]. The ventral anlage forms the head of the pancreas and has pancreatic polypeptide-rich islets with few if any A cells. The dorsal anlage forms the major portion of the pancreas, that being the tail, body, and part of the head; here the islets are glucagon-rich and pancreatic polypeptide-poor. Roughly the A and PP cells substitute for each other in number (15%–25% of the islet cells) while the percentages of β cells (70%–80%) and D cells (5%) remain the same.

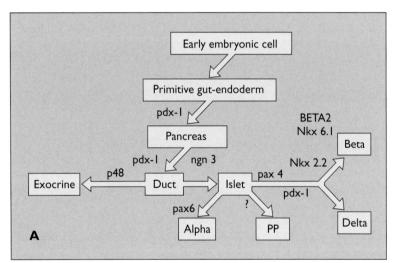

B. UNIQUE β-CELL DIFFERENTIATION	
Increased Expression	**Decreased Expression**
GLUT2	Glucose-6-phosphatase
Glucokinase	Hexokinase
mGPDH	Lactate dehydrogenase
Pyruvate carboxylase	PEPCK
Insulin	c-myc
IAPP	
PDX-1	
Nkx 6.1	

FIGURE 1-2. Pancreatic and islet differentiation. The complex control of differentiation of the pancreas and its three major components, exocrine acinar cells, ducts, and islets of Langerhans are being elucidated by genetic analysis (**A** and **B**) [1–3]. At present only some of the transcription factors involved in the transition from endoderm to pancreas and then to the final mature pancreatic cell types are known; several of them (BETA 2, Nkx 2.2, Nkx 6.1, ngn 3) are also involved in the development of the nervous system. One that is clearly necessary, but not sufficient, is pdx-1(ipf-1/stf-1/idx-1); without it no pancreas is formed and later it seems to be needed for β-cell differentiation. Both exocrine and islet cells differentiate from the pancreatic ductal epithelium, but whether they arise from the same precursor pool or even whether all the islet cells share a cell lineage remains unanswered. PP—pancreatic polypeptide. (*Adapted from* Edlund [1].)

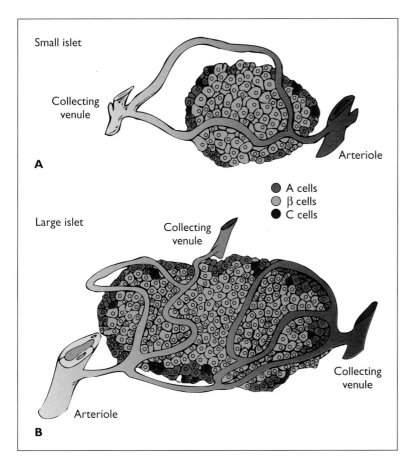

FIGURE 1-3. Islet vasculature and core/mantle relations. A diagrammatic summary of combined data from corrosion casts and the serial reconstructions of rat islets [2]. In both small and large islets, β cells make up the central core while the non–β cells (A, pancreatic polypeptide, and D cells) form the surrounding mantle. The A cells containing glucagon are found mainly in islets of the dorsal lobe of the pancreas, pancreatic polypeptide cells are found mainly in ventral lobe islets, and D cells containing somatostatin are found in islets of both lobes of the pancreas.

Short arterioles enter an islet at discontinuities of the non–β cell mantle and branch into capillaries that form a glomerular-like structure. After traversing the β-cell mass, capillaries penetrate the mantle of non-β cells as the blood leaves the islet. In small islets (less than 160 μm in diameter) (**A**), efferent capillaries pass through exocrine tissue before coalescing into collecting venules. In large islets (greater than 260 μm diameter) (**B**), capillaries coalesce at the edge of the islet and run along the mantle as collecting venules.

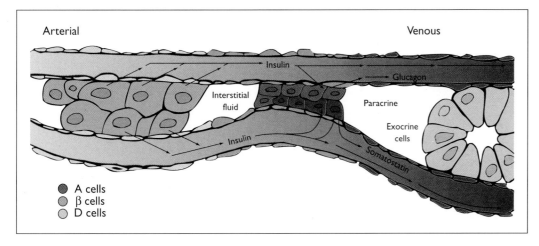

FIGURE 1-4. The relationship between islet core and mantle, indicating potential intra-islet portal-flow and paracrine interactions. This formulation is based on the known vascular anatomy and studies with passive immunization [4,5]. These relationships suggest that β cells, being upstream, are unlikely to be very much influenced by the glucagon and somatostatin produced by the A cells and D cells of the islet mantle, respectively. The downstream A cells, however, may be strongly influenced by insulin from the upstream β cells, which have a suppressive influence upon glucagon secretion. This helps explain why glucagon secretion cannot be suppressed by the hyperglycemia of diabetes, which means that glucagon is secreted in excessive amounts, thus contributing further to the hyperglycemia of diabetes. This vascular pattern is known as the islet-acinar portal circulation, which means that islet hormones are released downstream directly onto exocrine cells; insulin in particular is thought to have a trophic effect upon the exocrine pancreas.

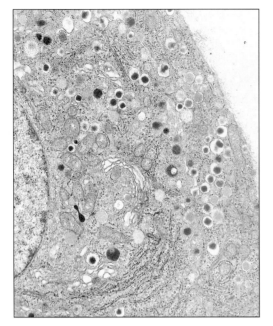

FIGURE 1-5. Electron micrograph of a β cell. There are four major endocrine cell types in mammalian islets: the insulin-producing β cell, the glucagon-producing A cell, the somatostatin-producing D cell, and the pancreatic polypeptide-producing PP cell. Ultrastructural and immunocytochemical techniques are used to distinguish these cell types. β cells are polyhedral, being truncated pyramids about 10 x 10 x 8 μm, and are usually well granulated with about 10,000 secretory granules. There are two forms of insulin granules (250–350 nm in diameter): mature granules with an electron-dense core that is visibly crystalline in some species and a loosely fitting granule-limiting membrane giving the appearance of a spacious halo, and immature granules with little or no halo and moderately electron-dense contents. Immature granules have been shown to be the major, if not the only, site of proinsulin to insulin conversion [6]. In each granule, besides insulin, there are at least 100 other peptides, including IAPP/amylin [7].

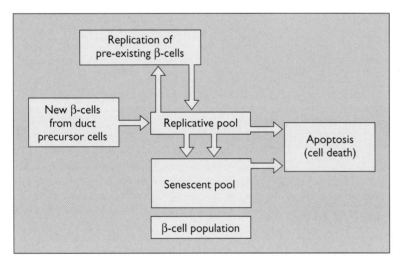

FIGURE 1-6. Mechanisms responsible for maintenance of β-cell mass. Both in normal development and in experimental studies it has become apparent that the population of β cells within an adult pancreas is dynamic and responds to metabolic demand with changes in mass and function in an effort to maintain euglycemia. The mass of β cells can change by cell number and/or cell size. Two mechanisms add new β cells: differentiation from precursor/stem cells in the ducts (often called neogenesis) and replication from pre-existing β cells [8]. It has been suggested that most cell types have a limited number of replications after which the ability to respond to replication signals is lost, so they are then considered to be senescent cells (terminally differentiated). These senescent cells can be long-lived and functional, probably functioning in some ways differently than younger replicative cells. Additionally, as with all cell types, β cells must have a finite lifespan and die by apoptosis [9]. The turnover of β cells implies that there are β cells of differing age at any stage of development. Adult β cells have only a low basal rate of replication, but this rate coupled with birth of new β cells from ducts must be enough to counterbalance cell loss and to accommodate functional demand.

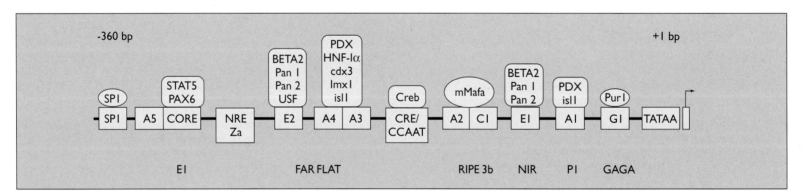

FIGURE 1-7. The promoter region of the insulin gene showing key enhancer elements and known binding transcription factors. Insulin gene expression is regulated by sequences at least 4 kb upstream from the transcription start site (represented by an arrow and designated as +1 bp) of the insulin gene. In adult mammals, insulin is selectively expressed in pancreatic β cells. A small (less than 400 bp) region of insulin promoter that is highly conserved in various mammalian species can regulate this selective expression and contains the major glucose control elements. This region can also recapitulate glucose responsive insulin gene expression.

In the figure, the organization of the proximal portion (-360 to +1 bp) of the insulin promoter is shown. Functionally conserved enhancer elements are illustrated as boxes. New names for these elements are shown within the boxes, while old names are shown below each box. Above the boxes are shown the names of cloned transcription factors that can bind corresponding elements. Enhancer elements E1, A2-C1, A4-A3, and E2 have been implicated in β-cell–specific expression of the insulin gene. The cell type-specific expression

is mediated by the restricted cellular distribution of the transcription factors (such as BETA2, mMafA, and PDX-1) that bind these elements [10]. Furthermore, these elements, along with element Za, are also responsible for glucose-regulated insulin gene expression. Other enhancer elements, CRE/CCAAT and CORE, regulate insulin gene expression in response to other signals such as cAMP (by regulating cAMP Regulatory Element Binding protein) and growth hormone or leptin (via signal transducer and activator of transcription [STAT] factor 5).

In addition to their role in regulating cell-specific and glucose responsive expression, insulin gene transcription factors are involved in pancreatic development and differentiation of ß cells. Lack of transcription factors such as PDX-1, BETA2, PAX6, and HNF-1a and isl1 results in either complete absence of or abnormal pancreatic development. Interestingly, humans with a mutant allele for PDX-1, BETA2, or HNF-1a develop maturity-onset diabetes of youth, whereas individuals with mutations in both PDX-1 alleles show pancreatic agenesis. (*Adapted from* Sander and German [11].)

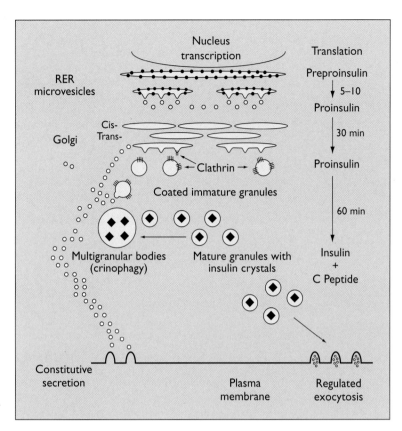

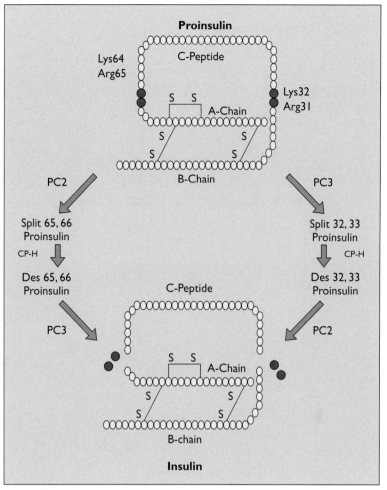

FIGURE 1-8. Pathways of insulin biosynthesis. Glucose stimulates the production of preproinsulin through effects on transcription and even stronger influences on translation. Shortly after its inception preproinsulin is cleaved to proinsulin which is then transported through the Golgi and packaged into clathrin-coated immature granules, where proinsulin is further processed to proinsulin-like peptides, insulin, and c-peptide. Granules containing crystallized insulin can either remain in a storage compartment, be absorbed into multigranular bodies where they are degraded by the process of crinophagy, or be secreted via the regulated pathway of secretion, the final event being exocytosis. Although the vast majority of insulin is secreted through the regulated pathway, a small amount can be released from microvesicles through the pathway of constitutive secretion. (See references 12 and 13 for more details).

FIGURE 1-9. Proinsulin processing. Proinsulin is cleaved by endopeptidases contained in secretory granules which act at the two dibasic sites, Arg31,Arg32 and Lys64,Arg65. PC2 also is known as type II proinsulin-processing endopeptidase and PC3 is the type I endopeptidase. Following cleavage by either PC2 or PC3, the dibasic amino acids are removed by the exopeptidase carboxypeptidase H (CP-H). Insulin and C-peptide are usually released in equimolar amounts. Of the secreted insulin immunoreactivity, about 2%–4% consists of proinsulin and proinsulin-related peptides. Because the clearance of these peptides in the circulation is considerably slower than insulin, they account for 10%–40% of circulating insulin immunoreactivity. About one third of proinsulin-like immunoreactivity is accounted for by proinsulin and most of the rest by des 32-33 split proinsulin, with only small amounts of des 65-66 split proinsulin being present. In type 2 diabetes the ratio of proinsulin-like peptides to insulin is increased, while in IGT this finding is less consistent. The increased proportion of secreted proinsulin-like peptides is thought to be due to depletion of mature granules from the increased secretory demand by hyperglycemia, leading to the release of the incompletely processed contents of the available immature granules [12,13]. (*Adapted from* Rhodes [12].)

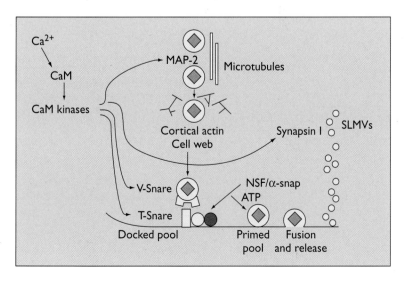

FIGURE 1-10. Distal steps of secretion. Insulin-containing secretory granules are associated with microtubules and the move to the cell surface via further interactions with the microfilaments of the cortical actin web. Increased cytosolic calcium plays a key role in several distal steps. Initially calcium binds to calmodulin (CaM), which can bind the CaM kinases. CaM kinase II has been localized to insulin secretory granules. These kinases can then phosphorylate proteins such as microtubule-associated protein-2 (MAP-2) and synapsin I, which may be involved in the exocytosis of synaptic-like microvesicles (SLMV). They may also regulate the key proteins involved in the docking of granules, v-SNARES (synaptobrevin [VAMP] and cellubrevin) and t-SNARES (SNAP-25 and syntaxin). The docking complex binds to α-SNAP (soluble NSF attachment protein) and NSF (N-ethyl-maleimide-sensitive fusion protein), the latter having ATPase activity which probably allows the formation of fusion competent granules that are primed for release as the first phase of insulin secretion. (*Adapted from* Easom [14].)

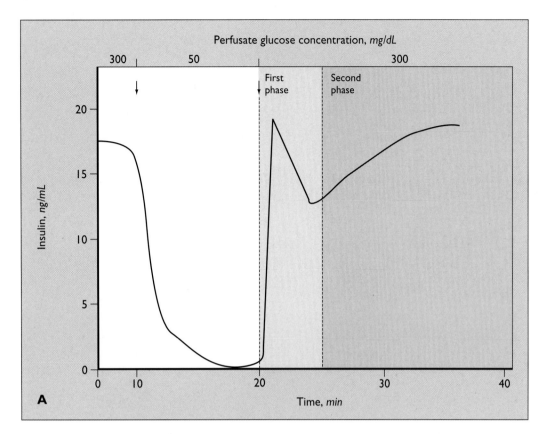

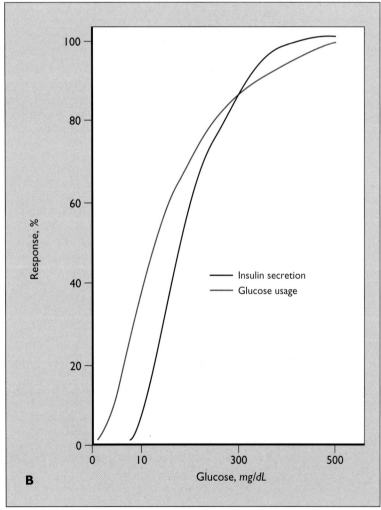

FIGURE 1-11. Glucose stimulation of insulin secretion. **A,** Insulin secretion from the isolated perfused rat pancreas. At glucose concentrations at 50 mg/dL or below, insulin secretory rates are very low. Challenge with a high concentration of glucose provokes a biphasic pattern of insulin response [15]. **B,** Comparative rates of insulin secretion and glucose utilization in isolated rat islets. Glucose utilization was measured by the conversion of 5-tritiated glucose to tritiated H_2O [16]. The curves show the close relationship between the two except at glucose concentrations below 4 mmol. Similar relationships are found between insulin secretion and glucose oxidation as measured by conversion of labeled glucose to carbon dioxide. (*Adapted from* Leahy *et al.* [15].)

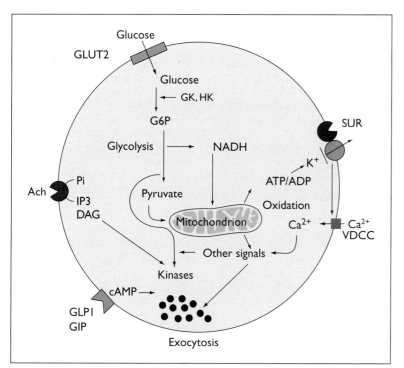

FIGURE 1-12. Mechanisms of β-cell secretion. Glucose enters the β cell through a facultative glucose transporter that allows rapid equilibration between extra- and intracellular glucose concentrations. Although GLUT2 is dominant in many species, GLUT1 may be more important in humans. Glucose is phosphorylated mainly by glucokinase (GK) rather than hexokinase (HK). Metabolism increases the ATP/ADP ratio both through oxidation via pyruvate and by NADH that is brought by shuttles into mitochondria [17]. The increases in the ATP/ADP ratio inhibit the ATP-sensitive potassium channel, which leads to depolarization and opening of voltage-dependent calcium channels (VDCC), with a resultant major increase in cytosolic calcium which triggers exocytosis. Glucose-stimulated insulin secretion is caused by two mechanisms: the triggering pathway, which is potassium channel ATP-dependent, and the amplifying pathway, which is potassium channel ATP-independent [17,18]. The molecular basis of the latter pathway is unknown. Cytosolic calcium levels can also be increased by release of calcium from the endoplasmic reticulum. Glucose has stimulatory effects on insulin secretion that are separate from depolarization, but poorly understood. Insulin secretion can also be stimulated by agents such as acetylcholine (Ach) that, via muscarinic receptors, work through lipid mediators such as inositol 1,4,5-triphosphate (IP3) and diacylglycerol (DAG). Glucagon-like peptide 1 (GLP-1) and gastric inhibitory peptide (GIP) are hormones released from gut with meals that stimulate secretion via adenylate cyclase and cAMP. There are many other agents that influence insulin secretion.

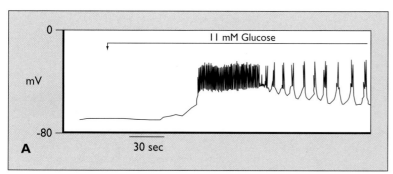

A

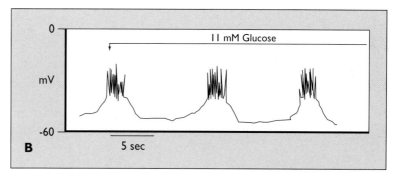

B

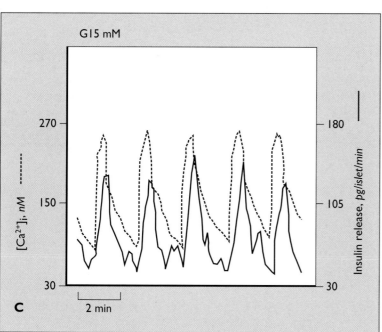

C

FIGURE 1-13. Glucose-induced electrical activity of the mouse β cell. **A**, The electrical activity of a mouse β cell contained in an isolated islet induced by stimulation with 11 mM glucose. When the membrane depolarizes to about -50 mV, bursting occurs, which is periodic electrical activity. Note the biphasic pattern of electrical activity, which may be related to the first phase of insulin secretion but is shorter in duration and unlikely to be the full explanation. When depolarization reaches about -35 mV, action potentials, or spikes, occur, which are best seen in the expanded scale in **B**. When glucose levels are very high (>22 mM), continuous spiking activity is observed. **C**, Comparison of the oscillations of insulin release and calcium in a single pancreatic mouse islet during steady state stimulation with 15 mM glucose, suggesting a cause and effect relationship. Calcium was measured with fluorescence of fura-2 loaded into islets. Increased calcium spikes come mainly from entrance of extracellular calcium through L-type voltage gated calcium channels. The depolarization is mainly caused by closure of ATP-regulated potassium channels [19]. (Panels A and B adapted from Atwater et al. [20]; panel C adapted from Gilon et al. [21].)

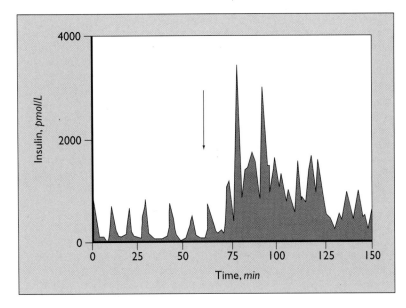

FIGURE 1-14. Pulsatile insulin secretion. Insulin is normally secreted in coordinated secretory bursts. In humans, pulses occur about every 10 minutes. In dogs they occur somewhat more rapidly, at about 7-minute intervals in a basal state. Although the variations in peripheral insulin levels are modest, marked variations can be found in the portal vein [22]. Basal pulsation is depicted during the 60-minute period. After oral ingestion of glucose (*arrow*), which produces both a glucose stimulus and an incretin effect, an increase in the amplitude of the bursts is seen, as well as an increase in frequency, with intervals falling from about 7 to 5 minutes. The mechanisms controlling the oscillations are uncertain. Metabolic oscillation of glycolysis must play a key role, but there may also be some kind of neural network that can coordinate communication between islets in different parts of the pancreas. (*Adapted from* Porksen *et al.* [23].)

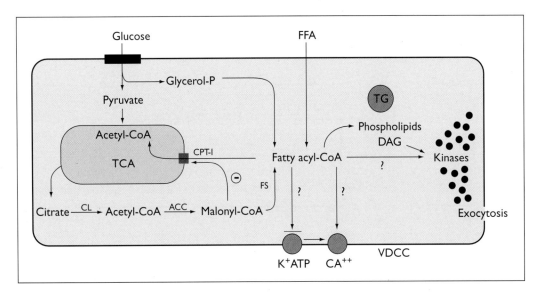

FIGURE 1-15. Fatty acid influence upon β-cell function. Fat metabolism is likely to have important influences upon insulin secretion, but the mechanisms responsible for these effects are still not well understood. It appears that the modest elevations of free fatty acids (FFAs) of obesity contribute to the hyperinsulinemia of that state. Depletion of circulating FFAs during prolonged fasting when glucose levels are low and β-cell lipid stores depleted results in impairment of insulin secretion. Excessive elevations of FFAs can have an inhibitory influence upon insulin secretion.

Some of glucose-stimulated insulin secretion could be mediated not only by glucose metabolism, but also by fatty acid mediators. Thus, increases in glucose metabolism could produce increased cytosolic concentrations of citrate, which can be converted by citrate lyase (CL) to acetyl-CoA, which can be turned into malonyl-CoA by acetyl-CoA carboxylase (ACC). Malonyl-CoA, can inhibit carnitine palmitoyltransferase I (CPT I), which helps control the entrance of fatty acyl-CoA into the fatty acid oxidation pathways of mitochondria. By inhibiting the entrance of fatty acyl-CoA into mitochondria, fatty acid mediators could be generated in the cytoplasm that might influence insulin secretion.

Fatty acids that enter the β cell could be converted to fatty acid mediators, which can act upon ion channels, kinases, or through other mechanisms to stimulate the exocytosis of insulin. Some of the lipid mediators include the phospholipid inositol 1,4,5-triphosphate (IP3) and diacylglycerol (DAG), which can act via protein kinase C. Alternatively, fatty acids could be stored as triglycerides (TG) for use during times of fuel deprivation. Fatty acid oxidation may under some circumstances contribute to ATP formation and thus help close the ATP-sensitive potassium channel (K+ATP) resulting in depolarization and opening of the voltage dependent calcium channels (VDCC). TCA—tricarboxylic acid cycle. (*Adapted from* McGarry and Dobbins [24] and Prentki and Corkey [22].)

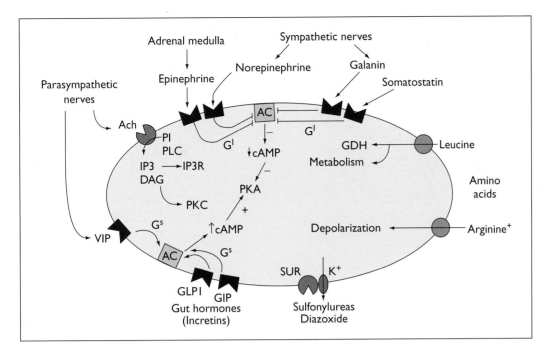

FIGURE 1-16. Effects upon insulin secretion by the autonomic nervous system, gut hormones, amino acids, and drugs. The parasympathetic arm of the autonomic nervous system has a stimulatory influence upon insulin secretion exerted by acetylcholine acting mainly through phospholipase C (PLC) to generate

inositol phosphate mediators and diacylglycerol (DAG). Parasympathetic stimulation also leads to release of the peptide mediator vasoactive intestinal peptide (VIP), which enhances secretion via stimulatory G proteins (G^s) acting through adenylate cyclase (AC). The sympathetic nervous system inhibits insulin secretion, with epinephrine and norepinephrine having a negative effect on AC through inhibitory G proteins (G^i). The sympathetic peptide mediator galanin and somatostatin have inhibitory effects on insulin secretion through similar mechanisms. The gut hormones GLP-1 and gastric inhibitory peptide (GIP) stimulate insulin secretion through cAMP and protein kinase A (PKA). Sulfonylureas stimulate insulin secretion by acting on the sulfonylurea receptor (SUR) to close the ATP-sensitive potassium channel, which causes depolarization. Diazoxide has an opposite effect leading to hyperpolarization, which is inhibitory. Amino acids stimulate insulin secretion by several mechanisms. Arginine is positively charged, producing depolarization when transported into β cells, but this is not an important mechanism at physiologic concentrations of arginine. Leucine can influence insulin secretion by being oxidized via acetyl CoA or through a more complex metabolic effect mediated by glutamate dehydrogenase (GDH). IP3—inositol 3 phosphate; IP3R—inositol 3 phosphate receptor.

Insulin Secretion in Type 2 Diabetes

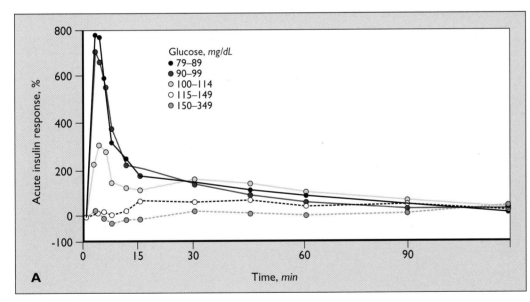

FIGURE 1-17. Insulin secretory characteristics in type 2 diabetes. **A,** Loss of early insulin secretory response to an intravenous glucose challenge as fasting plasma glucose rises in subjects progressing from the normal state towards type 2 diabetes [25]. It should be noted that impaired insulin responses to glucoses can even be seen before glucose levels rise to levels required for the diagnosis of impaired glucose tolerance (fasting glucose levels 110 mg/dL or above).

B, Preservation of acute insulin secretion in response to an intravenous pulse of arginine in type 2 diabetes [26]. The acute insulin responses to glucose were lost in these subjects. Insulin responses are also preserved for a variety of other secretagogues including isoproterenol, sulfonylureas, and the gut hormone glucagon-like peptide 1.

(Continued on next page)

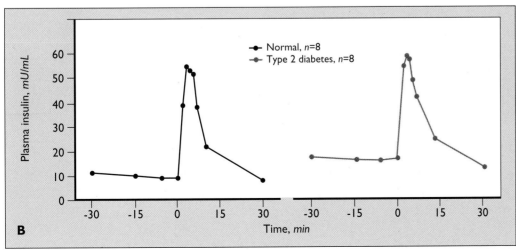

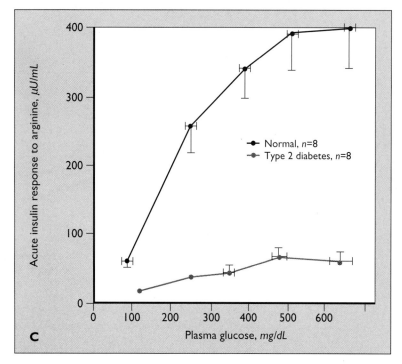

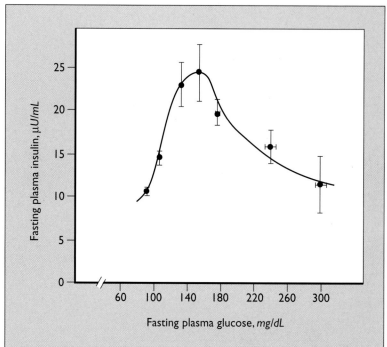

FIGURE I-17. (*Continued*) **C,** Loss of glucose influence upon arginine-stimulated insulin secretion in type 2 diabetes [27]. The insulin secretory responses to a 350 mg/dL glucose concentration in subjects with type 2 diabetes were similar to the responses to an 80 mg/dL glucose concentration in control subjects. However, when the glucose concentrations in control subjects were raised with glucose infusions, the insulin responses far exceeded those of subjects with type 2 diabetes. Because individuals with type 2 diabetes have been found to have a β-cell mass approximately 50% of normal, the response in these subjects, which is only about 15% of controls, suggests that the secretory capacity for a given β-cell mass is severely impaired. (*Adapted from* Ward *et al.* [27].)

FIGURE I-18. Inverted U-shaped curve of insulin secretion during progression from normal state to type 2 diabetes. Fasting plasma insulin levels rise as fasting glucose levels climb into the range of impaired glucose tolerance but then fall as diabetes develops and worsens. A similar pattern can be seen for plasma insulin levels obtained after an oral glucose or meal challenge. The rising insulin levels are likely to reflect a compensatory response to increasing insulin resistance, while the falling levels are indicative of β-cell failure, probably through a combination of impaired function and reduced β-cell mass. (*Adapted from* DeFronzo *et al.* [28].)

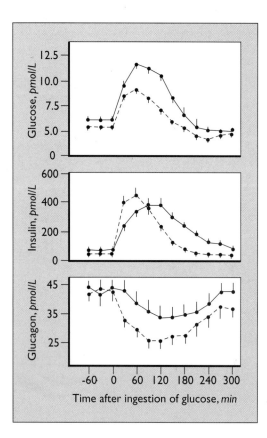

FIGURE I-19. Insulin secretory profiles in the state of impaired glucose tolerance (IGT) (*solid line*) during an oral glucose tolerance test (OGTT). The insulin responses at 60 and 90 minutes may be higher than those found in control patients (*broken line*), which probably reflects the combined influence of higher glucose levels at these time points and insulin resistance. Importantly, the insulin responses at 30 minutes in IGT are typically lower than normal, indicating the presence of a reduction in early impairment of glucagon suppression leading to an inefficient suppression of hepatic glucose output, which contributes to the higher glucose levels found in the latter stages of OGTT. The early insulin responses found after oral glucose are higher than those seen after an intravenous glucose challenge. This is thought to be due to the insulinotropic effects of the gut peptides GLP-1 and GIP, and possibly to some influence from activation of the parasympathetic nervous system. (*Adapted from* Mitrakou *et al.* [29].)

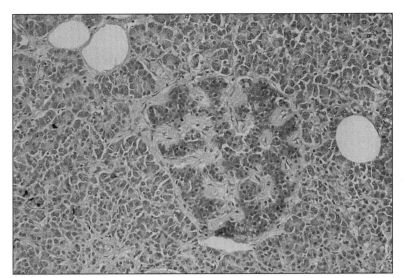

FIGURE 1-20. (See Color Plate) Amyloid deposits in islets in type 2 diabetes. In this photomicrograph of an islet, insulin-containing cells are immunostained and amyloid deposition can be seen in the pericapillary space. The amyloid found in a high proportion of the islets of people with type 2 diabetes consists of β-pleated sheets of the peptide islet-associated polypeptide (IAPP, amylin), which consists of 37 amino acids. The sequence between positions 20 and 29 is important for the ability of this peptide to form amyloid. Production of IAPP is restricted to β cells and its content is only about 1% that of insulin. Amyloid deposition adjacent to β cells is found in diabetes and some insulinomas, but not in the normal state or in obesity with its insulin resistance and high rates of insulin secretion [30]. The mechanisms responsible for its deposition are not known. It is also unclear whether this amyloid formation contributes to the pathogenesis of type 2 diabetes, but it has been shown that human IAPP fibrils have a toxic effect on islet cells [31].

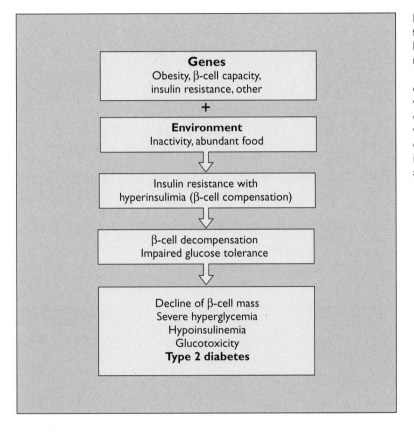

FIGURE 1-21. Pathogenesis of type 2 diabetes. This schema shows the various factors that contribute to the pathogenesis of type 2 diabetes [30]. Genes are likely to determine how well β cells can function over a lifetime. For example, most of the gene defects of maturity-onset diabetes of youth (MODY) (MODY 1, 3, and 4) and some mutations of mitochondrial DNA lead to diabetes, which often does not become manifest until middle age. There are probably genes which limit the ability of β-cell mass to compensate for insulin resistance over decades and even lead to a critical reduction in β-cell mass. Everything is made worse by the challenges of Western lifestyle with its plentiful food and lack of exercise. Once hyperglycemia develops, glucose toxicity can produce further impairment of β-cell function and worsen insulin resistance. Lipotoxicity also appears to have adverse effects on the same two sites.

STAGES OF β-CELL DECOMPENSATION IN DIABETES

Compensation for insulin resistance

β-cell hypertrophy

β-cell hyperplasia

Shift to the left of glucose dose-response curve

(Increased secretion per cell at given glucose level)

"Normal" or increased glucose-induced insulin secretion

Decompensation: mild hyperglycemia

Loss of glucose-induced insulin secretion

Preservation of responses to nonglucose secretagogues (arginine, etc.)

Normal insulin stores

Early β-cell dedifferentiation

Decreased gene expression of GLUT2, glucokinase, mGAPDH, pyruvate carboxylase, VDCC, SERCA3, IP3R-II, and transcription factors (PDX-1, HNFs, Nkx 6.1, pax6)

Increased gene expression of LDH, hexokinase, glucose-6-phosphatase, and the transcription factor c-myc

Decompensation: severe hyperglycemia

Loss of glucose-induced insulin secretion

Impairment of responses to nonglucose secretagogues (arginine, etc.)

Increased ratio of secreted proinsulin to insulin

Reduced insulin stores (degranulation)

More severe β-cell dedifferentiation

Decrease gene expression of insulin, IAPP, glucokinase, Kir6.2, SERCA2B, and transcription factor BETA 2

Increased gene expression of glucose-6-phosphatase, 12-lipoxygenase, fatty acid synthase, and the transcription factor C/EBPβ

FIGURE 1-22. Stages of β-cell decomposition in diabetes [3,25,32].

β-CELL GLUCOTOXICITY AND LIPOTOXICITY

Abnormal β-cell function in diabetes: β-cell function in diabetes is abnormal, whether in type 2 diabetes, early type 1 diabetes, or with an inadequate number of transplanted islets. A variety of secretory abnormalities have been identified, most notably loss of glucose-induced insulin secretion (GIIS), thought to be caused by exposure of β cells to the diabetic milieu

Definition problem: Descriptive terms include: glucotoxicity, lipotoxicity, exhaustion, excess demand, decreased reserve, fatigue, overwork, desensitization, stress, dysfunction, and others

Glucotoxicity

Loss of GIIS tightly tied to modest climb of glucose levels

Reduction of GIIS can be seen with fasting plasma glucose (FPG) of 100 mg/dL

Complete loss usually when FPG above 115 mg/dL

Abnormal GIIS in a diabetic state can be seen in absence of FFA increase

Lipotoxicity (contributions unclear)

Free fatty acids (FFAs) important for β-cell function, at least as permissive factor

Increased FFAs of obesity associated with high GIIS

Close correlation between FFAs of mild diabetes and loss of GIIS not well established

Very high FFAs inhibit GIIS

Synergy between FFAs and hyperglycemia not yet understood

FFAs important for maintaining insulin secretion during a prolonged fast

FIGURE 1-23. β-cell glucotoxicity and lipotoxicity [17,22,25].

References

1. Edlund H: Transcribing pancreas. *Diabetes* 1998, 47:1817–1823.

2. Jonas JC, Sharma A, Hasenkamp W, et al.: Chronic hyperglycemia triggers loss of pancreatic beta cell differentiation in an animal model of diabetes. *J Biol Chem* 1999, 274(20):14112–14121.

3. Weir GC, Laybutt DR, Kaneto H, et al.: Beta-cell adaptation and decompensation during the progression of diabetes. *Diabetes* 2001, 50(Suppl 1):S154–S159.

4. Bonner-Weir S, Orci L: New perspectives on the microvasculature of the islets of Langerhans in the rat. *Diabetes* 1982, 31:883–939.

5. Weir GC, Bonner-Weir S: Islets of Langerhans: the puzzle of intraislet interactions and their relevance to diabetes. *J Clin Invest* 1990, 85:983–987.

6. Orci L: The insulin factory: a tour of the plant surroundings and a visit to the assembly line. *Diabetologia* 1985, 28:528–546.

7. Guest PC, Bailyes EM, Rutherford NG, Hutton JC: Insulin secretory granule biogenesis. *Biochem J* 1991, 274:73–78.

8. Bonner-Weir S, Baxter LA, Schuppin GT, Smith FE: A second pathway for regeneration of the adult exocrine and endocrine pancreas: a possible recapitulation of embryonic development. *Diabetes* 1993, 42:1715–1720.

9. Finegood DT, Scaglia L, Bonner-Weir S: (Perspective) Dynamics of B-cell mass in the growing rat pancreas: estimation with a simple mathematical model. *Diabetes* 1995, 44:249–256.

10. Olbrot M, Rud J, Moss LG, Sharma A: Identification of beta-cell specific insulin gene transcription factor RIPE3b1 as a mammalian MafA. *Proc Natl Acad Sci USA* 2001. (In press.)

11. Sander M, German MS: The β-cell transcription factors and development of the pancreas. *J Mol Med* 1997, 75:327–340.

12. Rhodes CJ: Processing of the insulin molecule. In *Diabetes Mellitus*. Edited by LeRoith D, Taylor SI, Olefsky JM. Philadelphia: Lippincott-Raven; 1996:27–41.

13. Rhodes CJ, Alarcon C: What β-cell defect could lead to hyperproinsulinemia in NIDDM: Some clues from recent advances made in understanding the proinsulin conversion mechanism. *Diabetes* 1994, 43:511–517.

14. Easom RA: CaM kinase II: a protein kinase with extraordinary talents germane to insulin exocytosis. *Diabetes* 1999, 48(4):675–684.

15. Leahy JL, Cooper HE, Deal DA, Weir GC: Chronic hyperglycemia is associated with impaired glucose influence on insulin secretion: a study in normal rats using chronic in vivo glucose infusions. *J Clin Invest* 1986, 77:908–915.

16. Meglasson MD, Matschinsky FM: New perspectives on pancreatic islet glucokinase. *Am J Physiol* 1984, 246:E1–E13.

17. Henquin JC: Triggering and amplifying pathways of regulation of insulin secretion by glucose. *Diabetes* 2000, 49(11):1751–1760.

18. Weir GC, Bonner-Weir S: Insulin secretion in type 2 diabetes. In *Diabetes Mellitus: A Fundamental and Clinical Text*, edn 2. Edited by LeRoith D, Taylor SI, Olefsky JM. Philadelphia: Lippincott Williams & Wilkins; 2000:595–604.

19. Eto K, Tsubamoto Y, Terauchi Y, *et al.*: Role of NADH shuttle system in glucose-induced activation of mitochondrial metabolism and insulin secretion. *Science* 1999, 283:981–985.

20. Atwater I, Mears D, Rojas E: Electrophysiology of the pancreatic β-cell. In *Diabetes Mellitus*. Edited by LeRoith D, Taylor SI, Olefsky JM. Philadelphia: Lippincott-Raven; 1996:78–102.

21. Gilon P, Shepherd RM Henquin JC: Oscillations of secretion driven by oscillations of cytoplasmic Ca2 as evidenced in single pancreatic islets. *J Biol Chem* 1993, 268:22265–22268.

22. Prentki M, Corkey BE: Are the β-cell signaling molecules malonyl-CoA and cytosolic long-chain acyl-CoA implicated in multiple tissue defects of obesity and NIDDM? *Diabetes* 1996, 45:273–283.

23. Porksen N, Munn S, Steers J, *et al.*: Effects of glucose ingestion versus infusion on pulsatile insulin secretion. *Diabetes* 1996, 45:1317–1323.

24. McGarry JD Dobbins RL: Fatty acids, lipotoxicity and insulin secretion. *Diabetolgia* 1999, 42:128–138.

25. Brunzell JD, Robertson RP, Lerner RL, *et al.*: Relationships between fasting plasma glucose levels and insulin secretion during intravenous glucose tolerance tests. *J Clin Endocrinol Metab* 1976, 42:222–229.

26. Ward WK, Beard JC, Halter JB, *et al.*: Pathophysiology of insulin secretion in non–insulin-dependent diabetes mellitus. *Diabetes Care* 1984, 7:491–502.

27. Ward WK, Bolgiano DC, McKnight B, *et al.*: Diminished β-cell secretory capacity in patients with noninsulin-dependent diabetes mellitus. *J Clin Invest* 1984, 74:1318–1328.

28. DeFronzo RA, Ferrannini E, Simonson DC: Fasting hyperglycemia in noninsulin-dependent diabetes mellitus: contributions of excessive hepatic glucose production and impaired tissue glucose uptake. *Metabolism* 1989, 38:387–395.

29. Mitrakou A, Kelley D, Mokan M, *et al.*: Role of suppression of glucose production and diminished early insulin release in impaired glucose tolerance. *N Engl J Med* 1992, 326:22–29.

30. Kahn SE, Andrikopoulos S, Verchere CB: Islet amyloid: A long-recognized but underappreciated pathological feature of type 2 diabetes. *Diabetes* 1999, 48:241–253.

31. Lorenzo A, Bronwyn R, Weir GC, Yankner BA: Pancreatic islet cell toxicity of amylin associated with type 2 diabetes mellitus. *Nature* 1994, 368:756–760.

32. Tokuyama Y, Sturis J, Depaoli AM, *et al.*: Evolution of β-cell dysfunction in the male Zucker diabetic fatty rat. *Diabetes* 1995, 44:1447–1457.

MECHANISMS OF INSULIN ACTION

Morris F. White and Tracey L. Fisher

2

The storage and release of energy during feeding and fasting, as well as somatic growth, is regulated by the insulin/*IGF* signaling system. Insulin is best known for its role in the regulation of blood glucose, because it suppresses hepatic gluconeogenesis and promotes glycogen synthesis and storage in liver and muscle, triglycerides synthesis in liver and storage in adipose tissue, and amino acid storage in muscle [1]. However, the insulin signaling system has a broader role in mammalian physiology because it is shared with the insulin-like growth factor-1 receptor (IGFr1). During development, the insulin/*IGF* signaling system promotes somatic growth [2,3], and after birth it promotes growth and survival of many tissues, including pancreatic β cells, bone, neurons, and retina, to name a few [4–8]. Except for insulin, which can be replaced by injection as a treatment for diabetes, the complete dysfunction of essential components in the insulin/*IGF* signaling system is rare and invariably lethal. By contrast, partial failure of the insulin/*IGF* signaling system, frequently called insulin resistance, is associated with many metabolic disorders including dyslipidemia, hypertension, female infertility, and glucose intolerance that eventually progresses to diabetes [9].

Diabetes is an epidemic disorder that arises when insulin secretion from pancreatic β cells fails to maintain blood glucose levels in the normal range, especially when exacerbated by peripheral insulin resistance. The underlying pathophysiology of diabetes is diverse, but pancreatic β-cell failure is the common theme [10]. Type 2 diabetes is the most common form, which arises when pancreatic β-cell insulin secretion fails to compensate for peripheral insulin resistance [11]. Cline *et al.* [12] suggest that type 2 diabetes begins with skeletal muscle insulin resistance; however, peripheral insulin resistance might not be enough, as transgenic mice lacking muscle insulin receptors or patients with muscle insulin resistance owing to defective mRNA splicing do not ordinarily develop diabetes [13,14]. Despite incontrovertible evidence of genetic links for type 2 diabetes, diabetes is not a Mendelian disorder, so the genes responsible have been difficult to identify [15]. Consequently, linkage analysis with well-defined populations has made slow progress, although a possible role for the serine protease CAPN10 was recently revealed [16,17].

The mechanism by which insulin regulates energy metabolism and promotes cell growth has been studied extensively. In the 1950s, the pioneering work of Levine and coworkers led to the hypothesis that the effect of insulin on glucose utilization was due to increased glucose transport across the plasma membrane. In 1971, Roth *et al.* [18] discovered the insulin receptor, which led to identification of its tyrosine kinase activity a decade later and, ultimately, to the discovery of the insulin receptor substrate (IRS) proteins and the mechanism of insulin action.

Insulin exerts its diverse actions by inducing tyrosine phosphorylation of its cell surface receptor, which promotes the activity of the intracellular catalytic domain that phosphorylates tyrosine residues on other intracellular proteins [19]. Autophosphorylation further activates the receptor as a tyrosine-specific protein kinase, allowing the activated receptor to phosphorylate a host of cytosolic and membrane-bound proteins. Phosphorylation of protein substrates is required to mediate insulin action. The proximal effectors of insulin action have been convincingly identified; they include IRS proteins and several others [20]. IRS proteins serve an important function as "docking" molecules, favoring the assembly of multiprotein complexes and generation of intracellular signals. Much work remains to be done to understand how these intracellular signals coordinate biologic effects.

Understanding the molecular basis of insulin action will reveal the pathophysiology of diabetes. It is firmly established that patients with type 2 diabetes have defects of insulin action, commonly referred to as insulin resistance. Our approach to understanding diabetes has been based on the hypothesis that common signaling pathways might mediate both peripheral insulin action and pancreatic β-cell function. When elements of these pathways fail, owing to a combination of genetic variation and epigenetic challenge, diabetes might ensue. Evidence supporting this hypothesis emerged from our work on the insulin receptor substrates (IRS proteins). Disruption of the gene for *Irs2* in mice causes diabetes due to peripheral insulin resistance and dysregulated hepatic gluconeogenesis that is exacerbated by pancreatic β-cell failure [21]. Although all the experimental evidence is not yet available, failure of components that are regulated by the IRS2-branch of the insulin/*IGF* signaling pathway might be an important cause of diabetes.

Overview of Insulin Effects

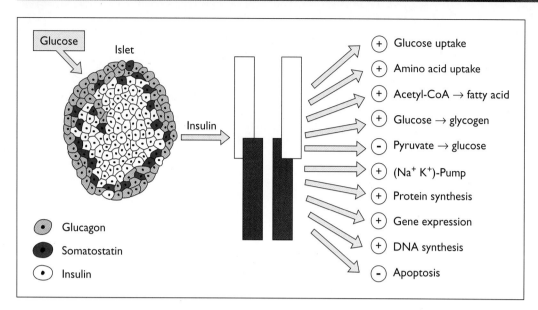

FIGURE 2-1. Insulin actions in peripheral tissues. Protein phosphorylation is required to mediate insulin action. After receptor autophosphorylation, the β subunit becomes active as a tyrosine-specific kinase and catalyzes phosphorylation of several intracellular proteins. This event promotes the multifaceted actions of insulin. Insulin stimulates glucose turnover by favoring its transport across the plasma membrane followed either by oxidative or nonoxidative disposal, the latter being associated with glycogen synthesis. The effect of insulin on glucose transport is observed only in skeletal muscle, adipose cells, and heart. Insulin promotes protein synthesis in almost all tissues by virtue of a combined effect on gene transcription, messenger RNA translation, and amino acid uptake. Insulin also has a mitogenic effect that is mediated through increased DNA synthesis and prevention of programmed cell death, or apoptosis. In addition, insulin stimulates ion transport across the plasma membrane of multiple tissues. Finally, insulin stimulates lipid synthesis in fat cells, skeletal muscle, and liver while preventing lipolysis by inhibiting hormone-sensitive lipase. There is increasing evidence for a direct role of insulin, acting through the insulin or insulin-like growth factor (IGF) receptors, to regulate pancreatic β-cell growth, survival, and insulin release from the pancreatic β cells [21,22]. Different tissues are known to respond differently to insulin. While tissue sensitivity to insulin correlates with the levels of insulin receptors expressed on the plasma membrane, it is clear that the assembly of different components of the insulin signaling pathway also confers specificity of insulin signaling on target cells. Thus, insulin-dependent glucose transport is only observed in skeletal muscle and adipose cells because these cells possess the insulin-dependent glucose transporter GLUT4. Likewise, the effect of insulin to inhibit gluconeo-genesis is specific to liver and kidney. In contrast, the effects on gene expression and protein synthesis might be ubiquitous.

Insulin Receptor

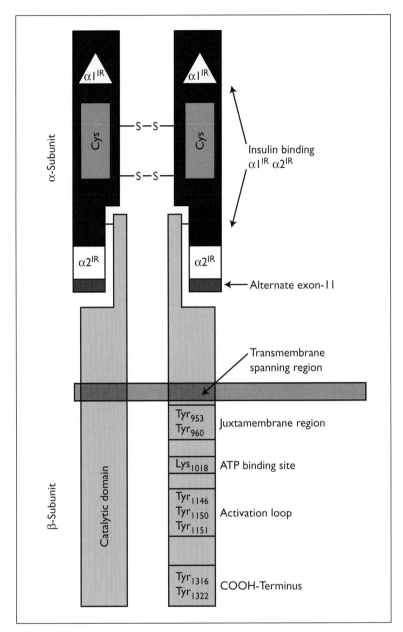

FIGURE 2-2. Insulin-receptor structure. The insulin receptor is required to mediate insulin action. The product of a single copy gene located on the short arm of chromosome 19 (cytogenetic band 19p13), the insulin receptor is synthesized as a single-chain polypeptide precursor that undergoes post-translational cleavage forming separate α and β subunits, which form heterodimers that are exported to the plasma membrane. During maturation, the receptor is glycosylated and acylated, and forms a heterotetramer composed of two α and two β subunits ($\alpha 2$–$\beta 2$). The α subunit is completely extracellular and contains high- and low-affinity binding sites for insulin ($\alpha 1$–$\alpha 2$). The asymmetric insulin molecules interact with the α subunits by binding to an $\alpha 1$ and $\alpha 2$ site on adjacent subunits. The β subunit spans the plasma membrane once and is linked to the α subunit through disulfide bridges and noncovalent interactions. The intracellular part of the β subunit contains a tyrosine-specific protein kinase domain. Insulin binding to the extracellular domain causes a conformational modification in the intracellular domain such that the receptor undergoes autophosphorylation and can bind adenosine triphosphate (ATP). Several tyrosine residues are phosphorylated, including tyrosine 972, which promotes substrate binding and phosphorylation [20,23]. Specific phosphorylation sites in the catalytic domain (tyrosine 1158, 1162, and 1163) are essential to promote the kinase activity of the receptor toward other protein substrates [24]. The role of the carboxy-terminal phosphorylation sites (tyrosine 1328 and 1334) is more controversial, with some investigations suggesting these sites may play a role in stimulating the mitogenic activity of the receptor. The insulin receptor is expressed as two variably spliced isoforms, resulting from inclusion (isoform B) or exclusion (isoform A) of exon-11 during processing of messenger RNA (mRNA). Exon-11 encodes a peptide with 12 amino acids located at the carboxy-terminal end of the α subunit of the receptor, which decreases the affinity for insulin [25]. Dysregulation of insulin receptor gene splicing alters fetal growth patterns and contributes to insulin resistance in adults [14,25].

Role of Insulin Receptor Substrate Proteins in Insulin Signaling

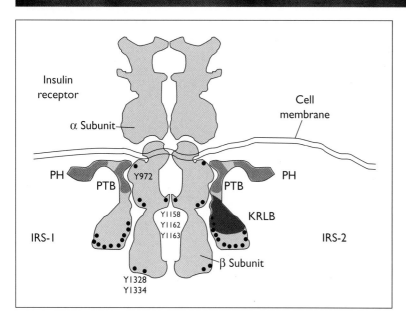

FIGURE 2-3. Model for the interaction of insulin receptors (IR) and insulin receptor substrate (IRS) molecules. IRS proteins were identified as tyrosine-phosphorylated proteins in cells treated with insulin [26–28]. In addition to insulin, other agents such as insulin-like growth factors and interleukins stimulate IRS protein phosphorylation [20]. After activation of the IR kinase, the phosphotyrosine-binding (PTB) domain of IRS becomes closely associated with the juxtamembrane region of the IR. This interaction requires phosphorylation of tyrosine 972 in the IR. In addition, it is possible that the pleckstrin homology (PH) domain stabilizes this interaction. The PH domain is located at the amino-terminal end of the IRS protein, which might promote interaction with the membrane bilayer. Many PH domains bind phospholipids. In addition, there exists at least one additional domain that interacts with the IR, called the kinase regulatory loop-binding (KRLB) domain. Its interaction with the IR requires phosphorylation of tyrosine residues in the catalytic domain of the receptor (tyrosines 1158, 1162, and 1163). Since the KRLB is only present in Irs-2, it might determine specificity of the interaction between the IR and its substrates [29,30]. Gene ablation experiments in mice indicate that various IRS proteins have unique functions. Mice lacking Irs-1 are growth-retarded and mildly insulin resistant, suggesting that Irs-1 plays an important role in both insulin and insulin-like growth factor-I receptor function; mice lacking Irs-2 develop insulin resistance and impaired β-cell development, suggesting that Irs-2 is important for metabolic regulation in response to insulin [4,21].

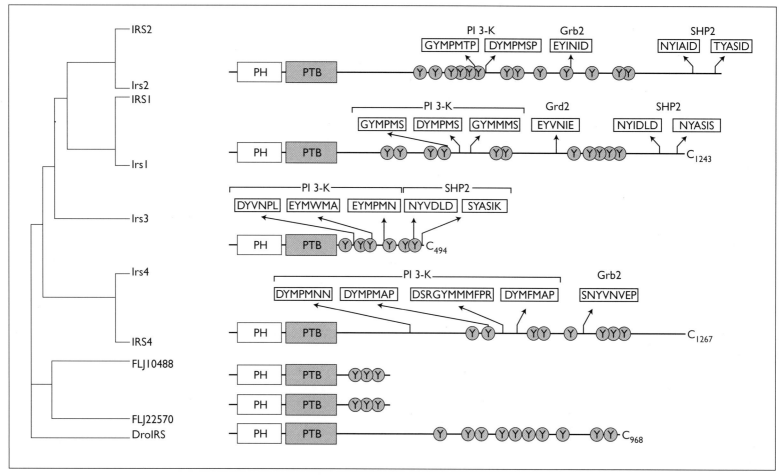

FIGURE 2-4. Structure of the insulin receptor substrate (IRS) proteins. The IRS proteins lack intrinsic catalytic activities, but are composed of multiple interaction domains and phosphorylation motifs. At least three IRS proteins occur in mice and people, including widely expressed IRS1 and IRS2 while IRS4 is limited to the thymus, brain, kidney, and possibly pancreatic β cells [31]. Rodents also express Irs3, which is largely restricted to adipose tissue and displays activity similar to Irs1; however, this short ortholog might not occur in people [32]. Phylogenetic analysis reveals a close evolutionary relation between *IRS1/Irs1* and *IRS2/Irs2* from people/mice, which might have diverged from *IRS4/Irs4*. The Drosophila IRS protein, Chico, is weakly related to its mammalian orthologs as it contains few COOH-terminal tyrosine phosphorylation sites. Finally, analysis of the human genome sequence reveals at least 2 putative IRS proteins recognized by adjacent pleckstrin homology (PH) and phosphotyrosine-binding (PTB) domains; however, they contain very short COOH tails with a few

tyrosine phosphorylation sites, so their function remains unknown (see Fig. 2-2). All IRS proteins are characterized by the presence of an NH2-terminal PH domain adjacent to a PTB domain, followed by a variable length COOH-terminal tail that contains numerous tyrosine and serine phosphorylation sites. The PH and PTB domains mediate specific interactions with the insulin and insulin-like growth factor-I (IGF-I) receptor kinases [33,34]. The PTB domain binds to phosphorylated NPXY motifs in the receptors for insulin, IGF-I, or interleukin-4; however, other receptors that promote IRS protein tyrosine phosphorylation do not contain NPXY motifs [35]. Candidate PH domain binding partners might include phospholipids, acidic peptides, or specific proteins such as PHIP [36,37]. Among the proteins that have been shown to bind to IRS1, the most prominent is the p85 subunit of phosphatidylinositol 3-kinase (PI 3-K), the enzymatic activity of which is thought to be crucial in stimulating many biologic actions of insulin.

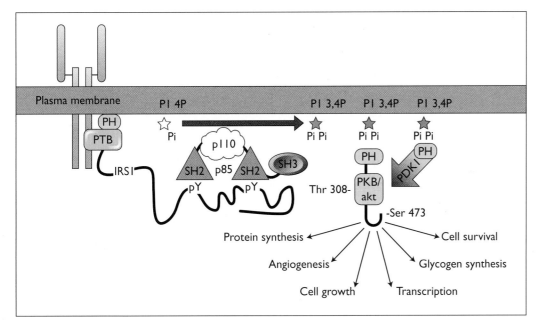

domains in the regulatory subunit (p85) of phosphatidylinositol 3-kinase (PI 3-K), resulting in activation of the p110 catalytic subunit. The p110 subunit catalyzes phosphorylation of phosphatidylinositol (PI) on the D3 position of the inositol ring, leading to the generation of PI 3-phosphate from PI, PI 3,4-bisphosphate from PI 4-phosphate, and PI 3,4,5-trisphosphate from PI 4,5-bisphosphate. There is increasing evidence that D3-phosphorylated inositides act as intracellular messengers leading to activation of PI-dependent kinases, changes in intracellular trafficking, and growth stimulation [39]. Products of the PI 3-kinase interact with cytosolic serine kinases (PDK, PKB and others) to generate a membrane-bound signaling system that mediates various biological processes, including glycogen synthesis and glucose transport. The PH domain of PKB binds to the PI 3-phosphate, whereas maximal enzyme activity requires PDK-mediated phosphorylation of Thr308 and Ser473 [40]. In addition to its role in metabolic regulation, PKB promotes insulin-like growth factor I-mediated inhibition of apoptosis, as well as the activation of the p70S6k kinase with attendant protein synthesis, regulation of entry into the cell cycle, and cellular differentiation [41]. PKB—protein kinase B; PDK—phosphoinositide-dependent protein kinase.

FIGURE 2-5. Tyrosine phosphorylation occurs in various amino acid sequence motifs that create binding sites for so-called SH2 (for src homology 2) motifs [38]. SH2 motifs are 50 to 100 amino acids long that bind with high affinity to phosphotyrosine residues in various intracellular signaling molecules. During insulin stimulation, tyrosine phosphorylated insulin receptor substrate (IRS) proteins bind to both SH2

Downstream Signaling Pathways

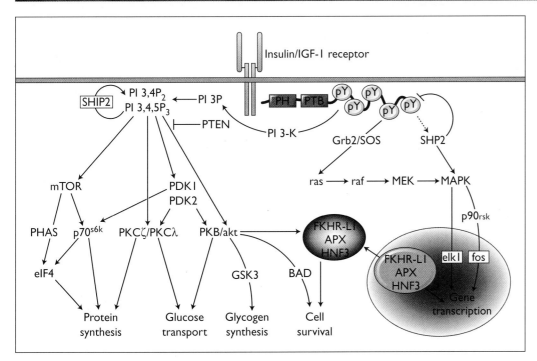

activated protein (MAP) kinase cascade. SHP2 feeds back to inhibit IRS protein phosphorylation by directly dephosphorylating the IRS protein, but might also transmit an independent signal to activate MAP kinase. The activated MAP kinase phosphorylates p90rsk, which itself phosphorylates the transcription factor c-fos, increasing its transcriptional activity. MAP kinase likewise phosphorylates elk1, increasing its transcriptional activity. The activation of PI 3-K by IRS protein recruitment results in the generation of PI 3,4P2 and PI 3,4,5P3 (antagonized by the action of PTEN or SHIP2). Together, PI 3,4P2 and PI 3,4,5P3 activate various kinases, including mTOR, atypical PKC isoforms, and phosphoinositide-dependent protein kinase (PDK1). PDK1 is upstream of PKB, which promotes glucose transport; the atypical PKC isoforms also play a role. PKB also regulates GSK3, which might regulate glycogen synthesis, and a variety of regulators of cell survival; PKB-mediated BAD phosphorylation inhibits apoptosis. PKB also phosphorylates the forkhead transcription factors (such as Foxo1), which restricts their location to the cytoplasm and inhibits their transcriptional activity. PKB—protein kinase B; GAP—guanosine triphosphatase-associated protein; GLUT4—glucose transporter 4; GRB-2—growth factor receptor binding protein 2; GSK3—glycogen synthase kinase 3; MAPKK—MAP kinase kinase; PKC—protein kinase C; SOS—son-of-sevenless.

FIGURE 2-6. Insulin receptor substrate (IRS) proteins coordinate multiple downstream signaling pathways. The diversity of insulin action in different tissues is partly explained by the different outputs coupled to the pathways activated by the hormone. There are two main limbs that propagate the signal generated through the insulin receptor, including the phosphatidyl 3-kinase (PI 3-K) branch and the Ras/mitogen-activated protein kinase branch. The IRS proteins bind PI 3-K, Grb2/SOS, and SHP-2. The GRb2/SOS complex mediates the activation of p21ras, thereby activating the ras→raf→methylethylketone (MEK)→mitogen-

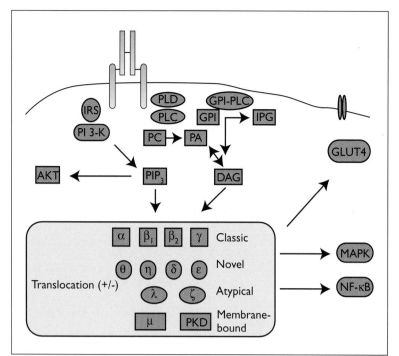

FIGURE 2-7. Members of the PKC family of serine/threonine kinases are implicated in several insulin actions. There are two subgroups of PKCs. The "classic" PKC isoforms bind calcium for activation. The atypical PKCs are activated by diacylglycerol (DAG) binding or by other phospholipids such as phosphatidylinositol 3,4,5-trisphosphate (PIP3). Insulin activates different members of this kinase family through formation of DAG and PIP3. Insulin stimulates DAG formation through phosphatidylcholine (PC) hydrolysis into DAG and phosphatidic acid (PA), or through activity of a glycosyl-phosphatidylinositol-specific phospholipase C (GPI-PLC), leading to the formation of DAG and inositol-phosphoglycan (IPG). Different isoforms of PKC have been shown to undergo translocation from the cytosol to the membrane in response to insulin stimulation in different tissues. Evidence exists that this process may be important for the biologic activity of PKCs [42]. It is known that PKCs can directly activate the MAP kinase pathway and the transcription factor NF-κB, leading to increased gene expression and protein synthesis. More recently, evidence has emerged that activation of atypical PKCs by PIP3 may be important in the process of insulin-dependent glucose transport [43].

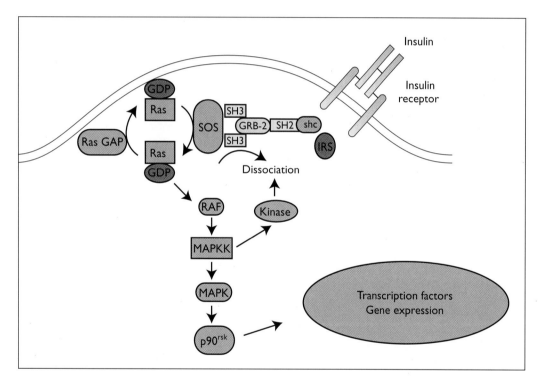

FIGURE 2-8. The Ras signaling pathway plays an important role in cellular growth and transformation [38]. Insulin activates the Ras pathway, leading to increased protein synthesis and mitogenesis. Activation of Ras in response to insulin requires formation of a signaling complex between insulin receptor substrate (IRS) or shc (src homology 2/collagen homology-containing protein) and growth factor receptor binding protein 2 (GRB-2). GRB-2 consists of one SH2 domain that binds the phosphorylated tyrosine residues in IRS or shc, and two SH3 (src homology 3 motif) domains that recognize proline-rich motifs on the exchange factor son-of-sevenless (SOS). SOS catalyzes the conversion of Ras from an inactive form (guanosine diphosphate-bound) to an active form (guanosine triphosphate-bound). A rasGAP catalyzes the reverse reaction forming inactive Ras. Ras-GTP activates the Raf kinase, which phosphorylates mitogen-activated protein kinase kinase (MAPKK). MAPKK phosphorylates extracellular-regulated kinases Erk1/2, which stimulate other kinases, including p90rsk, which promote protein synthesis and gene expression. On activation, MAPKK also activates additional pathways that catalyze the dissociation of GRB-2 from SOS, which terminates the signal. It appears that the relative roles of IRS and shc in activating SOS through GRB-2 vary in different tissues [44].

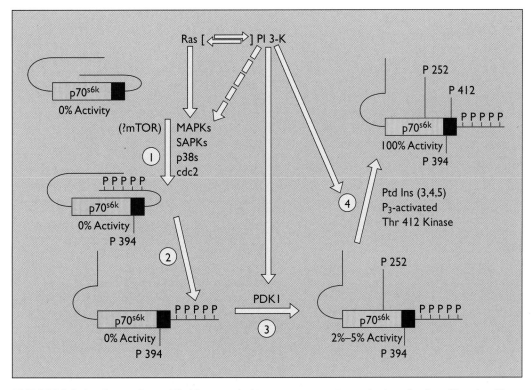

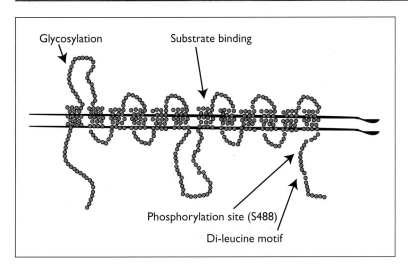

S6K1 inhibits insulin signaling [45]. S6K1 is activated in vivo through multisite phosphorylation events in response to insulin and other mitogens if a sufficient supply of amino acids is available or in response to high concentrations of amino acids alone [46]. Thus p70s6k is thought to be a nutrient sensor [47]. A variety of proline-directed kinases, including Erk, Cdc2 and mTOR, phosphorylate several sites in p70s6k, including Ser/Thr-Pro sites in the pseudosubstrate autoinhibitory domain of the carboxyl-terminal tail (Ser434, Ser441, Thr444, Ser447, and Ser452) as well as sites in the catalytic domain extension (Thr390 and Ser394) [46]. Phosphorylation of the pseudosubstrate autoinhibitory domain serves to disengage the carboxyl-terminal tail enabling access to Thr252 and Thr412. PDK1 catalyzes phosphorylation of Thr252 in the activation loop of the catalytic domain, which increases kinase activity slightly and facilitates PtdIns (3,4,5)P3-stimulated phosphorylation of Thr412, which is the rate-limiting step in activation. The concurrent phosphorylation of Thr252 and Thr412 increases p70s6k activity by 20- to 30-fold [39]. The deactivation of p70s6k that occurs on withdrawal of insulin or inhibition of PI 3 kinase results from the complete dephosphorylation of Thr412, with residual phosphorylation remaining at Thr252, reflecting the requirement for dual (412/252) phosphorylation for complete kinase activity.

FIGURE 2-9. Insulin regulates p70s6 kinase, which promotes protein synthesis and cell proliferation. The p70s6k occurs as two isoforms called S6K1 and S6K2. Disruption of *s6k1* causes glucose intolerance due to reduced size of islet β cells; by contrast, peripheral insulin action might be enhanced suggesting that

The Regulation of Glucose Transport and Metabolism

cial loop contains glycosylation sites, whereas the cytoplasmic carboxy-terminal domain contains a putative phosphorylation site (serine 488) and a di-leucine motif thought to play a role in the rapid endocytosis of GLUT4. The proposed substrate-binding site also is shown [48]. There is evidence for eight different members of the glucose transporter gene family. GLUT1 is expressed in all tissues and cell lines, and accounts for most basal (insulin-independent) glucose uptake. GLUT2 is mainly expressed in liver and pancreatic β cells; because of its relatively low affinity and high capacity for glucose, it serves to provide a constant flux of glucose into these organs at physiologic plasma glucose concentrations (5 mM). In the β cell, the uptake of glucose through GLUT2 is the first step in the detection of circulating glucose levels. GLUT3 is expressed ubiquitously and possesses a relatively high affinity for glucose. Interestingly, GLUT3 is abundant in the central nervous system, where glucose concentrations are lower than in the bloodstream. The presence of a high-affinity glucose transporter provides a mechanism for efficient glucose uptake by neurons. GLUT4 is the prototypical insulin-responsive glucose transporter. GLUT4 is found in intracellular vesicles in insulin-responsive tissues including skeletal muscle, adipose cells, and heart. Evidence now exists for the presence of an additional insulin-responsive glucose transporter, GLUT8. GLUT5 is a fructose transporter expressed in the intestinal epithelial membrane and kidney. GLUT6 is a nonfunctional pseudogene. GLUT7 is a microsomal glucose transporter that is part of the glucose-6-phosphatase complex thought to play a role in glucose release from the endoplasmic reticulum [48].

FIGURE 2-10. Glucose transporters. Glucose transport is mediated by a family of facilitative glucose carriers, or glucose transporters. These proteins have a typical structure, including a cytoplasmic amino-terminus followed by 12 membrane-spanning domains and a cytoplasmic tail. The proposed structure of the insulin-responsive glucose transporter 4 (GLUT4) is shown. The first exofa-

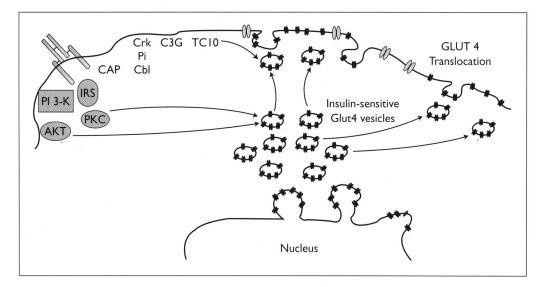

the effect of insulin to stimulate glucose uptake in muscle and fat can be accounted for in its entirety by the translocation hypothesis. Other factors, such as an increase in the activity of glucose transporters, might play a role. Substantial evidence exists to suggest that phosphatidylinositol 3-kinase (PI 3-K) activity mediates the effect of insulin on glucose transport. In addition to PI 3-K activity, other signals seem to be required for insulin-stimulated glucose uptake, including a second pathway involving tyrosine phosphorylation of the Cbl proto-oncogene [49]. In most insulin-responsive cells, Cbl is associated with the adapter protein CAP, which binds to proline-rich sequences in Cbl through its carboxyl-terminal SH3 domain. Upon phosphorylation, the Cbl–CAP complex associates with flotillin in plasma membrane lipid rafts where phospho-Cbl recruits the CrkII-C3G complex. CrkII forms a constitutive complex with C3G, a guanyl nucleotide-exchange protein that catalyzes the exchange of GTP for GDP in the G-protein TC10. Activated TC10 may contribute to stabilization of cortical actin and provide a second signal to the GLUT4 protein that functions in parallel with the activation of the PI 3-K pathway.

FIGURE 2-11. Insulin action on glucose transport. In tissues that are insulin-responsive for glucose uptake, GLUT4 exists under basal conditions in intracellular vesicles. GLUT4-containing vesicles are released from their intracellular storage compartment and reach the cell surface during insulin stimulation. The mechanism of insulin-induced redistribution of glucose transporters is referred to as translocation. It is not clear whether

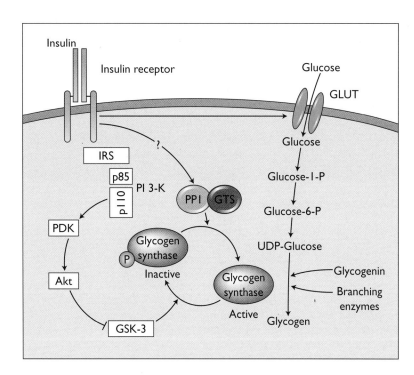

FIGURE 2-12. Insulin stimulation of glycogen synthesis. Insulin plays an essential role in stimulating glycogen synthesis in many tissues. This process involves the regulation of multiple enzymatic activities. Glycogen synthase (GS) activity is regulated by phosphorylation. This crucial enzyme is inactive when phosphorylated [50]. Glycogen synthase kinase-3 (GSK-3) is one enzyme that catalyzes the phosphorylation and inactivation of glycogen synthase. GSK-3 itself is inactivated by phosphorylation. Insulin stimulates GSK-3 phosphorylation through activation of the Akt kinase (product of the akt proto-oncogene). Akt is activated in response to phosphatidylinositol 3-kinase (PI 3-K) through PI-dependent kinases 1 and 2 (PDK1 and PDK2). Akt can phosphorylate and inactivate GSK-3, thus decreasing the net rate of GS phosphorylation [51]. Additionally, insulin has been shown to increase the activity of the glycogen-bound form of the serine/threonine protein phosphatase-1 (PP1) which dephosphorylates and activates GS [52]. The exact mechanism of PP1 stimulation by insulin remains unclear [53]. Glycogen synthesis requires the assembly of a complex of proteins, including glycogenin, to provide a molecular scaffold, branching enzymes, and a variety of glycogen targeting subunits (GTS) that regulate PP1 localization and activity [54]. The extent to which insulin regulates GTS localization and/or function is currently under investigation. Insulin-stimulated glucose transport has also been shown to contribute to GS regulation [55].

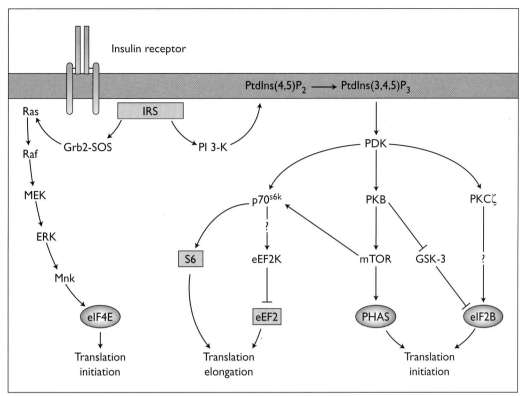

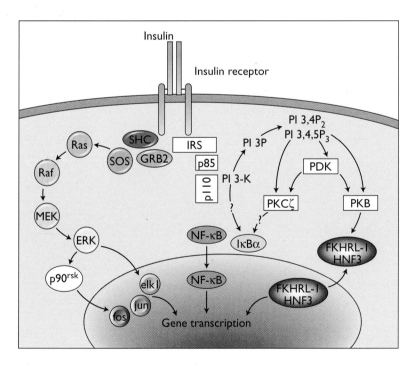

Glycogen synthase kinase-3 (GSK-3) phosphory-lates eIF2B at Ser540, keeping it inactive. Insulin stimulates the inhibition of GSK-3 in turn, leading to the activation of eIF2B [48,50]. Insulin also stim-ulates eIF2B activity through PI 3-kinase–dependent activation of the atypical protein kinase C, PKCζ [57]. This activation of eIF2B leads to an overall increase in translation initiation [58]. The mRNA cap-binding protein, eIF4E, is inactive when bound to PHAS-I. Insulin activates eIF4E by stimulating mTOR-mediated phosphorylation of PHAS-I, resulting in a dissociation of this complex [59]. Mnk is activated by insulin through the Ras/ERK cascade [60]. Mnk increases the affinity of eIF4E for caps via phosphorylation at Ser209 [61]. The phosphoryla-tion and subsequent affinity of eIF4G, another member of the active cap-binding complex for eIF4E, is also stimulated by insulin [62,63]. Formation of the active cap-binding complex leads to increased translation initiation. Insulin also stim-ulates elongation by phosphorylation of eEF1 and S6, the latter occurring by both multipotential S6 kinase and p70s6K. eEF2, an important factor in the elongation process, is inactive when phosphory-lated [64]. Insulin stimulates the dephosphorylation of eEF2 via a rapamycin-sensitive route possibly involving the phosphorylation and inactivation of eEF2 kinase by p70s6K [65]. Other growth factors acting through receptor tyrosine kinases produce similar changes in protein synthesis, eg, platelet-derived growth factor, nerve growth factor, and epidermal growth factor.

FIGURE 2-13. Regulation of protein synthesis by insulin. Insulin stimulates both initiation and elongation by changing the intrinsic activity or binding properties of certain key factors. This occurs via phosphoryla-tion or sequestration of repressive factors in an inactive complex. Components of the translational machinery that are targets of insulin regulation include eIF2B, eIF4E, eIF4G, S6, eEF1, and eEF2 [56].

FIGURE 2-14. Regulation of gene expression by insulin. Insulin effects target gene expression in a variety of cells and organs. Both the phosphatidlyinositol 3-kinase (PI 3-K) and the Ras/extracellular-regulated kinase (ERK) signaling pathways have been shown to mediate insulin action on gene transcription in different tissues. The Ras/ERK pathway activates p90rsk whereby individually ERK and p90rsk translocate into the nucleus and phosphorylate transcription factors including elk1 and fos. These phosphorylation events increase transcrip-tional activity mediated by such factors. The PI 3-K pathway activates protein kinase B (PKB) through PI-dependent protein kinase (PDK). Active PKB phos-phorylates members of the FKHR transcriptional enhancer family including FKHR-L1 and HNF3, which, under basal conditions, are localized to the nucleus. Phosphorylation of these FKHR factors leads to their nuclear exclu-sion and cytoplasmic retention, effectively inhibiting specific gene transcription [66]. Insulin also effects the inhibitory complex dissociation of IκB from NF-κB. NF-κB is then free to enter the nucleus and activate target gene transcription. The insulin stimulation of NF-κB has been shown to be sensitive to inhibitors of PI 3-K, implicating the involvement of the PI 3-K pathway [67]. Activation of atypical protein kinase C, such as PKCζ, may also contribute to activation of NF-κB. The regulation of NF-κB by insulin remains unclear.

Insulin Resistance

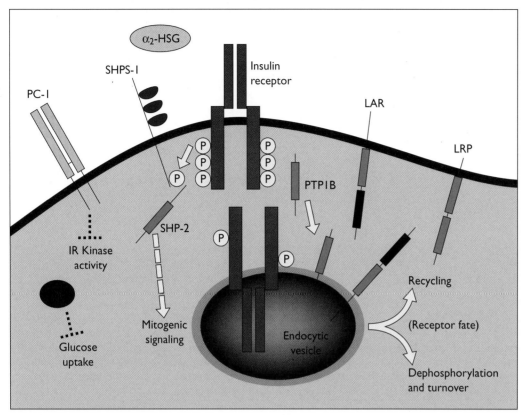

FIGURE 2-15. Modulators of insulin action. Multiple signals converge on the insulin receptor (IR) to modulate its function. Protein tyrosine phosphatases (PTP) appear to play an important role in deactivating the IR, providing a mechanism for regulating the insulin response. The endocytic step that follows insulin binding, with internalization of the ligand/receptor complex into clathrin-coated vesicles, may be another point for receptor dephosphorylation. The endosome has been identified as a major site of tyrosine phosphatase activity towards the IR [68]. Many studies of obese, insulin-resistant humans and rodents demonstrate alterations in the expression and/or activity of PTPs in insulin-responsive tissues [69–73]. There are

two major classes of tyrosine phosphatases: receptor-type (membrane-bound) and nonreceptor-type (cytosolic). Tyrosine phosphatases identified as IR phosphatases include LAR and LRP (receptor-type) as well as PTP1B (cytosolic). These phosphatases may also alter insulin signaling by targeting IR substrates for dephosphorylation. Transgenic mouse studies show overexpression of LAR in muscle results in whole-body insulin resistance [74]. PTP1B knockout mice are resistant to obesity and demonstrate increased insulin sensitivity [75,76]. A variety of other molecules affect insulin action. The membrane glycoprotein PC-1 has been proposed to exert a negative effect on IR function by dampening its kinase activity [77]. Studies indicate a correlation between PC-1 expression and insulin resistance in patients with type II diabetes [78]. Another inhibitor of the IR kinase is the serum glycoprotein α2-HSG. This 63-kDa protein has been reported to inhibit insulin-induced receptor autophosphorylation as well as phosphorylation of IR substrate-1 and the IR substrate Shc, with an associated decrease of the mitogenic actions of insulin. No effect of α2-HSG has been reported on the metabolic functions of insulin [79]. Rad (ras-like protein associated with diabetes) originally was identified by subtractive hybridization as a gene overexpressed in patients with diabetes. Although subsequent studies have failed to confirm this association, it is interesting that overexpression of Rad in transfected cells impairs insulin-dependent glucose uptake [80]. The transmembrane glycoprotein SHPS-1 is phosphorylated and forms a complex with SHP-2, a non-receptor PTP, in response to insulin. This complex appears to enhance ERK activity in response to insulin [81].

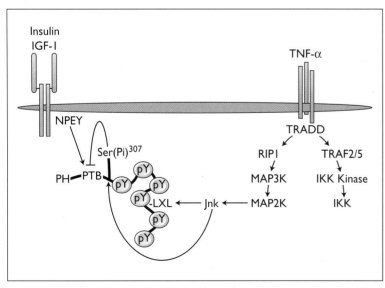

FIGURE 2-16. Tumor necrosis factor-α (TNF-α) as modulator of insulin action. The important idea that inflammation is associated with insulin resistance has

been known for a long time [82], and is consistent with the finding that stress-induced cytokines like TNF-α cause insulin resistance. The signaling cascades regulated by TNF-α are complex and involve many branch points, including the activation of various serine kinases and transcription factors that promote apoptosis or proliferation [83]. One of the branches of the TNF-α signaling pathway involves activation of the c-Jun N-terminal kinase (Jnk) [84–86]. Jnk is a prototype stress-induced kinase that is stimulated by many agonists during acute or chronic inflammation. Jnk phosphorylates numerous cellular proteins, including IRS-1 and IRS-2, Shc, and Gab1 [87]. A role for Jnk during insulin action is compelling, as both IRS-1 and IRS-2 contain Jnk binding motifs. This motif mediates the specific association of Jnk with IRS-1, which promotes phosphorylation of a specific serine residue that is located on the COOH-terminal side of the phosphotyrosine-binding (PTB) domain (Ser307 in murine IRS-1; Ser312 in human IRS-1). Phosphorylation of this residue inhibits the function of the PTB domain, which disrupts the association between the insulin receptor and IRS-1, and inhibits tyrosine phosphorylation [87]. In this model, TNF-α–binding to TNF–receptor type 1 (TNFR1) results in recruitment of TNF–receptor-associated factor 2/5 (TRAF2/5) and receptor-interacting protein 1 (RIP1) through the adaptor protein TRADD. TRAF2/5 and RIP1 promote activation of the protein kinases Jnk and IκB kinase (IKK). Activated Jnk associates with the Jnk binding LXL-motif in IRS-1, which promotes phosphorylation of Ser307. Phosphorylation of Ser307 inhibits PTB domain function and inhibits insulin/IGF- stimulated tyrosine phosphorylation and signal transduction.

References

1. DeFronzo RA, Ferrannini E: Regulation of intermediary metabolism during fasting and feeding. In *Endocrinology*. Edited by DeGroot LJ, Jameson JL. Philadelphia: WB Saunders; 2001:737–755.

2. Baker J, Liu JP, Robertson EJ, Efstratiadis A: Role of insulin-like growth factors in embryonic and postnatal growth. *Cell* 1993, 75:73–82.

3. Liu JP, Baker J, Perkins JA, et al.: Mice carrying null mutations of the genes encoding insulin-like growth factor I (Igf-I) and type 1 IGF receptor (Igf1r). *Cell* 1993, 75:59–72.

4. Withers DJ, Burks DJ, Towery HH, et al.: Irs-2 coordinates Igf-I receptor-mediated beta-cell development and peripheral insulin signalling. *Nat Genet* 1999, 23(1):32–40.

5. Lupu F, Terwilliger JD, Lee K, et al.: Roles of growth hormone and insulin-like growth factor 1 in mouse postnatal growth. *Dev Biol* 2001, 229(1):141–162.

6. Dudek H, Datta SR, Franke TF, et al.: Regulation of neuronal survival by the serine-threonine protein kinase Akt. *Science* 1997, 275:661–665.

7. Hellstrom A, Perruzzi C, Ju M, et al.: Low IGF-I suppresses VEGF-survival signaling in retinal endothelial cells: direct correlation with clinical retinopathy of prematurity. *Proc Natl Acad Sci U S A* 2001, 98(10):5804–5808.

8. Pete G, Fuller CR, Oldham JM, et al.: Postnatal growth responses to insulin-like growth factor I in insulin receptor substrate-1–deficient mice. *Endocrinology* 1999, 140(12):5478–5487.

9. Reaven GM: Banting Lecture 1988. Role of insulin resistance in human disease. 1988 [classical article]. *Nutrition* 1997, 13(1):65.

10. Halban PA, Kahn SE, Lernmark A, Rhodes CJ: Gene and cell-replacement therapy in the treatment of type 1 diabetes: how high must the standards be set? *Diabetes* 2001, 50(10):2181–2191.

11. DeFronzo RA: Pathogenesis of type 2 diabetes: Metabolic and molecular implications for identifying diabetes genes. *Diabetes Rev* 1997, 5(3):177–269.

12. Cline GW, Rothman DL, Magnusson I, et al.: 13C-nuclear magnetic resonance spectroscopy studies of hepatic glucose metabolism in normal subjects and subjects with insulin-dependent diabetes mellitus. *J Clin Invest* 1994, 94:2369–2376.

13. Bruning JC, Michael MD, Winnay JN, et al.: A muscle-specific insulin receptor knockout exhibits features of the metabolic syndrome of NIDDM without altering glucose tolerance. *Mol Cell* 1998, 2(5):559–569.

14. Savkur RS, Philips AV, Cooper TA: Aberrant regulation of insulin receptor alternative splicing is associated with insulin resistance in myotonic dystrophy. *Nat Genet* 2001, 29(1):40–47.

15. Burghes AH, Vaessin HE, de La Chapelle A: Genetics. The land between Mendelian and multifactorial inheritance. *Science* 2001, 293(5538):2213–2214.

16. Sreenan SK, Zhou YP, Otani K, et al.: Calpains play a role in insulin secretion and action. *Diabetes* 2001, 50(9):2013–2020.

17. Horikawa Y, Oda N, Cox NJ, et al.: Genetic variation in the gene encoding calpain-10 is associated with type 2 diabetes mellitus. *Nat Genet* 2000, 26(2):163–175.

18. Freychet P, Roth J, Neville DM, Jr: Insulin receptors in the liver: specific binding of [125I] insulin to the plasma membrane and its relation to insulin bioactivity. *Proc Natl Acad Sci U S A* 1971, 68:1833–1837.

19. White MF, Kahn CR: The insulin signaling system. *J Biol Chem* 1994, 269(1):1–4.

20. Yenush L, White MF: The IRS-signaling system during insulin and cytokine action. *Bio Essays* 1997, 19(5):491–500.

21. Withers DJ, Gutierrez JS, Towery H, et al.: Disruption of IRS-2 causes type 2 diabetes in mice. *Nature* 1998, 391(6670):900–904.

22. Kulkarni RN, Bruning JC, Winnay JN, et al.: Tissue-specific knockout of the insulin receptor in pancreatic beta cells creates an insulin secretory defect similar to that in type 2 diabetes. *Cell* 1999, 96(3):329–339.

23. White MF, Livingston JN, Backer JM, et al.: Mutation of the insulin receptor at tyrosine 960 inhibits signal transmission but does not affect its tyrosine kinase activity. *Cell* 1988, 54:641–649.

24. White MF, Shoelson SE, Keutmann H, Kahn CR: A cascade of tyrosine autophosphorylation in the beta-subunit activates the insulin receptor. *J Biol Chem* 1988, 263:2969–2980.

25. Frasca F, Pandini G, Scalia P, et al.: Insulin receptor isoform A, a newly recognized, high-affinity insulin-like growth factor II receptor in fetal and cancer cells. *Mol Cell Biol* 1999, 19(5):3278–3288.

26. White MF, Maron R, Kahn CR: Insulin rapidly stimulates tyrosine phosphorylation of a Mr 185,000 protein in intact cells. *Nature* 1985, 318:183–186.

27. Sun XJ, Rothenberg PL, Kahn CR, et al.: The structure of the insulin receptor substrate IRS-1 defines a unique signal transduction protein. *Nature* 1991, 352:73–77.

28. Sun XJ, Wang LM, Zhang Y, et al.: Role of IRS-2 in insulin and cytokine signalling. *Nature* 1995, 377:173–177.

29. Sawka-Verhelle D, Tartare-Deckert S, White MF, Van Obberghen E: Insulin receptor substrate-2 binds to the insulin receptor through its phosphotyrosine-binding domain and through a newly identified domain comprising amino acids 591-786. *J Biol Chem* 1996, 271(11):5980–5983.

30. He W, Craparo A, Zhu Y, et al.: Interaction of insulin receptor substrate-2 (IRS-2) with the insulin and insulin-like growth factor I receptors. Evidence for two distinct phosphotyrosine-dependent interaction domains within IRS-2. *J Biol Chem* 1996, 271(20):11641–11645.

31. Uchida T, Myers MG Jr, White MF: IRS-4 mediates activation of PKB/Akt during insulin stimulation without inhibition of apoptosis. *Mol Cell Biol* 2000, 20(1):126–138.

32. Xu P, Jacobs AR, Taylor SI: Interaction of insulin receptor substrate 3 with insulin receptor, insulin receptor-related receptor, insulin-like growth factor-1 receptor, and downstream proteins. *J Biochem* 1999, 274:15262–15270.

33. Yenush L, Zanella C, Uchida T, et al.: The pleckstrin homology and phosphotyrosine binding domains of insulin receptor substrate 1 mediate inhibition of apoptosis by insulin. *Mol Cell Biol* 1998, 18(11):6784–6794.

34. Burks DJ, Pons S, Towery H, et al.: Heterologous PH domains do not mediate coupling of IRS-1 to the insulin receptor. *J Biol Chem* 1997, 272(44):27716–27721.

35. Wolf G, Trub T, Ottinger E, et al.: The PTB domains of IRS-1 and Shc have distinct but overlapping specificities. *J Biol Chem* 1995, 270:27407–27410.

36. Burks DJ, Wang J, Towery H, et al.: IRS pleckstrin homology domains bind to acidic motifs in proteins. *J Biol Chem* 1998, 273(47):31061–31067.

37. Farhang-Fallah J, Yin X, Trentin G, et al.: Cloning and characterization of PHIP, a novel insulin receptor substrate-1 pleckstrin homology domain interacting protein. *J Biol Chem* 2000, 275(51):40492–40497.

38. Pawson T, Scott JD: Signaling through scaffold, anchoring, and adaptor proteins. *Science* 1997, 278(5346):2075–2080.

39. Toker A, Cantley LC: Signalling through the lipid products of phosphoinosite-3-OH kinase. *Nature* 1997, 387:673–676.

40. Cross DAE, Alessi DR, Cohen P, et al.: Inhibition of glycogen synthase kinase-3 by insulin mediated protein kinase B. *Nature* 1996, 378:785–787.

41. Brazil DP, Hemmings BA: Ten years of protein kinase B signalling: a hard Akt to follow. *Trends Biochem Sci* 2001, 26(11):657–664.

42. Farese RV: Insulin-sensitive phospholipid signaling systems and glucose transport. Update II. *Exp Biol Med* 2001, 226(4):283–295.

43. Standaert ML, Bandyopadhyay G, Kanoh Y, et al.: Insulin and PIP3 activate PKC-zeta by mechanisms that are both dependent and independent of phosphorylation of activation loop (T410) and autophosphorylation (T560) sites. *Biochemistry* 2001, 40(1):249–255.

44. Ceresa BP, Pessin JE: Insulin regulation of the Ras activation/inactivation cycle. *Mol Cell Biochem* 1998; 182(1–2):23–29.

45. Pende M, Kozma SC, Jaquet M, *et al.*: Hypoinsulinaemia, glucose intolerance and diminished beta-cell size in S6K1-deficient mice. *Nature* 2000, 408(6815):994–997.

46. Isotani S, Hara K, Tokunaga C, *et al.*: Immunopurified mammalian target of rapamycin phosphorylates and activates p70 S6 kinase alpha in vitro. *J Biol Chem* 1999, 274(48):34493–34498.

47. Avruch J, Belham C, Weng Q, *et al.*: The p70 S6 kinase integrates nutrient and growth signals to control translational capacity. *Prog Mol Subcell Biol* 2001, 26:115–154.

48. Czech MP: Molecular actions of insulin on glucose transport. *Annu Rev Nutr* 1995, 15:441–471.

49. Saltiel AR, Kahn CR: Insulin signalling and the regulation of glucose and lipid metabolism. *Nature* 2001, 414(6865):799–806.

50. Roach PJ: Control of glycogen synthase by hierarchal protein phosphorylation. *FASEB J* 1990, 4(12):2961–2968.

51. Cross DA, Alessi DR, Cohen P, *et al.*: Inhibition of glycogen synthase kinase-3 by insulin mediated by protein kinase B. *Nature* 1995, 378(6559):785–789.

52. Haystead TAJ, Sim AT, Carling D, *et al.*: Effects of the tumour promoter okadaic acid on intracellular protein phosphorylation and metabolism. *Nature* 1989, 337:78–81.

53. Brady MJ, Saltiel AR: The role of protein phosphatase-1 in insulin action. *Recent Prog Horm Res* 2001, 56:157–173.

54. Newgard CB, Brady MJ, O'Doherty RM, Saltiel AR: Organizing glucose disposal: emerging roles of the glycogen targeting subunits of protein phosphatase-1. *Diabetes* 2000, 49(12):1967–1977.

55. Brady MJ, Kartha PM, Aysola AA, Saltiel AR: The role of glucose metabolites in the activation and translocation of glycogen synthase by insulin in 3T3-L1 adipocytes. *J Biol Chem* 1999, 274(39):27497–27504.

56. Rhoads RE: Signal transduction pathways that regulate eukaryotic protein synthesis. *J Biol Chem* 1999, 274(43):30337–30340.

57. Mendez R, Kollmorgen G, White MF, Rhoads RE: Requirement of protein kinase C zeta for stimulation of protein synthesis by insulin. *Mol Cell Biol* 1997, 17(9):5184–5192.

58. Proud CG, Denton RM: Molecular mechanisms for the control of translation by insulin. *Biochem J* 1997, 328(Pt 2):329–341.

59. Brunn GJ, Hudson CC, Sekulic A, *et al.*: Phosphorylation of the translational repressor PHAS-I by the mammalian target of rapamycin. *Science* 1997, 277(5322):99–101.

60. Waskiewicz AJ, Johnson JC, Penn B, *et al.*: Phosphorylation of the cap-binding protein eukaryotic translation initiation factor 4E by protein kinase Mnk1 in vivo. *Mol Cell Biol* 1999, 19(3):1871–1880.

61. Minich WB, Balasta ML, Goss DJ, Rhoads RE: Chromatographic resolution of in vivo phosphorylated and nonphorphorylated eukaryotic translation initiation factor eIF-4E: Increased cap affinity of the phosphorylated form. *Proc Natl Acad Sci U S A* 1994, 91:7668–7672.

62. Morley SJ, Dever TE, Etchison D, Traugh JA: Phosphorylation of eIF-4F by protein kinase C or multipotential S6 kinase stimulates protein synthesis at initiation. *J Biol Chem* 1991, 266(8):4669–4672.

63. Sinaud S, Balage M, Bayle G, *et al.*: Diazoxide-induced insulin deficiency greatly reduced muscle protein synthesis in rats: involvement of eIF4E. *Am J Physiol* 1999, 276(1 Pt 1):E50–E61.

64. Redpath NT, Price NT, Severinov KV, Proud CG: Regulation of elongation factor-2 by multisite phosphorylation. *Eur J Biochem* 1993, 213(2):689–699.

65. Proud CG, Wang X, Patel JV, *et al.*: Interplay between insulin and nutrients in the regulation of translation factors. *Biochem Soc Trans* 2001, 29(Pt 4):541–547.

66. Kilberg MS, Handlogten ME, Christensen HN: Characteristics of an amino acid transport system in rat liver for glutamine, asparagine, histidine, and closely related analogs. *J Biol Chem* 1980, 255(9):4011–4019.

67. Pandey SK, He HJ, Chesley A, *et al.*: Wortmannin-sensitive pathway is required for insulin-stimulated phosphorylation of inhibitor kappaBalpha. *Endocrinology* 2002, 143(2):375–385.

68. Di Guglielmo GM, Drake PG, Baass PC, *et al.*: Insulin receptor internalization and signalling. *Mol Cell Biochem* 1998, 182(1–2):59–63.

69. Ahmad F, Azevedo JL, Cortright R, *et al.*: Alterations in skeletal muscle protein-tyrosine phosphatase activity and expression in insulin-resistant human obesity and diabetes. *J Clin Invest* 1997, 100(2):449–458.

70. Ahmad F, Considine RV, Bauer TL, *et al.*: Improved sensitivity to insulin in obese subjects following weight loss is accompanied by reduced protein-tyrosine phosphatases in adipose tissue. *Metabolism* 1997, 46(10):1140–1145.

71. Ahmad F, Goldstein BJ: Increased abundance of specific skeletal muscle protein-tyrosine phosphatases in a genetic model of insulin-resistant obesity and diabetes mellitus. *Metabolism* 1995, 44(9):1175–1184.

72. Ahmad F, Considine RV, Goldstein BJ: Increased abundance of the receptor-type protein-tyrosine phosphatase LAR accounts for the elevated insulin receptor dephosphorylating activity in adipose tissue of obese human subjects. *J Clin Invest* 1995, 95(6):2806–2812.

73. McGuire MC, Fields RM, Nyomba BL, *et al.*: Abnormal regulation of protein tyrosine phosphatase activities in skeletal muscle of insulin-resistant humans. *Diabetes* 1991, 40:939–942.

74. Zabolotny JM, Kim YB, Peroni OD, *et al.*: Overexpression of the LAR (leukocyte antigen-related) protein-tyrosine phosphatase in muscle causes insulin resistance. *Proc Natl Acad Sci U S A* 2001, 98(9):5187–5192.

75. Elchebly M, Payette P, Michaliszyn E, *et al.*: Increased insulin sensitivity and obesity resistance in mice lacking the protein tyrosine phosphatase-1B gene [see comments]. *Science* 1999, 283(5407):1544–1548.

76. Klaman LD, Boss O, Peroni OD, *et al.*: Increased energy expenditure, decreased adiposity, and tissue-specific insulin sensitivity in protein-tyrosine phosphatase 1B-deficient mice. *Mol Cell Biol* 2000, 20(15):5479–5489.

77. Goldfine ID, Maddux BA, Youngren JF, *et al.*: Membrane glycoprotein PC-1 and insulin resistance. *Mol Cell Biochem* 1998, 182(1–2):177–184.

78. Frittitta L, Ercolino T, Bozzali M, *et al.*: A cluster of three single nucleotide polymorphisms in the 3'-untranslated region of human glycoprotein PC-1 gene stabilizes PC-1 mRNA and is associated with increased PC-1 protein content and insulin resistance-related abnormalities. *Diabetes* 2001, 50(8):1952–1955.

79. Srinivas PR, Deutsch DD, Mathews ST, *et al.*: Recombinant human alpha 2-HS glycoprotein inhibits insulin-stimulated mitogenic pathway without affecting metabolic signalling in Chinese hamster ovary cells overexpressing the human insulin receptor. *Cell Signal* 1996, 8:567–573.

80. Moyers JS, Bilan PJ, Reynet C, Kahn CR: Overexpression of Rad inhibits glucose uptake in cultured muscle and fat cells. *J Biol Chem* 1996, 271(38):23111–23116.

81. Takada T, Matozaki T, Takeda H, *et al.*: Roles of the complex formation of SHPS-1 with SHP-2 in insulin-stimulated mitogen-activated protein kinase activation. *J Biol Chem* 1998, 273(15):9234–9242.

82. Baron SH: Salicylates as hypoglycemic agents. *Diabetes Care* 1982, 5(1):64–71.

83. Baud V, Karin M: Signal transduction by tumor necrosis factor and its relatives. *Trends Cell Biol* 2001, 11(9):372–377.

84. Yuasa T, Ohno S, Kehrl JH, Kyriakis JM: Tumor necrosis factor signaling to stress-activated protein kinase (SAPK)/Jun NH2-terminal kinase (JNK) and p38. Germinal center kinase couples TRAF2 to mitogen-activated protein kinase/ERK kinase kinase 1 and SAPK while receptor interacting protein associates with a mitogen-activated protein kinase kinase kinase upstream of MKK6 and p38. *J Biol Chem* 1998, 273(35):22681–22692.

85. Kuan CY, Yang DD, Samanta Roy DR, *et al.*: The Jnk1 and Jnk2 protein kinases are required for regional specific apoptosis during early brain development. *Neuron* 1999, 22(4):667–676.

86. Rincon M, Whitmarsh A, Yang DD, *et al.*: The JNK pathway regulates the in vivo deletion of immature CD4(+)CD8(+) thymocytes. *J Exp Med* 1998, 188(10):1817–1830.

87. Aguirre V, Uchida T, Yenush L, *et al.*: The c-Jun NH2-terminal kinase promotes insulin resistance during association with insulin receptor substrate-1 and phosphorylation of Ser307. *J Biol Chem* 2000, 275(12):9047–9054.

CONSEQUENCES OF INSULIN DEFICIENCY

3

Abbas E. Kitabchi and Mary Beth Murphy

Diabetes [Mellitus] is a remarkable disorder, and not one very common to man...The disease is chronic in its character, and is slowly engendered, though the patient does not survive long when it is completely established, for the marasmus produced is rapid, and death speedy. Life too is odious and painful, the thirst is ungovernable, and the copious potations are more than equaled by the profuse urinary discharge; for more urine flows away, and it is impossible to put any restraint to the patient's drinking or making water. For if he stop for a very brief period, and leave off drinking, the mouth becomes parched, the body dry; the bowels seem on fire, he is wretched and uneasy, and soon dies, tormented with burning thirst.

Aretaeus of Cappodocia (ea. 120 A.D.–200 AD) [1]

Diabetes mellitus (type 1 or type 2) is the result of an absolute or relative insulin-deficient state that, if not corrected, gives rise to the acute metabolic decompensation of hyperglycemic crises so poignantly described above by Aretaeus of Cappodocia more than 1800 years ago. The two major hyperglycemic crises are diabetic ketoacidosis (DKA) and hyperglycemic hyperosmolar state (HHS). These two syndromes are the hallmark of insulin-deficient states. These crises continue to be important causes of mortality and morbidity among patients with diabetes. The annual incidence of DKA hospital admissions ranges from 4.6 to 8 episodes per 1000 patients with diabetes. It is estimated that DKA accounts for 4% to 9% of all hospital admissions for patients diagnosed with diabetes, whereas this figure for HHS is less than 1% [2,3].

The most common precipitating causes for these hyperglycemic emergencies are a) infection, b) undertreatment or omission of insulin, c) previously undiagnosed diabetes, and d) presence of comorbid conditions [4]. In addition, contributing factors for the development of HHS include decreased intake of fluid and electrolytes and excessive use of such drugs as glucocorticoids, diuretics, β-blockers, as well as the use of immunosuppressive agents and diazoxide [4]. Although DKA is most frequently seen in type 1 diabetes and HHS is often associated with type 2 diabetes, each of these conditions can be seen in both types because DKA and HHS have common underlying causes, ie, ineffective insulin concentration, dehydration, and increased counterregulatory (stress) hormones, but at different levels. DKA can also occur in young, obese, previously undiagnosed blacks who demonstrate the characteristics of type 2 diabetes [5].

It is important to note that some patients may present with an overlapping metabolic picture of both DKA and HHS. The incidence of combined HHS and DKA in some series has been noted to be as high as 30% [6]. Hyperglycemic hyperosmolar state and DKA can also occur in relatively pure form. Generally, in DKA, the insulin deficiency is absolute whereas in HHS, the insulin may be insufficient relative to the excessive levels of stress hormones (cortisol, glucagon, catecholamines, and growth hormone).

With better understanding of the pathogenesis of insulin-deficient states, the use of more physiologic doses of insulin, and frequent monitoring of such patients in the hospital, the mortality rate has been reduced to less than 5% for DKA and 15% for HHS [3,4,7,8]. Indications for hospitalization include loss of greater than 5% body weight during the crisis, respiration rate faster than 35 per minute, intractable elevation of blood glucose, changes in mental status, uncontrolled fever, and unresolved nausea and vomiting [4]. Poor prognostic signs for DKA and HHS include advanced age, lower degree of consciousness, and lower blood pressure. The cost of these crises, in one study, was estimated to be about $13,000 per episode [9]. The annual hospital cost for patients in hyperglycemic crisis may exceed billions of dollars per year [9]. Prevention of these metabolic emergencies, therefore, poses an important medical and social challenge. Preventive procedures should include extensive educational programs which review steps to be taken during sick days for patients with diabetes, including frequent monitoring of blood glucose and urine ketones. The use of a liquid diet, containing salt and carbohydrates, close contact with health care providers, and, above all, the use of short-acting insulin are important precautionary measures for prevention of recurrence of these crises. Injection of short-acting insulin should not be stopped during sick days in patients with diabetes. In addition to educational endeavors, improved access to a health care delivery system and the availability of affordable medication in less affluent segments of society are some of the most effective methods for prevention of such crises.

Structure of the Islets of Langerhans

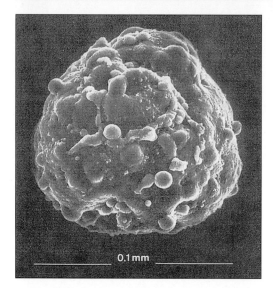

FIGURE 3-1. Surface topography of the periphery of the islet cell (× 900). (*From* Orci [10]; with permission.)

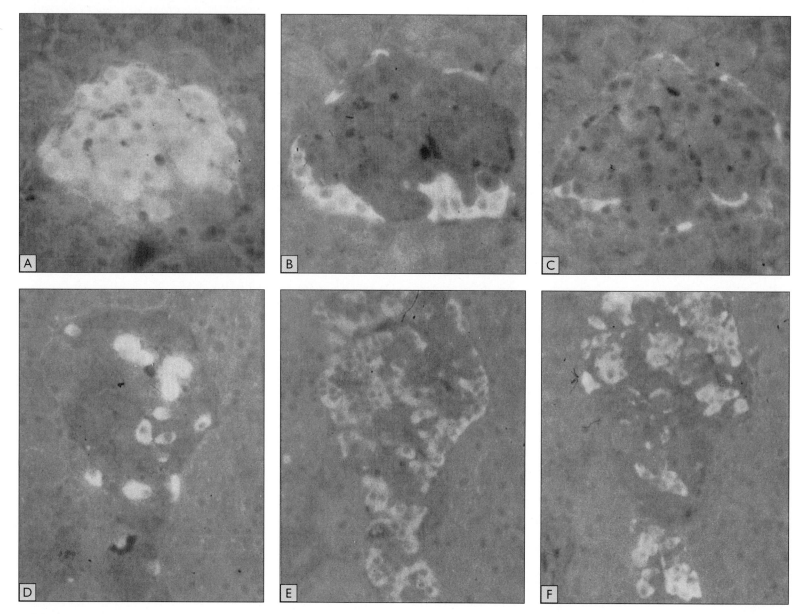

FIGURE 3-2. (See Color Plate) Consecutive serial sections of islets of Langerhans processed for indirect immunofluorescence. **A—C,** The location of insulin-, glucagon-, and somatostatin-containing cells, respectively, in the islet of a control rat. **D—F,** The profound perturbation of this normal distribution in the islet of a rat rendered experimentally diabetic for 17 months after a single intravenous injection of streptozotocin, 45 mg/kg. Note that the number of insulin-containing cells is strikingly reduced while that of glucagon- and somatostatin-containing cells is greatly increased. (*From* Orci et al. [11]; with permission.)

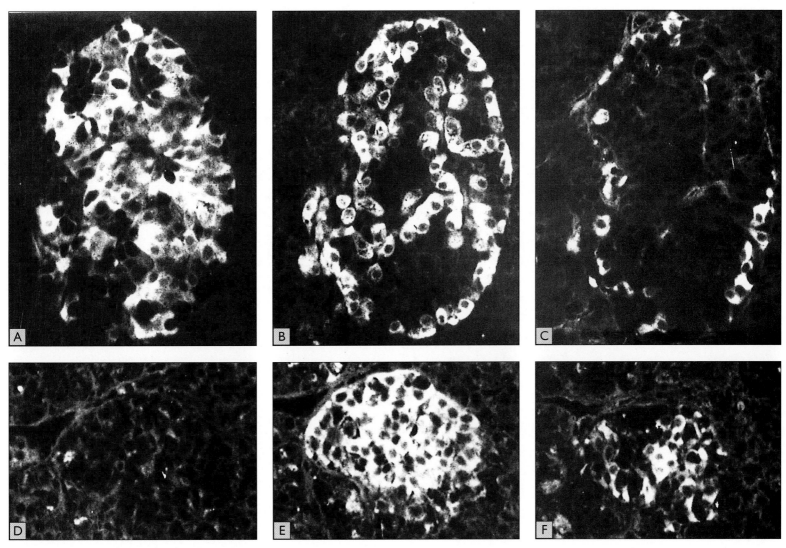

FIGURE 3-3. Distribution of β-, α-, and Δ-cells on serial sections of an islet from an adult nondiabetic subject. The indirect immunofluorescent technique demonstrates insulin (**A**), glucagon (**B**), and somatostatin (**C**). **D—F**, Serial sections of the islet of Langerhans in a patient with type 1 diabetes treated with the indirect immunofluorescent technique against insulin, glucagon, and somatostatin, respectively. The only detectable immunofluorescent cells within the islet are the numerous glucagon- and somatostatin-containing cells (× 200). (*From* Orci *et al.* [11]; with permission.)

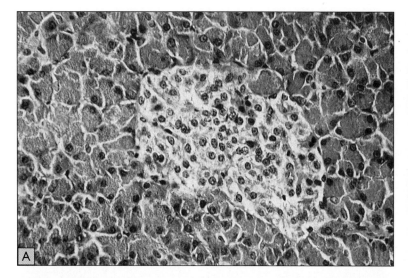

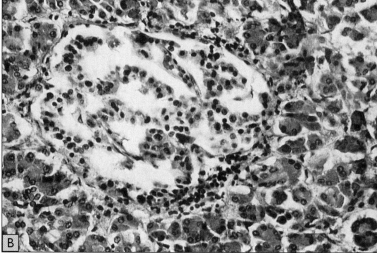

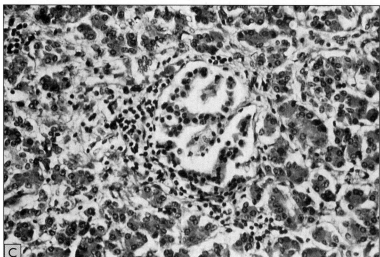

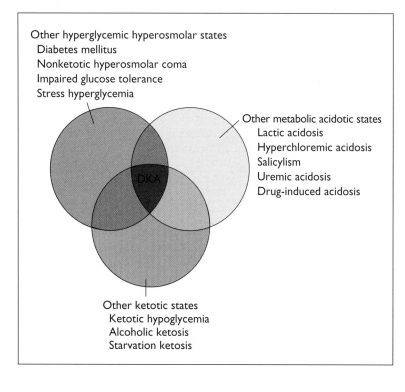

FIGURE 3-4. (See Color Plate) Islet cell necrosis and lymphocyte infiltration. **A,** Pancreatic islet section from normal, nondiabetic control patient. **B,** Pancreatic islet section from patient with type 1 diabetes. Lymphocytic infiltration can be seen throughout the pancreatic islets with residual islet cells. **C,** Pancreatic islet section from patient with type 1 diabetes showing lymphocytic infiltration in the pancreatic islets, particularly the peripheral islets. (*Courtesy of* J.W. Yoon.)

Definition and Criteria for Insulin-deficient State

Other hyperglycemic hyperosmolar states
Diabetes mellitus
Nonketotic hyperosmolar coma
Impaired glucose tolerance
Stress hyperglycemia

Other metabolic acidotic states
Lactic acidosis
Hyperchloremic acidosis
Salicylism
Uremic acidosis
Drug-induced acidosis

DKA

Other ketotic states
Ketotic hypoglycemia
Alcoholic ketosis
Starvation ketosis

FIGURE 3-5. Other conditions in which the components of the diagnostic triad for diabetic ketoacidosis (DKA) (hyperglycemia, ketosis, and acidosis) may be found. (*Adapted from* Kitabchi and Wall [12].)

Pathophysiology of Insulin-deficient State

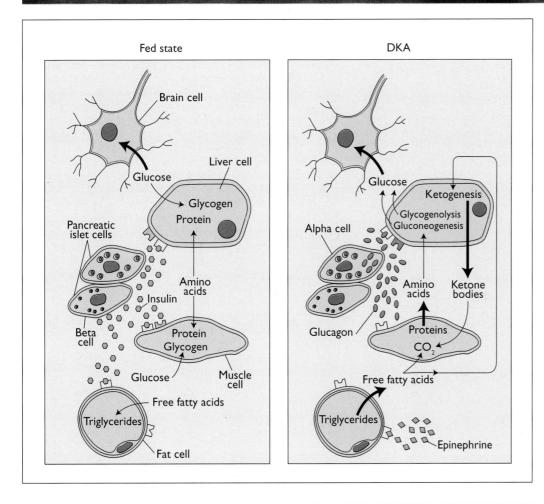

Fed state · DKA

FIGURE 3-8. Mechanisms of glucose regulation. Glucose supply to the brain can be maintained for days and even weeks when the body has been deprived of caloric intake. In the fed state (*left*), assimilation of metabolic fuels and substrates is promoted by insulin in tissues sensitive to the hormone. In diabetic ketoacidosis (DKA) (*right*), counterregulatory hormones (notably glucagon and epinephrine) reverse these processes, promoting glycogenolysis and creating substrates for ketogenesis and gluconeogenesis [14–17]. Denial of glucose to insulin-sensitive tissues preserves it for the brain. (*Adapted from* Kitabchi and Rumbak [17].)

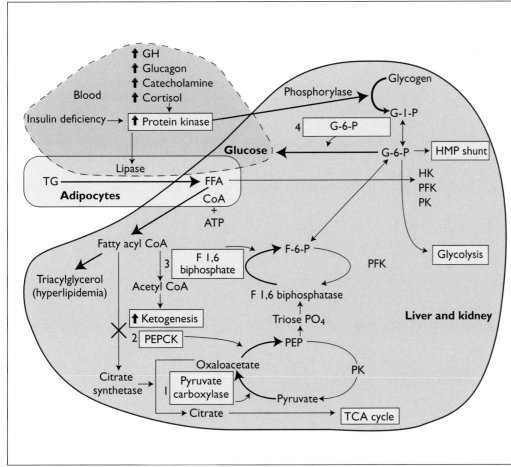

FIGURE 3-9. Proposed biochemical changes that occur during diabetic ketoacidosis. These alterations lead to increased gluconeogenesis and lipolysis and decreased glycolysis. *Note:* Lipolysis occurs mainly in adipose tissue. Other events occur primarily in the liver (except some gluconeogenesis in the kidney) [18]. *Thick arrows* indicate stimulated pathways in diabetic ketoacidosis, which consists of rate-limiting enzymes of gluconeogenesis, whereas *thin arrows* indicate inhibitory pathway in glycolysis. The tricarboxylic acid (TCA) cycle is inhibited by fatty and acyl coenzyme A (CoA)-induced inhibition of citrate synthesis, a rate-limiting enzyme in the TCA cycle. ATP—adenosine triphosphate; FFA—free fatty acids; F-6-P—fructose-6-phosphate; GH—growth hormone; G-1-P—glucose-1-phosphate; G-6-P—glucose-6-phosphate; HK—hexokinase; HMP—hexose monophosphate; PC—pyruvate carboxylase; PEP—phosphoenolpyruvate; PEPCK—phosphoenolpyruvate carboxykinase; PFK—phosphofructokinase; PK—pyruvate kinase; TG—triglycerides. (*Adapted from* Kitabchi et al. [8].)

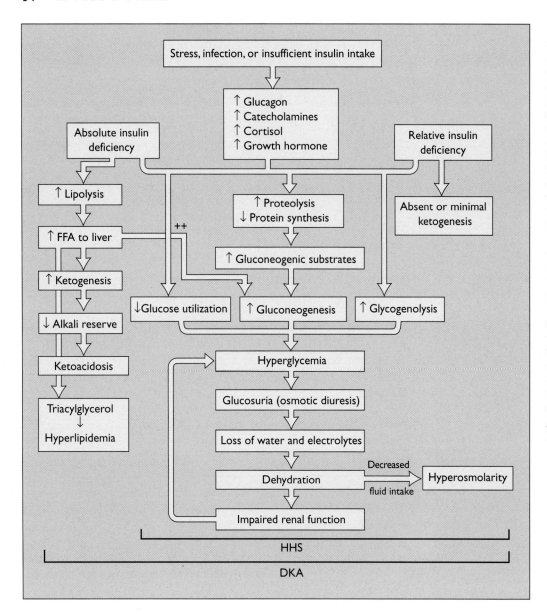

FIGURE 3-10. Pathogenesis of diabetic ketoacidosis (DKA) and hyperglycemic hyperosmolar syndrome (HHS). Alteration of fat, protein, and carbohydrate metabolism leads to metabolic changes toward catabolic states and symptoms of polyuria, polydipsia, polyphagia, osmotic diuresis, severe dehydration, and, if not treated, coma and death. The hallmark of these events is the insulin-deficient state and increased counterregulatory hormones. In HHS, in addition to the relative insulin deficiency and greater dehydration, there is also a greater amount of hyperglycemia (secondary to lower intake of fluid) than in DKA. Although the mechanism for the lack of a significant amount of ketosis and acidemia in HHS (as compared with DKA) is not entirely clear, in one study the level of C-peptide (as an indication of pancreatic insulin reserve) was shown to be five- to tenfold lower in DKA than in HHS [19]. This has been offered as a partial explanation for the lack of ketonemia in HHS. Since the required amount of insulin for its antilipolytic action is about five- to tenfold lower than for the glucose transport action [20], it follows that the larger amount of residual insulin (C-peptide) in HHS is sufficient to prevent lipolysis (thus no ketogenesis in HHS). This amount of insulin is not enough to promote glucose transport and its metabolism, thus the resultant hyperglycemia is noted in HHS without severe ketonemia. (*Adapted from* Kitabchi *et al.* [4].)

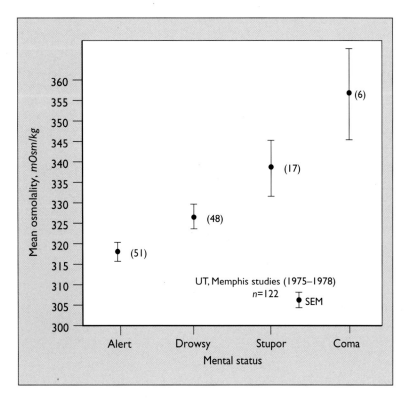

FIGURE 3-11. Calculated serum osmolality in 122 patients with diabetic ketoacidosis with relation to mental status. About one third of patients with hyperglycemic crises may present with altered mental status [6]. This can be correlated to serum osmolality but needs to be differentiated from various clinical conditions associated with altered mental status or coma (see Fig. 3-7), which may be present in diabetic patients. (*Adapted from* Kitabchi and Fisher [6].)

Treatment of Acute Diabetic Complications

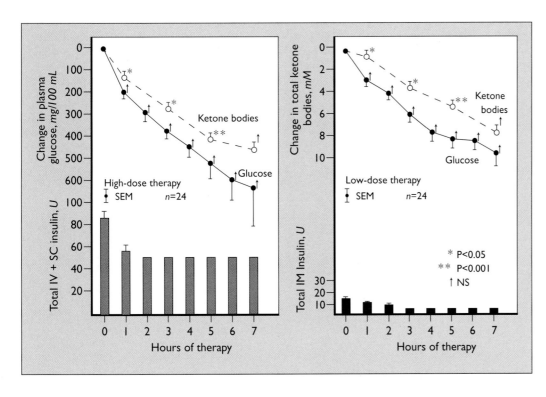

FIGURE 3-12. Efficacy of low-dose versus conventional therapy of insulin for treatment of diabetic ketoacidosis. Treatment of hyperglycemic crises has undergone numerous modifications since the discovery of insulin. In the early decades after the discovery of insulin, low-dose therapy was the norm due to the limited availability of insulin, but in subsequent decades, doses of insulin were modified from physiologic to pharmacologic and even suprapharmacologic doses until the mid-1970s. The initial observation of Alberti et al. [21] demonstrated the effectiveness of low-dose insulin and gave impetus to the first prospective randomized study, which is summarized here [22]. This study confirms the similarity of the responses to low-dose and high-dose insulin in diabetic ketoacidosis without the disadvantages of greater hypoglycemia and hypokalemia associated with high-dose insulin therapy. IV—intravenous; IM—intramuscular; SC—subcutaneous; NS—not significant. (*Adapted from* Kitabchi et al. [22].)

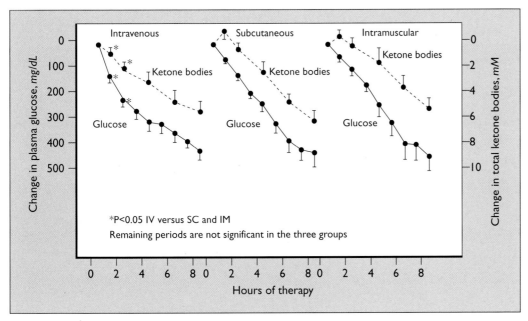

FIGURE 3-13. Comparison of the effects of randomized intravenous (IV), subcutaneous (SC), and intramuscular (IM) low-dose insulin regimens on changes in plasma glucose and total ketone bodies in patients with diabetic ketoacidosis (15 patients in each group). The low-dose insulin therapy was effective in lowering blood glucose in diabetic ketoacidosis therapy by any route of administration. (*Adapted from* Fisher et al. [23].)

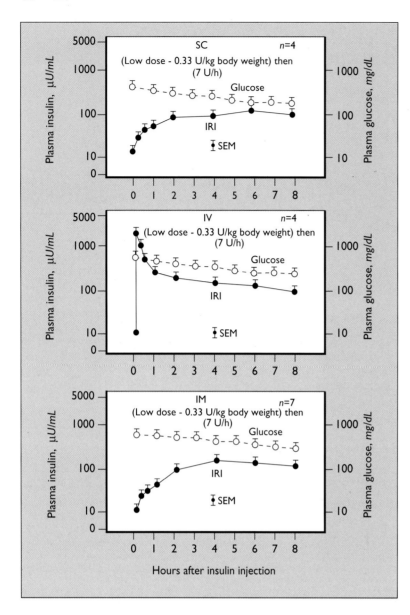

FIGURE 3-14. Comparison of the effect of low-dose insulin regimen (7 U/h) administered by subcutaneous (SC), intravenous (IV), and intramuscular (IM) injections on plasma immunoreactive insulin (IRI) levels (*closed circles*) and plasma glucose decrements (*open circles*) in three groups of diabetic ketoacidosis patients who had not previously been treated with insulin. In these patients, IV insulin caused serum insulin to rise immediately to supraphysiologic levels, whereas SC and IM injections of the same amount of insulin resulted in lower serum insulin concentrations, which reached near physiologic concentrations (postprandially) only after 2 to 3 hours. This low level of insulin may be the reason for the slow clearance of ketone bodies noted in Figure 3-13 for the IM and SC routes as compared to the IV route of the same amount of insulin injection (7 U/h). (*Adapted from* Kitabchi *et al.* [24].)

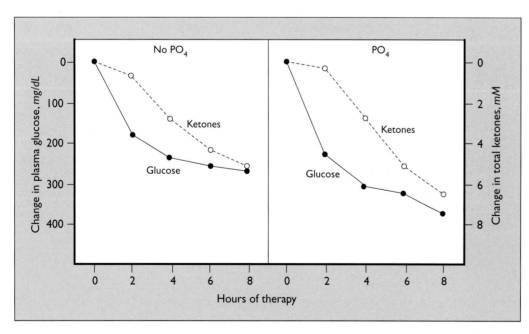

FIGURE 3-15. Use of phosphate in diabetic ketoacidosis. Another controversial issue in the management of diabetic ketoacidosis (DKA) prompted study on the use of phosphate (PO_4) replacement in DKA. This study shows that phosphate therapy does not affect the clinical and biochemical outcomes (plasma glucose and ketone bodies) of low-dose insulin therapy. However, the use of phosphate in DKA was associated with a certain degree of hypocalcemia. (*Adapted from* Fisher and Kitabchi [25].)

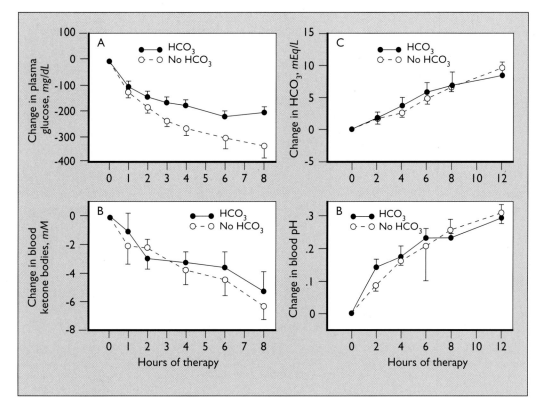

FIGURE 3-16. The role of bicarbonate therapy in the treatment of diabetic ketoacidosis [26]. This prospective randomized study shows the effect of bicarbonate (HCO₃) therapy on various recovery parameters of diabetic ketoacidosis (DKA), indicating that bicarbonate did not alter outcomes of DKA therapy on hours of recovery from hyperglycemia, acidosis, or hypocapnia [27]. There is, therefore, very little reason for the use of bicarbonate therapy in DKA, particularly when the pH level is greater than 7.0 [26]. [*Adapted from* Morris *et al.* [27].)

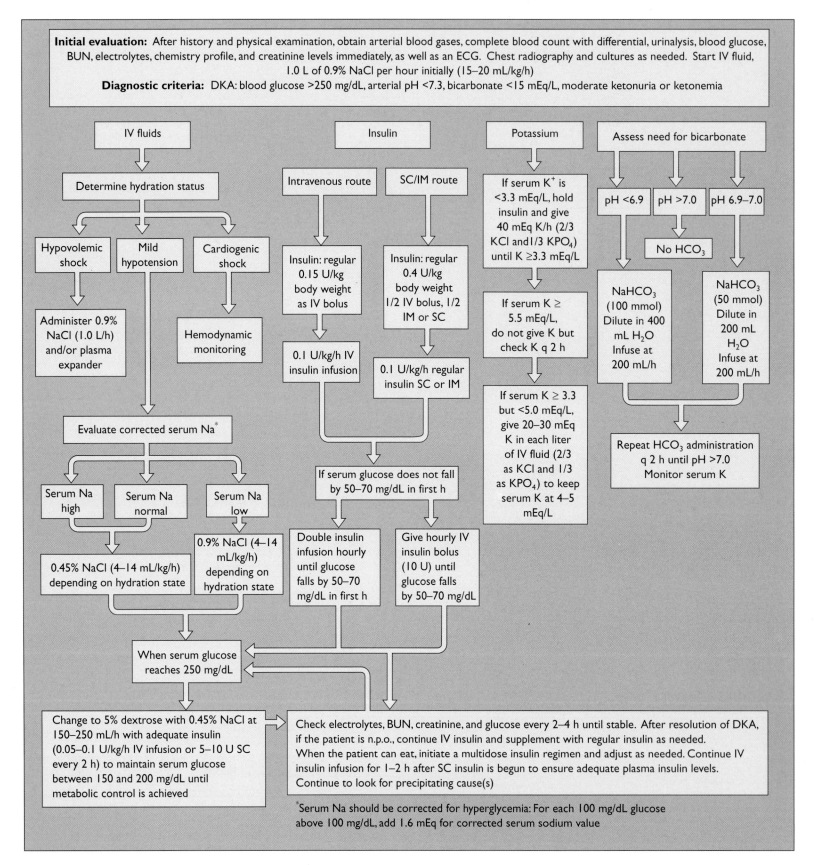

Initial evaluation: After history and physical examination, obtain arterial blood gases, complete blood count with differential, urinalysis, blood glucose, BUN, electrolytes, chemistry profile, and creatinine levels immediately, as well as an ECG. Chest radiography and cultures as needed. Start IV fluid, 1.0 L of 0.9% NaCl per hour initially (15–20 mL/kg/h)
Diagnostic criteria: DKA: blood glucose >250 mg/dL, arterial pH <7.3, bicarbonate <15 mEq/L, moderate ketonuria or ketonemia

IV fluids

Determine hydration status

Hypovolemic shock | Mild hypotension | Cardiogenic shock

Administer 0.9% NaCl (1.0 L/h) and/or plasma expander

Hemodynamic monitoring

Evaluate corrected serum Na*

Serum Na high | Serum Na normal | Serum Na low

0.9% NaCl (4–14 mL/kg/h) depending on hydration state

0.45% NaCl (4–14 mL/kg/h) depending on hydration state

Insulin

Intravenous route | SC/IM route

Insulin: regular 0.15 U/kg body weight as IV bolus

Insulin: regular 0.4 U/kg body weight 1/2 IV bolus, 1/2 IM or SC

0.1 U/kg/h IV insulin infusion

0.1 U/kg/h regular insulin SC or IM

If serum glucose does not fall by 50–70 mg/dL in first h

Double insulin infusion hourly until glucose falls by 50–70 mg/dL in first h

Give hourly IV insulin bolus (10 U) until glucose falls by 50–70 mg/dL

Potassium

If serum K$^+$ is <3.3 mEq/L, hold insulin and give 40 mEq K/h (2/3 KCl and 1/3 KPO$_4$) until K ≥3.3 mEq/L

If serum K ≥ 5.5 mEq/L, do not give K but check K q 2 h

If serum K ≥ 3.3 but <5.0 mEq/L, give 20–30 mEq K in each liter of IV fluid (2/3 as KCl and 1/3 as KPO$_4$) to keep serum K at 4–5 mEq/L

Assess need for bicarbonate

pH <6.9 | pH >7.0 | pH 6.9–7.0

No HCO$_3$

NaHCO$_3$ (100 mmol) Dilute in 400 mL H$_2$O Infuse at 200 mL/h

NaHCO$_3$ (50 mmol) Dilute in 200 mL H$_2$O Infuse at 200 mL/h

Repeat HCO$_3$ administration q 2 h until pH >7.0 Monitor serum K

When serum glucose reaches 250 mg/dL

Change to 5% dextrose with 0.45% NaCl at 150–250 mL/h with adequate insulin (0.05–0.1 U/kg/h IV infusion or 5–10 U SC every 2 h) to maintain serum glucose between 150 and 200 mg/dL until metabolic control is achieved

Check electrolytes, BUN, creatinine, and glucose every 2–4 h until stable. After resolution of DKA, if the patient is n.p.o., continue IV insulin and supplement with regular insulin as needed. When the patient can eat, initiate a multidose insulin regimen and adjust as needed. Continue IV insulin infusion for 1–2 h after SC insulin is begun to ensure adequate plasma insulin levels. Continue to look for precipitating cause(s)

*Serum Na should be corrected for hyperglycemia: For each 100 mg/dL glucose above 100 mg/dL, add 1.6 mEq for corrected serum sodium value

FIGURE 3-17. Protocol for the therapeutic management of patients with diabetic ketoacidosis (DKA). Important interventions include the use of insulin, adequate hydration, and frequent monitoring of patients [4,6,13].

BUN—blood urea nitrogen; ECG—electrocardiogram; IM—intramuscular; IV—intravenous; n.p.o.—nothing by mouth; SC—subcutaneous. (*Adapted from* [28].)

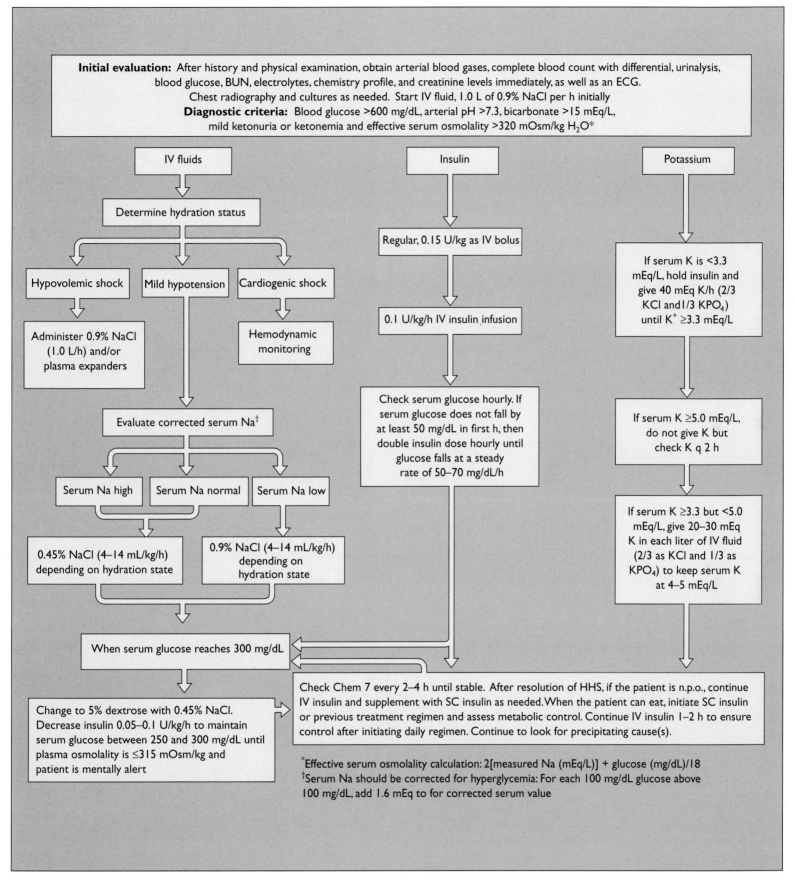

FIGURE 3-18. Protocol for the therapeutic management of patients with hyperglycemic hyperosmolar syndrome (HHS). These patients may require a greater amount of hydration as well as a slower rate of glucose decrement.

Chem 7—electrolytes, blood urea nitrogen (BUN), creatinine; ECG—electrocardiogram; IV—intravenous; n.p.o.—nothing by mouth; SC—subcutaneous. (*Adapted from* Kitabchi *et al.* [8].)

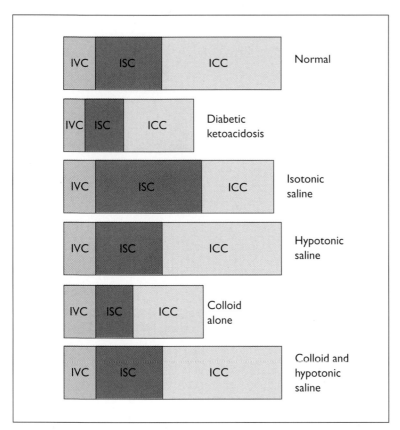

FIGURE 3-19. Use of hypotonic versus isotonic saline and plasma expanders. This figure demonstrates the effect of these solutions in various cellular compartments. The diagram depicts the decreased intravascular (IVC), interstitial (ISC), and intracellular (ICC) compartments present in patients with diabetic ketoacidosis (DKA), as compared with control patients. Subsequent panels show the effects of fluid resuscitation of DKA with different solutions. Isotonic solutions replete only IVC and ISC compartments, whereas hypotonic solutions replete all compartments. However, larger volumes of hypotonic solutions are required to produce equivalent increases in IVC. Colloid alone is restricted to the IVC; therefore, combined use of colloid plus hypotonic solution can lead to a rapid increase in IVC, followed by more gradual replacement of the other compartments. It is also important to remember that hydration in DKA and hyperglycemic hyperosmolar syndrome dilutes concentrations of the stress hormones and thus makes peripheral tissues more sensitive to lower doses of insulin [29]. (*Adapted from* Hillman [30].)

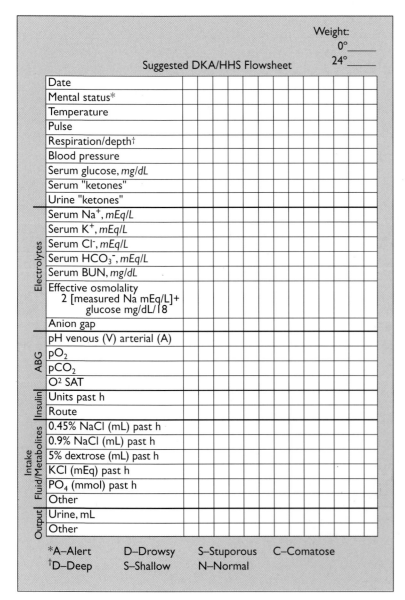

FIGURE 3-20. Flow sheet to document serial changes in laboratory/clinical values and supplementary measures during recovery from diabetic ketoacidosis (DKA). ABG—arterial blood gases; BUN—blood urea nitrogen; HHS—hyperglycemic hyperosmolar syndrome; SAT—saturation. (*Adapted from* Kitabchi *et al.* [8].)

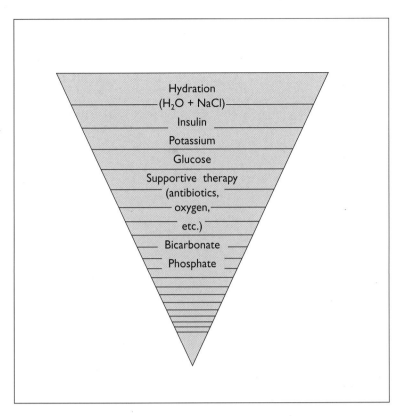

FIGURE 3-21. Treatment of hyperglycemic crisis. This figure summarizes the importance of documentation of various modalities of therapy and responses to treatment of hyperglycemic crises. The importance of frequent monitoring of patients by health care providers cannot be overemphasized. Precipitating causes of these crises must be sought while the patient is being managed, and the patient should be referred to an educational program, as discussed earlier, for prevention of future recurrence of such events. (*Adapted from* Kitabchi *et al.* [31]).

References

1. Turnebum A: Of the causes and signs of acute and chronic disease, 1554. Reynolds TF, translator. London: William Pickering, 1837.

2. Faich GA, Fishbein HA, Ellis SE: The epidemiology of diabetic acidosis: a population-based study. *Am J Epidemiol* 1983, 117:551.

3. Fishbein HA, Palumbo PJ: *Acute Metabolic Complications in Diabetes.* Diabetes in America (National Diabetes Data Group). Bethesda, MD: National Institutes of Health; 1995. NIH Publication 95-1468.

4. Kitabchi AE, Umpierrez GE, Murphy MB, *et al.*: Management of hyperglycemic crises in patients with diabetes. *Diabetes Care* 2001, 24:131–153.

5. Umpierrez GE, Kelly JP, Navarrete JE, *et al.*: Hyperglycemic crises in urban blacks. *Arch Int Med* 1997, 157:669–675.

6. Kitabchi AE, Fisher JN: Insulin therapy of diabetic ketoacidosis: physiologic versus pharmacologic doses of insulin and their routes of administration. In *Handbook of Diabetes Mellitus*, vol 5. Edited by Brownlee M. New York: Garland ATPM Press; 1981:95–149.

7. Carroll P, Matz R: Uncontrolled diabetes mellitus in adults: experience in treating diabetic ketoacidosis and hyperosmolar coma with low-dose insulin and uniform treatment regimen. *Diabetes Care* 1983, 6:579–585.

8. Kitabchi AE, Fisher JN, Murphy MB, Rumbak MJ: Diabetic ketoacidosis and the hyperglycemic hyperosmolar nonketotic state. In *Joslin's Diabetes Mellitus*, edn 13. Edited by Kahn CR, Weir GC. Philadelphia: Lea & Febiger; 1994:738–770.

9. Javor KA, Kotsanos JG, McDonald RC, *et al.*: Diabetic ketoacidosis charges relative to medical charges of adult patients with type 1 diabetes. *Diabetes Care* 1997, 20:349–354.

10. Orci L: *A fresh look at the interrelationships within the islets of Langerhans.* Diabetes Research Today. Stuttgart: Meeting of the Minkowski Prizewinners. Symposium Capri, FK Schattauer, Verlag; 1976.

11. Orci L, Baetens D, Rufener C, *et al.*: Hypertrophy and hyperplasia of somatostatin-containing D-cells in diabetes. *Proc Natl Acad Sci USA* 1976, 73:1338–1342.

12. Kitabchi AE, Wall BM: Diabetic ketoacidosis. *Med Clin North Am* 1995, 79:9–37.

13. Morris LE, Kitabchi AE: Coma in the diabetic. In *Diabetes Mellitus: Problems in Management.* Edited by Schnatz JD. Menlo Park, CA: Addison-Wesley; 1982:234–251.

14. DeFronzo RA, Matsuda M, Barrett E: Diabetic ketoacidosis. A combined metabolic-nephrologic approach to therapy. *Diabetes Review* 1994, 2:209–238.

15. Miles JM, Rizza RA, Haymond MW, Gerich JE: Effects of acute insulin deficiency on glucose and ketone body turnover in man: evidence for the primacy overproduction of glucose and ketone bodies in the genesis of diabetic ketoacidosis. *Diabetes* 1980, 29:926–930.

16. McGarry JD, Woeltje KF, Kuwajima M, Foster DW: Regulation of ketogenesis and the renaissance of carnitine palmitoyl transferase. *Diab Metab Rev* 1989, 5:271–284.

17. Kitabchi AE, Rumbak MJ: Management of diabetic emergencies. *Hosp Pract* 1989, 24:129–160.

18. Myer C, Stumvolle M, Nadkarni V, *et al.*: Abnormal renal and hepatic glucose metabolism in type 2 diabetes mellitus. *J Clin Invest* 1998, 102:619–624.

19. Chupin M, Charbonnel B, Chupin F: C-peptide levels in ketoacidosis and in hyperosmolar non-ketotic diabetic coma. *Acta Diabet* 1981, 18:123–128.

20. Schade DS, Eaton RP: Dose response to insulin in man: differential effects on glucose and ketone body regulation. *J Clin Endocrinol Metab* 1977, 44:1038–1053.

21. Alberti KGMM, Hockaday TDR, Turner RC: Small doses of intramuscular insulin in the treatment of diabetic coma. *Lancet* 1973, 5:515–522.

22. Kitabchi AE, Ayyagari V, Guerra SMO, Medical House Staff: The efficacy of low dose versus conventional therapy of insulin for treatment of diabetic ketoacidosis. *Ann Intern Med* 1976, 84:633–638.

23. Fisher JN, Shahshahani MN, Kitabchi AE: Diabetic ketoacidosis: low-dose insulin therapy by various routes. *N Engl J Med* 1977, 297:238–247.

24. Kitabchi AE, Young RT, Sacks HS, Morris L: Diabetic ketoacidosis: reappraisal of therapeutic approach. *Ann Rev Med* 1979, 30:339–357.

25. Fisher JN, Kitabchi AE: A randomized study of phosphate therapy in the treatment of diabetic ketoacidosis. *J Clin Endocrinol Metab* 1983, 57:177–180.

26. Matz R: Diabetic acidosis: rationale for not using bicarbonate. *NY State J Med* 1977, 76:1299–1303.

27. Morris LR, Murphy MB, Kitabchi AE: Bicarbonate therapy in severe diabetic ketoacidosis. *Ann Intern Med* 1986, 105:836–840.

28. Hyperglycemic crises in patients with diabetes mellitus. American Diabetes Association position statement. *Diabetes Care* 2002, 25:5100–5108.

29. Waldhausl W, Kleinberger G, Korn A, *et al.*: Severe hyperglycemia: effects of hydration on endocrine derangements and blood glucose concentration. *Diabetes* 1979, 28:577–584.

30. Hillman K: Fluid resuscitation in diabetic emergencies: a reappraisal. *Intensive Care Med* 1987, 13:4–8.

31. Kitabchi AE, Matteri R, Murphy MB: Optimum insulin delivery in diabetic ketoacidosis and hyperglycemic hyperosmolar nonketotic coma. *Diabetes Care* 1982, 5:78–87.

TYPE 1 DIABETES

Mark A. Atkinson

4

Type I diabetes is a chronic disorder resulting from autoimmune destruction of the insulin-producing pancreatic β cells. The epidemiologic features of type 1 diabetes are described, and the possible contributions of genetics and environment to its development are illustrated. In addition, based on improved knowledge of the immunopathogenesis of this disorder, we report on work that holds promise for future interventions aimed at prevention.

The exact cause or causes of type 1 diabetes remain unclear [1]. It occurs most frequently in whites of Northern European descent, with more than a 40-fold difference observed in disease incidence rates based on geographic location. Environmental factors such as diet, stress, and viruses have been proposed to play a modifying and perhaps even a primary role in the development of type 1 diabetes. Thus, these factors may contribute to its varying prevalence. The disorder was once termed *juvenile diabetes* and thought to occur predominantly in persons under 18 years of age. However, more recent evidence suggests that the number of new cases may be equal in those over and under 30 years of age.

Susceptibility to type 1 diabetes is inherited, and increased risk is associated with being a first-degree relative to a person with a diabetic proband. However, approximately 85% of new cases show no such familial lineage. The major genetic region associated with predisposition to the disease is the one that encodes genes for the highly polymorphic human leukocyte antigens (HLAs). However, nearly 20 other loci have been proposed as contributing from 50% to 70% of the total genetic susceptibility.

Multiple lines of evidence support the theory that type 1 diabetes has an autoimmune nature. The evidence includes the aforementioned association with HLA, presence of a lymphocytic infiltrate within the pancreatic islet cells (*ie*, insulitis), and expression of islet reactive autoantibodies. Although once viewed as an acutely developing illness, today it is known that the natural history of type 1 diabetes is that of a chronic autoimmune process. In most patients the disease exists for months to years in a preclinical, asymptomatic phase. Many improvements in our knowledge of the pathogenesis of type 1 diabetes derive from investigations of two spontaneous animal models for the disease (*ie*, BioBreeding rats and nonobese diabetic mice).

Although it remains unclear which immune system component or mechanism plays the major role in β-cell destruction, most studies point toward the cellular immune system as providing a key role. Furthermore, multiple interrelated flaws in immunoregulation may underlie the failure to form a tolerance to self-antigens that results in type 1 diabetes. A large number of islet cell antigens have been associated with type 1 diabetes. Their biochemical identification has led to improved markers for predicting future cases and provided the potential to design antigen-specific therapies aimed at prevention. Numerous intervention studies have been directed toward patients with new-onset type 1 diabetes (predominantly involving immunosuppression), with disappointing degrees of success in terms of disease reversal. Improvements have been made in the ability to predict future cases of type 1 diabetes and assess metabolic activity. Therefore, the more recent clinical trials have sought to use alternatives such as nicotinamide and insulin that are much less likely to have such serious side effects as immunosuppressive agents, thus providing a safe and effective means of disease prevention.

Clinical Description

COMPARISON OF CLINICAL, GENETIC, AND IMMUNOLOGIC FEATURES OF TYPE 1 AND TYPE 2 DIABETES

Characteristic	Type 1	Type 2
Onset	Abrupt	Progressive
Endogenous insulin	Low to absent	Normal, elevated, or depressed
Ketosis	Common	Rare
Age at onset	Any age	Vast majority in adults
Body mass	Usually nonobese	Obese or nonobese
Treatment	Insulin	Diet, oral hypoglycemics, insulin
Family history	10%–15%	30%
Twin concordance	30%–50%	70%–90%
Human leukocyte antigen (HLA) association	HLA-DR, HLA-DQ	Unrelated
Autoantibodies	Present in most (>85%)	Absent, except in patients with coincident type 1 disease

FIGURE 4-1. Comparison of features of type 1 diabetes. The terms applied to the subgroup of disorders known collectively as diabetes mellitus are useful. However, they often break down in practice owing to confusion regarding the age at diagnosis or to an overlap or absence of the indicated features normally associated with the specific disorder. In many instances, the terms *type 1 diabetes* and *insulin-dependent diabetes* are used interchangeably, as are the terms *type 2 diabetes* and *non–insulin-dependent diabetes*. However, enthusiasm has grown for the terms *type 1 diabetes* or *immune-mediated diabetes* (IMD) to identify the forms of diabetes involving an autoimmune destruction of the insulin-producing pancreatic β cells.

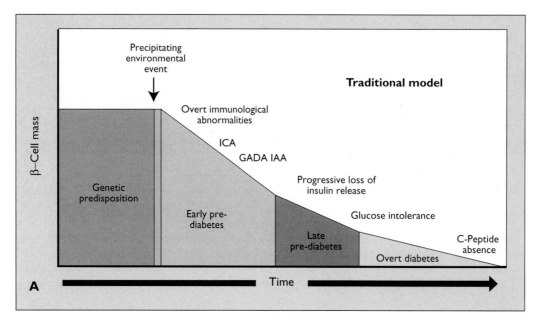

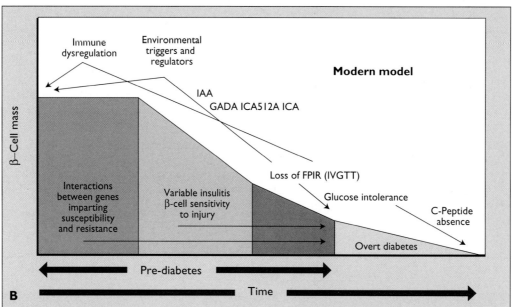

FIGURE 4-2. Traditional and modern models of the pathogenesis and natural history of type 1 diabetes. The traditional model provided represents common features cited in numerous publications and presentations from 1986 to date. The modern model expands and updates the traditional model by inclusion of information gained through an improved understanding of the roles of genetics, immunology, and environment in the natural history of type 1 diabetes. In the modern model, the natural history of type 1 diabetes has been modeled into a disease comprised of four stages. Stage 1 includes genetic susceptibility and resistance (major histocompatibility complex [MHC] and non-MHC) with intact β-cell mass. The interaction between the genetics surrounding this disorder, immune dysregulation, and environmental encounters results in stage 2, a process that in some cases can begin in the first few months or years of life. At that time, insulitis is initiated and again, owing to a genetic predisposition that does not properly regulate immune responses, the process of β-cell destruction begins. Autoantibodies to islet cell antigens develop, marking the autoimmune disease process; however, no measurable β-cell dysfunction occurs at this stage. In stage 3, a gradual decline in β-cell mass occurs, with the slope being highly variable between persons (*ie,* months to years). Incipient β-cell damage is first detectable as an abnormal intravenous glucose tolerance test with a deficient first-phase insulin response. In stage 4, an advanced degree of β-cell damage, hyperglycemia symptomatic of type 1 diabetes onset (with minimal C peptide), and exogenous insulin dependence occur. With complete β-cell destruction, the C peptide becomes undetectable and autoantibody markers of disease disappear. IAA—insulin autoantibodies; ICA—islet cell autoantibodies; FPIR—first phase insulin response; GADA—glutamic acid decarboxylase autoantibodies; IVGTT—intravenous glucose tolerance test. (*Adapted from* Atkinson [1] and Eisenbarth [2].)

Epidemiology

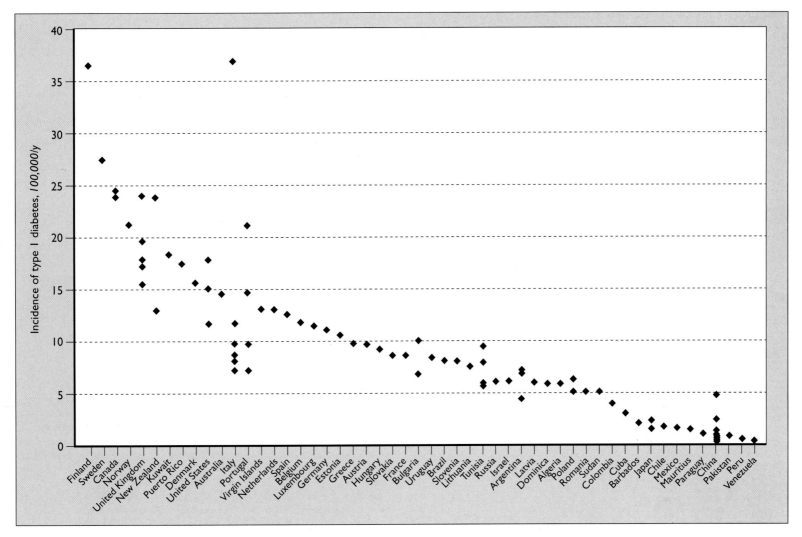

FIGURE 4-3. Variations in the incidence of type I diabetes based on geographic location. This disease predominantly affects populations with a substantial white genetic admixture. In Finland the incidence rate approaches 40 cases per 100,000 persons per year, whereas in Korea and Mexico the rate approximates 0.6 per 100,000 per year. In Europe the incidence is highest in the northern regions and generally declines in countries that lie in the south. Exceptions do exist, especially in the case of Sardinia, Italy, where the incidence rate approximates that of Finland. Furthermore, the disease incidence in Iceland is only one third that of Finland. Multiple studies suggest a continuing increase in the incidence of the disease, reporting regional increases of 6% to 20% per decade. (*Adapted from* Karvonen *et al.* [3].)

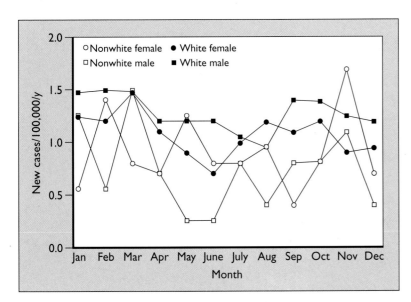

FIGURE 4-4. Variations in the frequency of diagnosing type I diabetes as a function of season. Data from Allegheny County, Pennsylvania, show a decline in newly diagnosed cases in the summer months. Additional studies confirm and expand on this finding, with reports of bimodal peaks in the late winter and early spring. Historically, such findings often have been considered as supporting an environmental agent in the pathogenesis of this disease. (*Adapted from* LaPorte *et al.* [4].)

ENVIRONMENTAL AGENTS AND LIFESTYLE PRACTICES PURPORTED TO INFLUENCE THE INCIDENCE OF HUMAN TYPE I DIABETES

Class	Specific Agent
Viruses	Coxsackie B
	Cytomegalovirus
	Echo
	Encephalomyocarditis
	Epstein-Barr
	Mumps
	Rotaviruses
	Rubella (congenital)
Diet	Cow's milk and cow's milk–based infant formulas
	Caffeine
	Nitrates (N-nitroso compounds)
	Duration of breast-feeding
Lifestyle	Exposure to β-cell toxins (eg, pyriminil)
	Stress
	Quantitative or qualitative exposure to viral and bacterial agents

FIGURE 4-5. Environmental agents and practices purported to influence the incidence of type I diabetes. Numerous epidemiologic studies and case reports have associated viral infections or local epidemics with type I diabetes. Likewise, epidemiologists have provided conflicting reports associating specific dietary practices with the disorder. However, when these practices are identified, their association (in terms of relative risk) usually is modest. Indeed, the collective literature to date has not demonstrated a diabetogenic agent that would represent a single major agent responsible for type I diabetes.

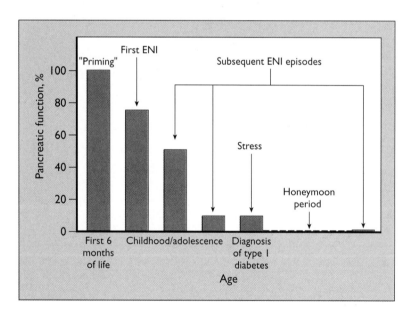

FIGURE 4-6. Multihit nature of action in type I diabetes. Thus far, no single agent has been associated exclusively with the disorder. Therefore, recent models associating environmental agents with type I diabetes have proposed a multihit nature of action. The primary "triggers" for type I diabetes could be those involving a yet to be identified interaction between an enterovirus and a nutritional factor. Subsequent enteroviral-nutritional interactions (ENI) could lead to further destruction of the pancreas. This situation would go unnoticed until there is not enough insulin-producing capability to respond to stress. Indeed, a stressful life event (eg, trauma, other infection, pubescent growth spurt, pregnancy) could cause a person to exceed the insulin-producing capacity of the pancreas and lead to the clinical diagnosis of type I diabetes. (*Adapted from* Hawkins [5].)

Genetics

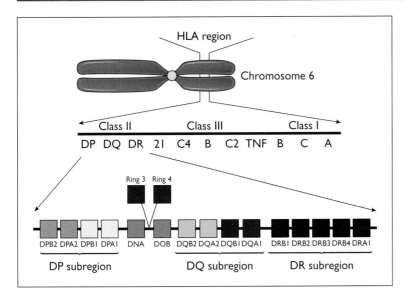

FIGURE 4-7. The human leukocyte antigen (HLA) region located on the short arm of chromosome 6. This region is approximately 3.5 centimorgans long and includes classes I, II, and III loci. Class I gene products (*ie*, HLA-A, HLA-B, and HLA-C) are expressed on all nucleated cells and serve as the classic transplantation antigens. These proteins present antigenic peptides to CD8+ T cells. Class II gene products are restricted in expression to antigen-presenting cells (*eg*, macrophages, dendritic cells, and B cells) and function to present peptides to CD4+ T cells. Class III gene products include complement proteins (*eg*, B, C2, and C4) and tumor necrosis factor (TNF).

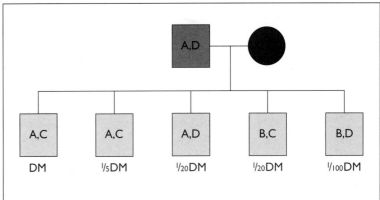

FIGURE 4-8. Familial risk of developing type I diabetes as a function of the relationship to the disease proband. The prevalence of disease (DM) is 30% to 50% in twins (not shown), 20% in human leukocyte antigen (HLA–) identical siblings (patient A,C), 5% in haploidentical siblings (A,D; B,C), and 1% in non-identical siblings (B,D). The mode of inheritance remains an enigma. Both dominant and recessive patterns of inheritance have been proposed; however, neither model adequately addresses type I diabetes. This line of investigation is further complicated by the potential interactions between genes and environmental factors, as well as evidence of the polygenic nature (*ie*, currently 20 additional loci) of the disorder. Furthermore, the risk of developing diabetes is higher in offspring of a father with type I diabetes than in offspring of a mother with the disorder. The lifetime risk for first-degree relatives is 5% to 8%. The probability is shown relative to inheritance of HLA haplotypes, which is indicated as A, B, C, D.

HLA-DR AND HLA-DQ TYPES AND THE RISK FOR TYPE I DIABETES	
Risk	**Genotype**
Susceptible	DR3
	DR4
	DR1 (<DR3 or DR4)
	DQA1*0301
	DQA1*0501
	DQB1*0201
	DQB1*0302
Resistant	DR2
	DR5 (< DR2)
	DQB1*0602
	DQB1*0301

FIGURE 4-9. HLA-DR and HLA-DQ types and the risk for type I diabetes. Note that these associations are representative of those most often observed in whites with a strong Northern European genetic influence. Interestingly, variance in susceptibility and resistance of human leukocyte antigen (HLA) types have been noted with type I diabetes in patients of different ethnic admixtures, especially those of Asian descent. Approximately 95% of whites with type I diabetes have either HLA-DR3 or HLA-DR4. However, susceptibility appears to reside predominantly in the HLA-DQ alleles under influence of HLA-DR. Furthermore, depending on the specific haplotype inherited, risk can be modified by the presence of a strong susceptibility or resistance allele, *eg*, DQB1*0602.

LOCATION AND MARKERS FOR REPORTED SUSCEPTIBILITY INTERVALS FOR HUMAN TYPE I DIABETES

Loci	Region	Markers
IDDM1	6p21.3	HLA-DRB1, DQB1, DQA1
IDDM2	11p15	INS VNTR
IDDM3	15q26	D15S107
IDDM4	11q13	D11S1337, FGF3
IDDM5	6q25	ESR
IDDM6	18q21	D18S487, JK
IDDM7	2q31	HOXD8, D2S152
IDDM8	6q27	D6S264, D6S446
IDDM9	3q21-q25	D3S1576
IDDM10	10p11-q11	D10S193
IDDM11	14q24.3-q31	D14S67
IDDM12	2q33	CTLA4
IDDM13	2q35	D2S164
IDDM15	6q21	D6S283
IDDM16	14q32.3	IGH, D14S542
IDDM17	10q25	D10S554
IDDM18	5q33-q34	IL12B
Unnamed	1q42	D1S1617
Unnamed	16q22-q24	D16S3098
Unnamed	19p13	D19S247
Unnamed	19q13	D19S225
Unnamed	Xp13-p11	DXS1068
Unnamed	7p13	GCK
Unnamed	12q14-q15	IFNG1

FIGURE 4-10. Location and markers for reported susceptibility intervals for human type I diabetes. Studies over the past 2 decades have suggested that a large number of genes or genetic intervals may be implicated in the pathogenesis of type I diabetes [6,7]. These genes are referred to as *susceptibility genes* that, by definition, increase or modify disease risk. Susceptibility genes are neither necessary nor sufficient for disease development. Therefore, some gene carriers may never develop the disease, whereas some noncarriers may develop type I diabetes. The IDDM1 loci (containing the HLA-DR and HLA-DQ regions) is the only major susceptibility interval, accounting for 30% to 50% of the total aggregated risk for type I diabetes.

Pathology

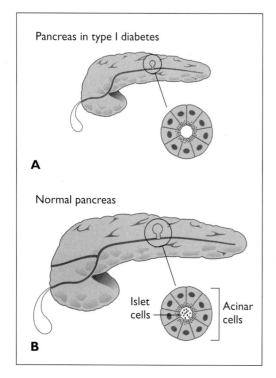

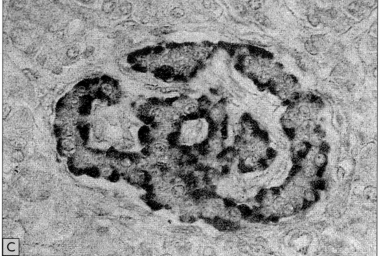

FIGURE 4-11. (See Color Plate) The effect of type I diabetes on the pancreas and islet cells. The pancreas of a person with type I diabetes (**A**) is often smaller and weighs less (ie, approximately 50% of total organ weight and 30% of endocrine weight) than its healthy counterpart (**B**). This difference is a consequence of the progressive atrophy of exocrine tissue that comprises about 98% of the total pancreatic volume. **C** and **D** demonstrate the pathology of pancreatic specimens from a patient with recent-onset type I diabetes. *Panel C,* Insulin-deficient islet stained for glucagon, somatostatin, and pancreatic polypeptide. All endocrine cells appear to have been stained, confirming the lack of β cells.

(Continued on next page)

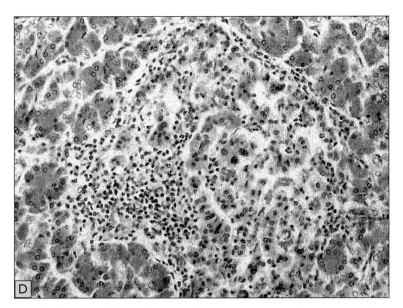

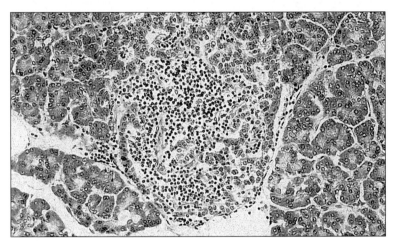

FIGURE 4-11. (*Continued*) Panel D, Insulitis. A chronic inflammatory cell infiltrate is centered on the islet. Insulitis is an elusive lesion to detect in the human pancreas, with only rare detection after 1 year of overt type I diabetes. With prolonged duration of disease, a progressive distortion of islet architecture develops, with a tendency for α and δ cells to leave the islet and spread as single cells into the exocrine parenchyma. (*Panel C,* immuno-alkaline phosphatase stain, ×1150; *panel D,* hematoxylin-eosin stain, ×300.) (*Panels C and D from* Foulis [8]; with permission.)

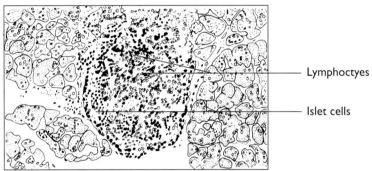

FIGURE 4-12. (*See* Color Plate) Islet of a patient recently diagnosed with type I diabetes demonstrating a diffuse lymphocytic infiltration (insulitis) with onset of atrophy of the islet cords. (Hematoxylin-eosin stain, ×300.) (*From* Foulis [8]; with permission.)

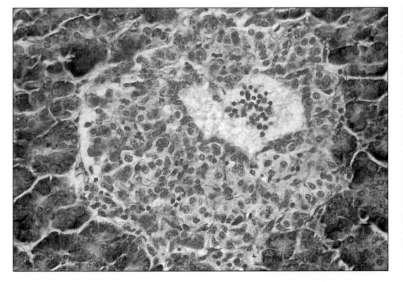

FIGURE 4-13. (*See* Color Plate) Pathology of a regenerating islet in the pancreas of a patient recently diagnosed with type I diabetes. Newly formed islet cells are derived from the epithelium of a duct. Lymphocytes are present in the lumen of the duct and in some places at the periphery. Evidence of such regeneration is rare in the pancreatic organs of patients with type I diabetes and is usually limited to those who die shortly after disease onset. (Hematoxylin-eosin stain, ×400.) (*From* Foulis [8]; with permission.)

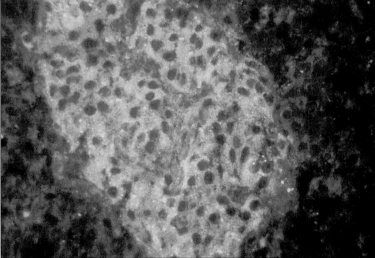

FIGURE 4-14. (*See* Color Plate) Islet cell autoantibodies (ICA). Islet cell autoantibodies are present in the serum of approximately 75% of persons at the onset of type I diabetes versus 0.4% of healthy persons. The first autoantibody ascribed to type I diabetes, the presence of islet cell autoantibodies is identified by indirect immunofluorescent assay using human blood group O pancreas. Islet cell autoantibodies specific for β cells have been identified. However, the autoantibodies react with all cells within the islet, including those that secrete insulin (β cells), glucagon (α cells), somatostatin cells (δ cells), and pancreatic polypeptide (PP cells). Autoantigens thus far ascribed to be responsible for the ICA reaction include sialoglycolipids, glutamic acid decarboxylase, and ICA512/IA-2.

AUTOANTIBODY MARKERS OF ISLET IMMUNITY IN HUMAN TYPE I DIABETES

Described in the 1970s
  Islet cell cytoplasmic autoantibodies
  Islet cell surface autoantibodies
Described in the 1980s
  64kD autoantibodies
  Carboxypeptidase-H autoantibodies
  Heat shock protein autoantibodies
  Insulin autoantibodies
  Insulin receptor autoantibodies
  Proinsulin autoantibodies
Described in the 1990s
  37kd/40kD tryptic fragment autoantibodies
  52kD rat insulinoma autoantibodies
  51kD aromatic-L-amino-acid decarboxylase autoantibodies
  128kD autoantibodies
  152kD autoantibodies
  Chymotrypsinogen-related 30 kD pancreatic autoantibodies
  DNA topoisomerase II autoantibodies
  Glucose transporter 2 autoantibodies
  Glutamic acid decarboxylase 65 autoantibodies
  Glutamic acid decarboxylase 67 autoantibodies
  Glima 38 autoantibodies
  Glycolipid autoantibodies
  GM2-1 islet ganglioside autoantibodies
  ICA512/IA-2 autoantibodies
  IA-2 autoantibodies
  Phogrin autoantibodies
Described in 2000s
  Carbonic anhidrase I autoantibodies
  Carbonic anhidrase II autoantibodies
  SOX-13 autoantibodies

FIGURE 4-15. Autoantibody markers of islet immunity in human type I diabetes. Since the first description of islet cell autoantibodies (ICAs) in 1974 (see Fig. 4-14), many new autoantibody markers of anti-islet immunity have been identified in patients with type I diabetes. In addition to their presence at disease onset, many of these markers have proved useful in identifying patients in the presymptomatic period, months to years before the clinical onset of type I diabetes. Of these, four markers have gained the most acceptance owing to scientific confirmation, high frequency of expression, and superior disease sensitivity and specificity: ICA, insulin autoantibodies, glutamic acid decarboxylase, and IA-2 autoantibodies.

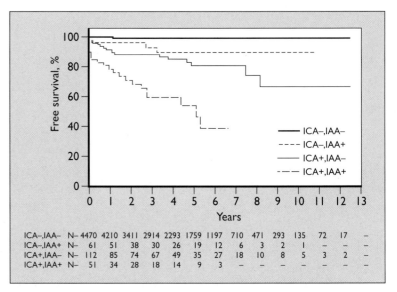

ICA–,IAA–	N–	4470	4210	3411	2914	2293	1759	1197	710	471	293	135	72	17	–
ICA–,IAA+	N–	61	51	38	30	26	19	12	6	3	2	1	–	–	–
ICA+,IAA–	N–	112	85	74	67	49	35	27	18	10	8	5	3	2	–
ICA+,IAA+	N–	51	34	28	18	14	9	3	–	–	–	–	–	–	–

FIGURE 4-16. Using autoantibodies to islet cell autoantigens to predict future cases of type I diabetes. This life-table analysis indicates the probability of remaining disease-free, stratified by the appearance of islet cell cytoplasmic autoantibodies (ICA) and insulin autoantibodies (IAA) in relatives of probands with the disease. The number of relatives followed since identification of the autoantibody is displayed at the bottom for each group. As can be observed, the probability of developing type I diabetes is highest in those persons with two autoantibodies, with approximately half of these persons developing the disease within 4 years. (*Adapted from* Krischer *et al.* [9].)

PREVALENCE OF GLUTAMIC ACID DECARBOXYLASE AUTOANTIBODIES AND THEIR POTENTIAL USE IN IDENTIFYING AUTOIMMUNE ACTIVITY

Subject Group	Autoantibody Frequency, %
Healthy control group	0.3–0.6
First-degree relatives of patients with type I diabetes	3–4
Patients with other autoimmune endocrine disorders	1–2
Patients with newly diagnosed type I diabetes	55–85
Patients with type 2 diabetes	10–15
Patients with gestational diabetes	10

FIGURE 4-17. Prevalence of glutamic acid decarboxylase autoantibodies and their potential use in identifying autoimmune activity. Glutamic acid decarboxylase (GAD) autoantibodies serve as a marker for predicting future cases and diagnosing new cases of type I diabetes. Recent investigations summarized in representative form here indicate that GAD autoantibodies may also be useful in identifying autoimmunity in persons diagnosed with other forms of diabetes. These identifications may be useful in terms of imparting appropriate diabetes management and clinical care.

THE NONOBESE DIABETIC MOUSE MODEL OF TYPE I DIABETES

Characteristic	Nonobese Diabetic Mice
Disease onset	Spontaneous, 13–30+ weeks of age
Gender bias	Female predominance
Disease frequency	Strong intercolony variation, 50%–80% female, 20%–50% male, typical rates at 26 weeks of age
Clinical presentation	Hyperglycemia, mild ketosis, polydipsia, polyuria, weight loss, insulin dependency
Additional disease model	Thyroiditis, sialoadenitis (Sjögren syndrome), deafness
Insulitis	Appears in nondestructive (5–12 wk) and destructive (13+ wk) phases; macrophages, dendritic cells, T and B lymphocytes, NK cells
Genetic susceptibility	Major histocompatibility complex (MHC) plus >15 non-MHC loci
Immune markers	Autoantibodies, autoreactive T cells

FIGURE 4-18. The nonobese diabetic mouse model of type I diabetes.

THE BIOBREEDING RAT MODEL OF TYPE I DIABETES

Characteristic	BioBreeding Rats
Disease onset	Spontaneous, 8–14 weeks of age
Gender bias	None
Disease frequency	Minor intercolony variation, 40%–70% at 12 weeks of age
Clinical presentation	Hyperglycemia, mild ketosis, polydipsia, polyuria, weight loss, insulin dependency
Additional disease model	Thyroiditis, T-cell lymphopenia
Insulitis	Rapidly progressive; appears near time of disease onset; macrophages, dendritic cells, T and B lymphocytes, NK cells
Genetic susceptibility	Major histocompatibility complex (MHC) plus *Lyp* (T-lymphopenia) locus (chromosome 4)
Immune markers	Autoantibodies, autoreactive T cells

FIGURE 4-19. The BioBreeding rat model of type I diabetes.

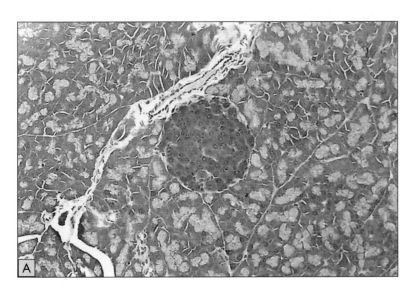

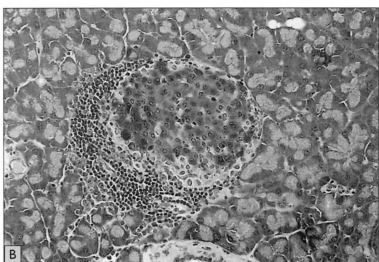

FIGURE 4-20. (See Color Plate) Developmental stages of the insulitis lesion in nonobese diabetic mice. Pathology of pancreatic specimens from a normal islet cell devoid of leukocytic infiltrate (**A**) and at various stages of infiltration (**B** to **H**).

(*Continued on next page*)

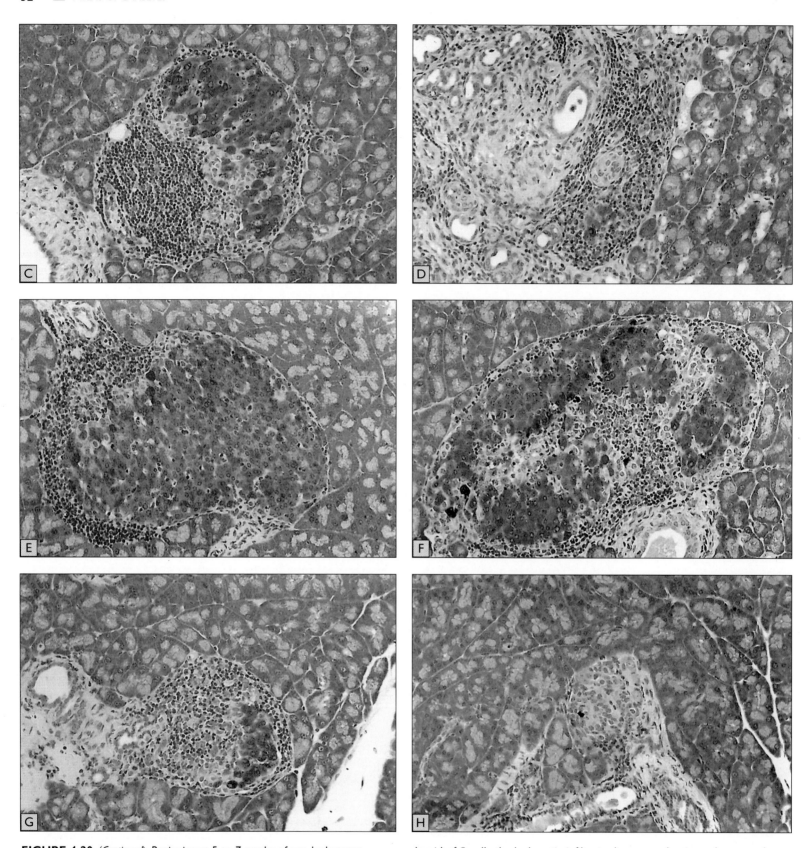

FIGURE 4-20. (*Continued*) Beginning at 5 to 7 weeks of age, leukocytes surround and eventually infiltrate the islets in increasing numbers. Beginning at 12 to 14 weeks, this early insulitis (often termed *nondestructive*) is replaced with an insulitis that destroys the insulin-producing β cells. When the islet is devoid of β cells the leukocytic infiltrate disappears, leaving only α, τ, and δ cells (*panel H*). (Hematoxylin-eosin stain followed by counterstaining with anti-insulin antibody and avidin-biotin, ×300.) (*Courtesy of* A. Peck, University of Florida.)

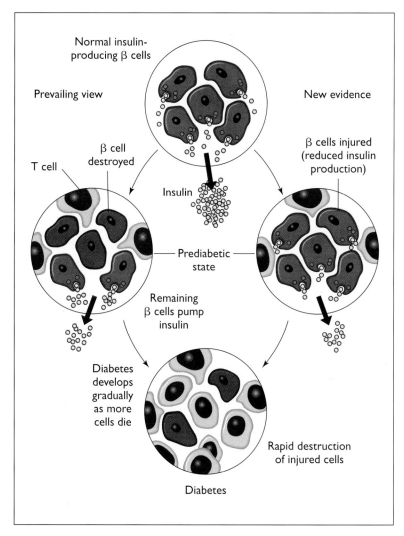

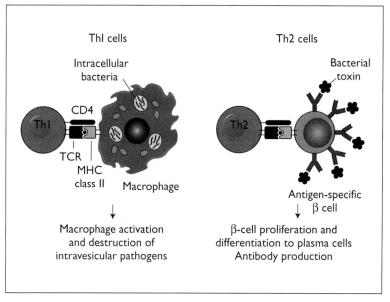

FIGURE 4-22. Th1/Th2 model for immune regulation. Both *in vivo* and *in vitro* studies have supported the notion that activities of CD4+ "helper-T" cells may directly or indirectly relate to the production of specific cytokines. Evolutionary immunologists indicate that the compartmentalization of such responses provides for a more efficient development of an immune response against pathogens of divergent origins and modes of evasion. Although somewhat of an overgeneralization, Th1 cytokines are viewed as enhancing cellular immune activities, whereas Th2 cytokines support those of humoral immunity. Specifically, Th1 activity appears to be enhanced by production of the lymphokines interferon γ (IFN-γ), interleukin 2 (IL-2), and IL-12. Conversely, Th2 augmentation of humoral immunity occurs through the release of IL-4 and IL-10. Note that IL-4 appears to be a strong inhibitor of Th1 immunity. The production of specific cytokines, both systemic and at the site of pancreatic inflammation, may have important implications for the pathogenesis of diabetes as well as the potential for developing methods aimed at disease prevention (*see* Fig. 4-30). MHC—major histocompatibility complex; TCR—T-cell receptor.

FIGURE 4-21. A new model showing rapid destruction of β cells in the pathogenesis of type 1 diabetes. Until recently, most models assessing the rate of β-cell destruction have presumed a gradual (*ie,* modified linear; *see* Fig. 4-2) endocrine cell loss characterized by small periods of "waxing and waning" in the immune response. However, recent investigations of nonobese diabetic mice have suggested that actual β-cell destruction occurs in a very limited time period immediately before symptomatic onset. The composition of the insulitic lesion, destructive activity, or both before this event would be of nondestructive or limited destructive capacity. Although limited evidence exists for this model in terms of human type 1 diabetes, it is the subject of ongoing investigation.

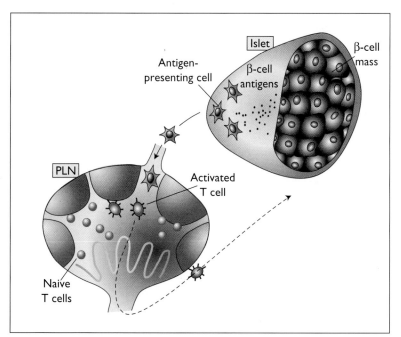

FIGURE 4-23. Hypothetical model for the initiation of type 1 diabetes. Native T cells circulate through the blood and lymphoid organs, including pancreatic lymph nodes (PLN). In the nodes, they encounter antigen-presenting cells (most likely mature dendritic cells) displaying on their surface major histocompatibility complex (MHC) molecules carrying antigens in the form of peptide fragments. In this case, the antigens derive from proteins synthesized by pancreatic islet β-cells, picked up (in soluble form, as cell bits or as apoptotic cells) when the antigen-presenting cells resided in the islets. A minute fraction of the naive T cells recognize MHC molecule/β-cell antigen complexes, become activated, and then access tissues including the pancreas, where they re-encounter cognate antigen, are reactivated, and are retained. (*Adapted from* Mathis *et al.* [10].)

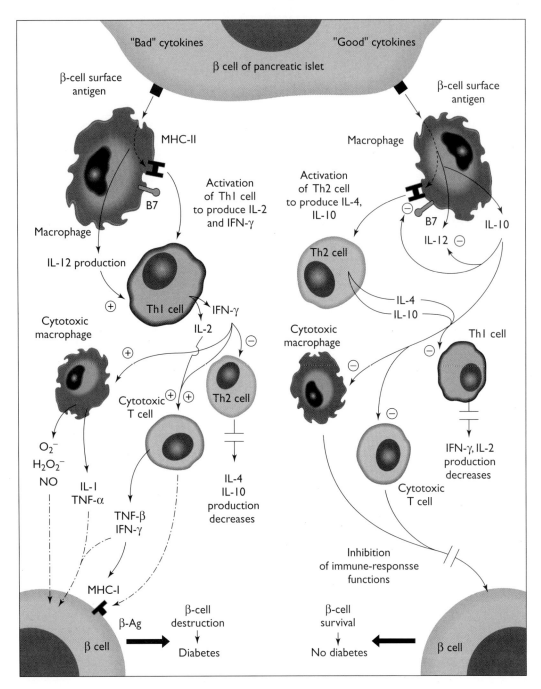

FIGURE 4-24. The "good and bad" cytokine model for the pathogenesis of type 1 diabetes. As modeled in accordance with Figures 4-22 and 4-23, production of Th2 cytokines would be viewed as providing a pathway of avoidance of β-cell destruction (hence the label "good" cytokine). Production of interleukin 4 (IL-4) and IL-10 would block the destructive actions of the cellular immune response. By contrast, immune responses characterized by "bad" Th1 cytokines would be considered as promoting β-cell destruction through enhancement of actions ascribed to cytotoxic T cells or macrophages (through oxygen radical–mediated damage). Ag—antigen; H_2O_2—hydrogen peroxide; IFN—interferon; MHC—major histocompatibility complex; minus sign—inhibitory pathway; NO—nitric oxide; O_2^-—oxygen free radical; plus sign—promoting pathway; TNF-α—tumor necrosis factor-α.

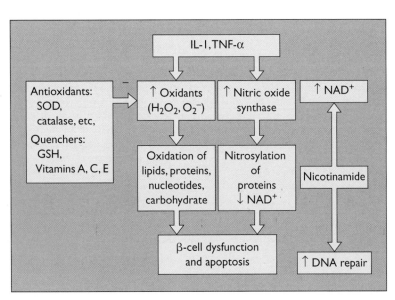

FIGURE 4-25. The lymphokine model for β-cell destruction in type 1 diabetes. Under this scenario, lymphokines produced in response to a nonspecific infection would, by their mode of action, impart a limited degree of initial β-cell destruction owing to an unusual susceptibility of β cells to such agents. The predominant lymphokines cited in this model are those produced by macrophages and include tumor necrosis factor-α (TNF-α) and interleukin 1 (IL-1). Despite the benefits of recovery from infection, this process of anti–β-cell immunity would result in those genetically susceptible to the disease. The continuing process of β-cell destruction would occur through the action of various cytotoxic agents (eg, oxidants and nitric oxide) as well as a lack of activity of numerous compounds associated with cellular or DNA repair mechanisms (eg, anti-oxidants). GSH—glomerulus-stimulating hormone; H_2O_2—hydrogen peroxide; NAD+—oxidized nicotinamide adenine dinucleotide; O_2^-—oxygen free radical; SOD—superoxide dismutase. (*Adapted from* Kolb and Kolb-Bachofen [11].)

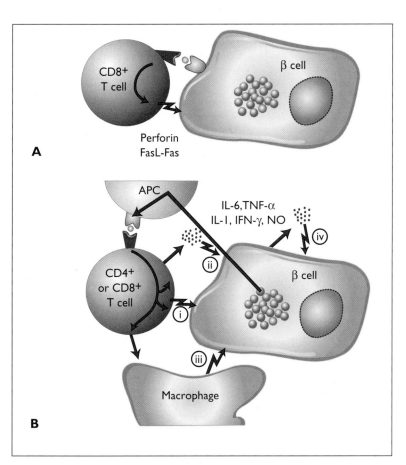

FIGURE 4-26. Proposed mechanisms of β-cell death. **A,** In a recognition-based model, a CD8⁺ T cell is activated by direct recognition of islet β-cell antigen (*circles*) presented by major histocompatibility complex molecules on β cells. Activation provokes killing of the β cell through cell/cell contact using various pathways (*eg,* Fas/FasL, perforin). **B,** In an activation-based model, a T cell (either CD4⁺ or CD8⁺) recognizes β-cell antigens presented indirectly by antigen-presenting cells (APC) located in the vicinity of the islet. The resulting activation provokes β-cell death by (*i*) surface receptors (*eg,* Fas/FasL), (*ii*) soluble mediators from T cells, (*iii*) activation of macrophage cytocidal activities, or (*iv*) activation of death signals in β cells. IFN—interferon; IL—interleukin; NO—nitric oxide. (*Adapted from* Mathis *et al.* [10].)

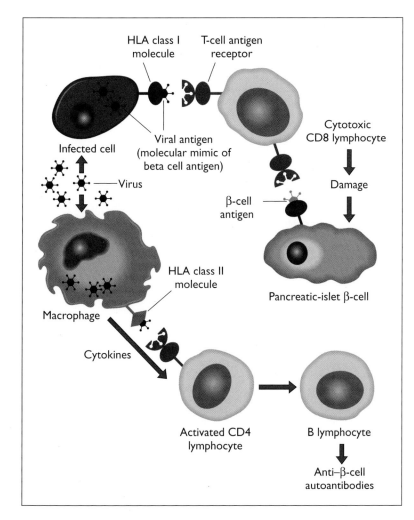

FIGURE 4-27. Potential role for viruses in the pathogenesis of type I diabetes: the molecular mimicry model. In this model, the autoimmune process begins after a "normal" immune response to a cell infected with a virus whose proteins share a similar sequence to that of a β-cell protein. The infected cells display processed viral antigens (by way of Class I molecules) to CD8+ T cells. Macrophages having phagocytosed and processed virus present the viral peptides to CD4+ T cells through Class II molecules. The CD4+ T cells amplify the actions of the CD8+ T cells to become cytotoxic effector cells that can kill β cells that express a peptide common to the viral protein. Despite exhaustive research efforts to demonstrate molecular mimicry as an underlying cause of type I diabetes, it remains an unproved model. Contemporary support predominantly derives from studies demonstrating amino acid sequence similarity between β-cell proteins (*eg,* glutamic acid decarboxylase and IA-2) with those of viruses (*eg,* Coxsackie and Rotavirus) and the ability of human lymphocyte antigen (HLA) molecules with susceptibility and resistance to type I disease to bind these regions of mimicry. Studies, in particular those of cellular immunity, of the natural history of diabetes in humans and nonobese diabetic mice have failed to elevate this model beyond the hypothetical stage. (*Adapted from* Atkinson and Eisenbarth [1].)

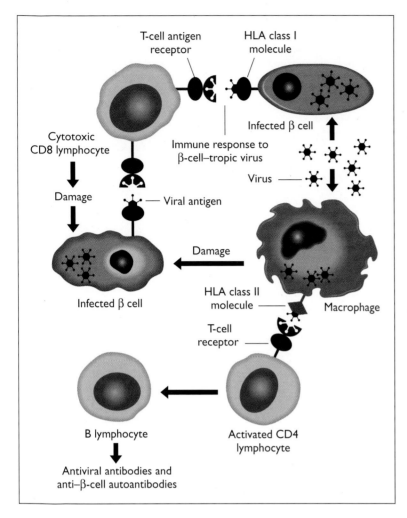

T-cell antigen receptor

HLA class I molecule

Cytotoxic CD8 lymphocyte

Immune response to β-cell–tropic virus

Infected β cell

Damage

Virus

Viral antigen

Damage

Infected β cell

HLA class II molecule

Macrophage

T-cell receptor

B lymphocyte

Activated CD4 lymphocyte

Antiviral antibodies and anti–β-cell autoantibodies

FIGURE 4-28. Potential role for viruses in the pathogenesis of type 1 diabetes: β-tropic virus–viral superantigen models. In these models, initiation of the autoimmune process follows direct viral infection of β cells or the expression in β cells of a virus acting as a superantigen. In both situations, leukocytes are recruited to pancreatic islets. Recruitment increases the release of cytokines (eg, interferon-α) and adhesion of leukocytes within the pancreatic islets. In the β-cell tropic model, the infected β cell is susceptible to direct attack by antiviral cytotoxic lymphocytes. In both models, cytokines and free radicals produced by macrophages activated within the islet cells may augment the cytotoxic response to the β cells; the cytokines also recruit CD4+ T cells to the lesion. Macrophages present autoantigens derived from virus-damaged β cells, thus leading to the development of lymphocytes and autoantibodies that react with β-cell proteins. Support for both of these models exists, yet they remain hypothetical. Whereas viruses capable of β-cell destruction have been isolated from an extremely limited number of human pancreatic organs, examination of a large number of these tissues from patients with type 1 diabetes has failed to reveal the presence of such viruses. Support for the superantigen model exists through the identification of T cells characteristic of superantigen activation in the pancreatic organs of a limited number of patients with new-onset type 1 diabetes. To date, however, no such viral superantigen has been unequivocally identified. HLA—human leukocyte antigen. (*Adapted from* Atkinson and Eisenbarth [1].)

Future Directions

THERAPIES DELAYING OR PREVENTING THE ONSET OF TYPE I DIABETES IN THE NONOBESE DIABETIC MOUSE MODEL

Androgens

Anesthesia

Azathioprine

Anti–B7-1

Bacille Calmette-Guérin

Baculofin

Anti-β 7 integrin

Blocking peptide of major histocompatibility complex (MHC) class II

Bone marrow transplantation

Castration

Anti-CD3

Anti-CD4

Anti-CD8

Anti-CD28

Cholera toxin–B subunit

Clip peptide

Cold exposure

Anti-complement receptor

Complete Freund adjuvant

Anti–CTLA4

Cyclosporin

Cyclosporin A

Deflazacort

Dendritic cells from pancreatic lymph node

Deoxyspergualin

Diazoxide

1,25-dihydroxyvitamin D$_3$

Elevated temperature

Escherichia coli extract

Encephalomyocarditis virus

Essential fatty acid-deficient diets

FK506

Gallium nitrate

Glucose (neonatal)

Glutamic acid decarboxylase: intraperitoneal, intrathymic, intravenous, oral

Glutamic acid decarboxylase peptides: intraperitoneal, intrathymic, intravenous, oral

Gonadectomy

Heat shock protein 65

Heat shock protein peptide (p277)

Anti–intracellular adhesion molecule 1

Immobilization

Immunoglobulin

Anti–integrin α 4

Inomide

Insulin: intraperitoneal, oral, subcutaneous, nasal

Insulin B chain, B chain amino acids 9-23: intraperitoneal, oral, subcutaneous, nasal

Interferon-γ

Anti–interferon-γ

Interleukin 1

Interleukin-1 receptor

Interleukin 2

Interleukin-2 fusion toxin

Interleukin 3

Interleukin 4

Interleukin 10

Interleukin 12 antagonist

Islet cells: intrathymic

Lactate dehydrogenase virus

Lazaroid

Linomide

Anti–lymphocyte function–associated antigen 1

Anti-L-selectin

Lymphocyte choriomeningitis virus

Anti–lymphocyte serum

LZ8

MDL 29311

Anti–MHC class I

Anti–MHC class II

Mixed allogeneic chimerism

Monosodium glutamate

Murine hepatitis virus

Mycobacterium

Natural antibodies

Nicotinamide

OK432

Overcrowding

Pancreatectomy

Pertussigen

Poly [I:C]

Pregestimil diet

Probucol

Prolactin

Rampamycin

Saline (repeated injection)

Semipurified diet (eg, AIN-76)

Silica

Sodium fusidate

Somatostatin

Nonspecific pathogen-free conditions

Streptococcal enterotoxins

Superantigens

Superoxide dismutase–desferrioxamine

Anti–T-cell receptor

Anti--thy-1

Thymectomy (neonatal)

Tolbutamide

Tumor necrosis factor-α

Vitamin E

Anti–VLA 4

FIGURE 4-29. Therapies delaying or preventing the onset of type I diabetes in the nonobese diabetic mouse model.

TREATMENTS AIMED AT INDUCING CLINICAL REMISSION OR PREVENTING HUMAN TYPE I DIABETES

Group Studied	Agent or Treatment
Patients with new-onset type I disease	Cyclosporine
	Azathioprine
	Anti-CD5 antibodies (CD5 plus)
	Intensive insulin therapy
	High-dose insulin therapy
	Antibody against interleukin 2 receptor
	Nicotinamide
	Intravenous immune globulin
	Plasmapheresis
	Anti–lymphocyte globulin
	Prednisone
	Bacille Calmette-Guérin
Persons at high risk for type I disease	Intensive therapy with intravenous insulin
	Prophylactic insulin therapy
	Nicotinamide
	Oral insulin
	Avoidance of cow's milk–based infant formulas

FIGURE 4-30. Treatments aimed at inducing clinical remission or preventing human type I diabetes. The identification of therapies capable of preventing type I diabetes in nonobese diabetic mice, combined with knowledge regarding the immunopathogenesis of the disease, have afforded the ability to attempt disease prevention and/or preservation of β-cell mass trials in humans. The figure provides a listing of agents that are undergoing active or planned clinical trial in humans.

References

1. Atkinson M, Eisenbarth G: Type I diabetes: new perspectives on disease pathogenesis and treatment. *Lancet* 2001, 358:221–229.
2. Eisenbarth GS: Type I diabetes mellitus. A chronic autoimmune disease. *N Engl J Med* 1986, 314:1360–1368.
3. Karvonen M, Tuomilehto J, Libman I, LaPorte R: WHO Diamond Project Group: a review of the recent epidemiological data on incidence of type I (insulin-dependent) diabetes mellitus worldwide. *Diabetologia* 36:883–892.
4. LaPorte RE, Matsushima M, Chang Y-F: Prevalence and incidence of insulin dependent diabetes. In *Diabetes in America*. Edited by Harris M. Bethesda, MD: NIH Publications; 1995:37–46.
5. Hawkins HW: Could the aetiology of IDDM be multifactorial? *Diabetologia* 1997, 40:1235–1240.
6. She JX: Susceptibility to type I diabetes: HLA-DQ and DR revisited. *Immunol Today* 1996, 17:323–329.
7. Field LL: Genetic linkage and association studies of Type I diabetes: challenges and rewards. *Diabetologia* 2002, 45:21–35.
8. Foulis AK: In *Textbook of Diabetes*. Vol. 1. Edited by Pickup J, Williams G. Oxford, England: Blackwell Scientific; 1991.
9. Krischer JP, Schatz D, Riley WJ, *et al.*: Insulin and islet cell autoantibodies as time-dependent covariates in the development of insulin-dependent diabetes. *J Clin Endocrinol Metab* 1993, 77:743–749.
10. Mathis D, Vence L, Benoist C: Beta-cell death during progression to diabetes. *Nature* 2001, 414:729798.
11. Kolb H, Kolb-Bachofen V: Nitric oxide in autoimmune disease: cytotoxic or regulatory mediator? *Immunol Today* 1998, 19:556-561.

MANAGEMENT AND PREVENTION OF COMPLICATIONS IN TYPE 1 DIABETES MELLITUS

David M. Nathan

5

Therapy for type 1 diabetes mellitus has a relatively short history that can be divided conveniently into three eras: pre-insulin, insulin, and the era after the Diabetes Control and Complications Trial (DCCT). Before the introduction of insulin therapy, persons with the form of diabetes we currently call type 1 had a mortality rate approaching 100% within the first 2 years of diagnosis. The existence of another distinct form of diabetes, now designated as type 2, was not well recognized until the mid-1930s. Considering the short life span of patients with type 1 diabetes, it is not surprising that the long-term complications of diabetes were virtually unknown. Two dramatic events accompanied the introduction of insulin therapy in 1922. First, type 1 diabetes was no longer an acutely fatal disease. Second, with longer survival, previously unheard of complications began to occur, including retinopathy, nephropathy, and neuropathy [1]. The consequences of these complications and the desire to prevent or delay them have been the focus of clinical care and research, culminating in the DCCT [2].

The DCCT and a series of smaller clinical studies, including the Kroc [3], Steno [4], Oslo [5], and Stockholm Diabetes [6] studies, examined whether the long-term complications of diabetes could be prevented or delayed by implementing therapies aimed at achieving blood glucose levels as close as possible to the normal range. These so-called intensive therapies were made possible by the development of self-glucose monitoring techniques and insights into the physiologic pattern of delivery of insulin necessary to achieve and maintain glucose levels in the near normal range [7]. Insulin therapy with long-acting and short-acting insulins was adjusted based on glucose self-monitoring results, meal content, and anticipated exercise. Short-acting insulins were given at least two to three times per day with multiple daily injection (MDI) therapy or with continuous subcutaneous insulin infusion (CSII) provided by an external pump. The development of an objective, accurate index of long-term glycemia, the *glycohemoglobin assay*, complemented these other developments and facilitated the performance of the clinical trials [8].

The DCCT was initiated in 1982 and completed in 1993. Patients with type 1 diabetes with either no retinopathy (primary prevention) or minimal to moderate nonproliferative retinopathy (secondary intervention) were randomly assigned to conventional or intensive therapy [2]. In conventional therapy, patients used one to two daily insulin injections and daily glucose monitoring. Conventional therapy was designed to avoid symptoms of hyperglycemia and hypoglycemia but had no specific blood glucose level goals. In contrast, intensive therapy was aimed at achieving blood glucose levels between 70 and 120 mg/dL before meals, under 180 mg/dL at 90 to 120 minutes after meals, and over 65 mg/dL at a weekly test performed at 3 AM to monitor and decrease the occurrence of nocturnal hypoglycemia. In addition, intensive therapy was aimed at achieving hemoglobin A_{1c} (HbA_{1c}) levels in the normal range (<6.05%).

A total of 1441 patients with type 1 diabetes, aged 13 to 40, were recruited between 1983 and 1990, and follow-up examinations were performed for a mean of 6.5 years. Intensive therapy resulted in a decrease in mean HbA_{1c} levels of 1.8% to 2.0% and a consistent and impressive reduction in the occurrence and progression of retinopathy, nephropathy, and neuropathy. When compared with conventional therapy, intensive therapy reduced the development of both early and later manifestations of retinopathy (three-step change, severe nonproliferative retinopathy, and the need for laser therapy), nephropathy (microalbuminuria and clinical grade albuminuria), and peripheral and autonomic neuropathy [2]. Included in the costs of intensive therapy were frequent supervision by a highly trained and expert staff and increased monitoring compared with conventional therapy. In addition, intensive therapy was accompanied by a threefold increased risk for severe hypoglycemia, including episodes that resulted in coma or seizure, and an increased risk for weight gain. No significant cognitive impairment occurred in the intensive treatment group, even in those patients who experienced repeated episodes of severe hypoglycemia.

The DCCT and other studies, especially the Stockholm Diabetes Study [6], have established intensive therapy as the standard of therapy for type 1 diabetes. Until new and improved therapies that are safer and more user-friendly supplant MDI and CSII, they will remain the staples for patients with type 1 diabetes. For those patients who cannot perform all of the myriad tasks intensive therapy requires, or who cannot achieve and maintain near-normal glycemia, any lowering of HbA_{1c} is likely to decrease the rate of development and slow the progression of long-term complications [9]. Note that intensive therapy has not been demonstrated to decrease the excessive cardiovascular disease (CVD) that affects patients with type 1 diabetes; however, longer-term studies may demonstrate a decrease in CVD owing to the decrease in renal failure, a major contributor to accelerated atherosclerosis.

Improvements in intensive therapy have been made in the relatively brief period of time since the completion of the DCCT. Improved glucose self-monitoring devices are now available. Better understanding of the pathogenesis of hypoglycemia and hypoglycemia unawareness may lead to strategies that decrease the risk of hypoglycemia accompanying intensive therapy [10–12]. The development of new insulin analogues, such as lispro, is now making physiologic replacement easier [13]. In addition, advances in whole-organ pancreas transplantation have made it an increasingly appropriate and acceptable procedure in the setting of kidney transplantation and, arguably, even as a solitary transplantation. Finally, progress in islet transplantation and the development of continuous and less invasive, or even noninvasive, monitoring technology may make these therapies a reality in the next decade.

For those patients who do not or cannot take advantage of the improvement in long-term outcome provided by intensive therapy, laser therapy, vitrectomy, renal replacement therapy, and treatments for painful neuropathy and the manifestations of autonomic neuropathy remain [14].

Herein, the seminal insights and developments that allowed physiologic replacement of insulin in type 1 diabetes, consequences of such therapy on long-term complications, and several new treatments are reviewed.

History of Type 1 Diabetes and Its Treatment

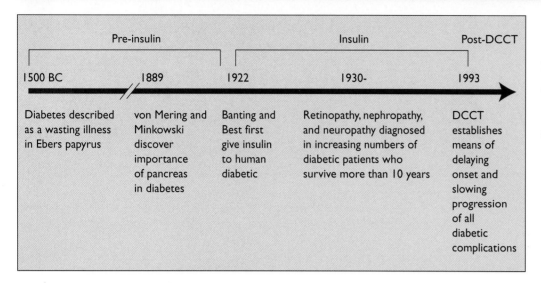

FIGURE 5-1. The history of type 1 diabetes can be divided conveniently into three eras. In the pre-insulin era, diabetes was usually fatal within 1 to 2 years of its development. In the insulin era, acute mortality was eliminated but chronic complications were first noted. The Diabetes Control and Complications Trial (DCCT) [2] proved that intensive therapy would decrease the development and progression of long-term complications.

Therapy for Type 1 Diabetes

FORMS OF MODIFIED INSULIN

Insulin form	Modification	Onset of Action	Duration of Activity
Very rapid acting		10–15 min	2–3 h
Lispro*	B-chain proline (amino acid 28) and lysine (amino acid 29) reversed		
Aspart	B-chain aspartate for proline (amino acid 28)		
Rapid-acting		30–45 min	4–6 h
Crystalline zinc insulin (CZI)†	Zinc		
Intermediate-acting		1–2 h	6–12 h
Neutral protamine Hagedorn (NPH)†	Protamine		
Lente†	Zinc		
Long-acting			
Ultralente*	Zinc	6–8 h	18 h
Glargine	A-chain glycine (amino acid 21)	Peakless	24 h
	B-chain arginine (amino acids 31 and 32)		
Premixed combinations			
70/30*	70% NPH and 30% CZI	30–45 min	6–12 h
50/50*	50% NPH and 50% CZI	30–45 min	6–12 h

*Available only as recombinant human insulin.
†Available as human, beef and pork, and pure pork. Effective January 1999, animal species insulins being phased out.

FIGURE 5-2. The available forms of modified insulin provide a spectrum of action that facilitates near normalization of glucose levels when used in conjunction with frequent monitoring of glucose levels. Selection of dose size and timing of administration are dependent on an understanding of the impact of exercise and meal size and composition on glucose fluctuations. Even with these tools, intensive therapy is imperfect. True normalization of glucose levels rarely, if ever, is achieved. Realistically, hemoglobin A_{1c} levels can be maintained at 4 to 5 standard deviations above the mean nondiabetic level, and then only with a substantial frequency of hypoglycemic reactions.

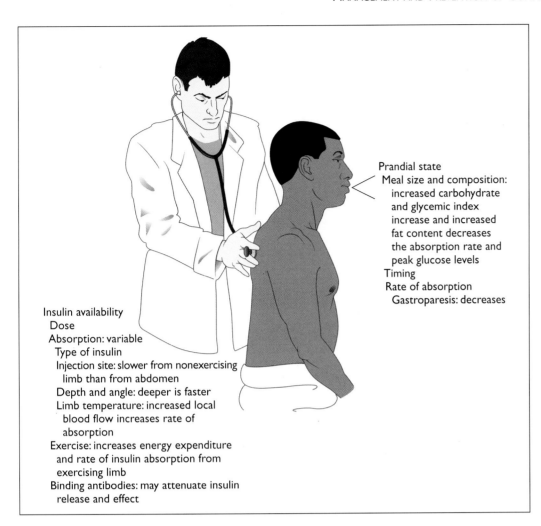

Prandial state
Meal size and composition:
  increased carbohydrate
  and glycemic index
  increase and increased
  fat content decreases
  the absorption rate and
  peak glucose levels
Timing
  Rate of absorption
  Gastroparesis: decreases

Insulin availability
  Dose
  Absorption: variable
    Type of insulin
    Injection site: slower from nonexercising
      limb than from abdomen
    Depth and angle: deeper is faster
    Limb temperature: increased local
      blood flow increases rate of
      absorption
  Exercise: increases energy expenditure
    and rate of insulin absorption from
    exercising limb
  Binding antibodies: may attenuate insulin
    release and effect

FIGURE 5-3. Causes of lability of glycemia in type I diabetes. After a variable but usually brief period of preserved insulin secretion, often called a honeymoon period, type I diabetes is characterized by a complete deficiency of endogenous insulin production. Whereas glucose levels in the nondiabetic state are maintained in a very limited range owing to the exquisite and coordinated responsiveness of the β cells (insulin) and α cells (glucagon) to ambient glucose levels and gut peptides, glucose levels are extremely labile once type I diabetes has been established. The patient with type I diabetes is entirely dependent on exogenous insulin delivery, which can be affected by many variables. In addition, the rate of increase in glucose levels is dictated by meal size and composition. Finally, a host of other factors, including exercise timing and intensity, can affect energy use and glucose levels.

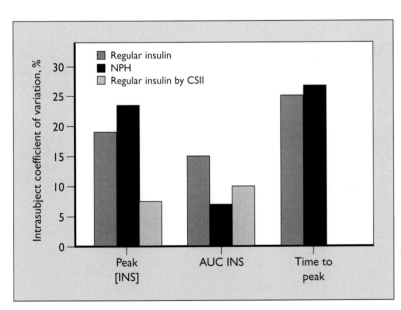

FIGURE 5-4. Variability (coefficients of variation) for insulin absorption. The absorption of insulin from the subcutaneous depot determines its delivery to its target tissues. Absorption is influenced by many factors (see Fig. 5-3), and it is highly variable. In the study results shown here, the same dose of subcutaneous insulin was administered repeatedly by nurses using the same anatomic site and standardized injection techniques. Alternatively, insulin was administered by continuous subcutaneous insulin infusion (CSII) with an external pump. The coefficients of variation within individuals for peak insulin level (Peak [INS]), area under the curve (AUC) for insulin levels, and time to peak level after a subcutaneous injection were as high as 25% to 30%. Variabilities in peak INS and AUC were somewhat less with CSII, suggesting that external pump therapy may provide more consistent insulin delivery than conventional subcutaneous insulin delivery therapy. (*Adapted from* Galloway *et al.* [15].)

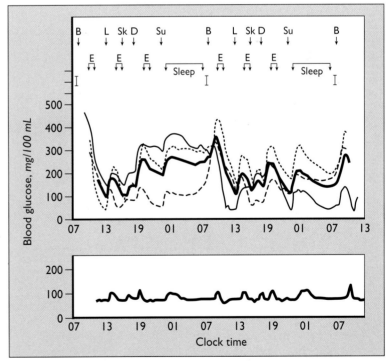

FIGURE 5-5. Daily blood glucose profiles in persons without diabetes and in patients with type I diabetes treated with nonphysiologic insulin replacement. Studies were performed in the highly regimented environment of an inpatient clinical research center, with standardized uniform meals and exercise. These studies demonstrate the relatively constant blood glucose levels maintained by persons without diabetes. In contrast, even in a highly regimented setting, patients with type I diabetes who are treated with a single dose of intermediate-acting insulin (I) have gross and seemingly unpredictable fluctuations in blood glucose levels. (*Adapted from* Molnar *et al.* [16].)

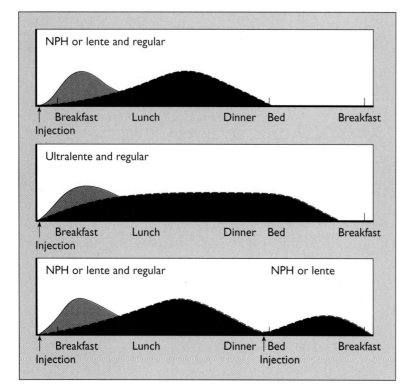

FIGURE 5-6. Insulin activity profiles and algorithms. Insulin profiles achieved with different injection regimens are shown. Minimal regimens are likely to be associated with intermittent symptoms of hyperglycemia and hemoglobin A_{1c} levels exceeding 10% (nondiabetic range, 4% to 6.1%). These relatively nondemanding insulin regimens will prevent ketosis most of the time. In addition to once or twice daily insulin injections, self-glucose monitoring should be performed daily. Patients should perform monitoring more often before traveling, with changes in schedule or regimen, and during illness. Urine ketone testing should be performed in the setting of unusually elevated glucose levels (>300 mg/dL) or in the presence of illness, especially when gastrointestinal symptoms are present.

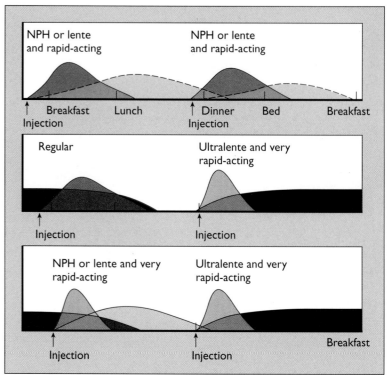

FIGURE 5-7. Moderate intensity regimens. These regimens include twice daily insulin injections coupled with glucose self-monitoring. Insulin doses are adjusted based on glucose levels and meal size. Such regimens are associated with hemoglobin A_{1c} levels of 8% to 9%. In general, patients should be asymptomatic, with infrequent symptoms of hyperglycemia.

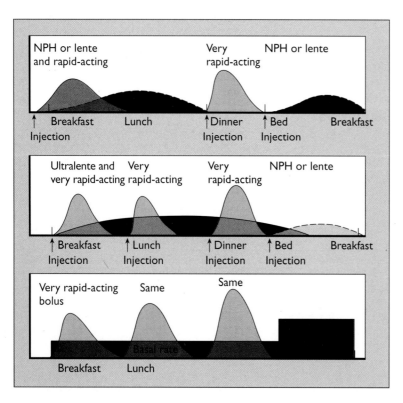

FIGURE 5-8. Intensive treatment regimens. These regimens include at least three injections of insulin daily or administration of insulin by an external pump. Self-monitoring of blood glucose levels is performed 4 times per day and at 3 AM once per week to detect and prevent episodes of otherwise unrecognized nocturnal hypoglycemia. Insulin doses, and especially the rapid or very rapid-acting insulins, are adjusted for each meal based on glucose level, meal size and composition, and anticipated exercise and activity. The basal delivery of insulin can be supplied with intermediate or long-acting (ultralente or glargine) insulins or with continuous rapid or very rapid-acting insulin infused with an external pump. Intensive regimens can achieve a hemoglobin A_{1c} of 7% or less but at a cost of a threefold increase in episodes of severe hypoglycemia. An episode of severe hypoglycemia is defined as requiring help for treatment. An expert team including a diabetologist, diabetes educator, and dietitian is helpful in implementing and supervising such regimens. Intensive regimens have been recommended as the standard of therapy since the Diabetes Control and Complications Trial demonstrated their efficacy in preventing the development of and slowing the progression of diabetic complications.

Results of Therapy: Glycemia

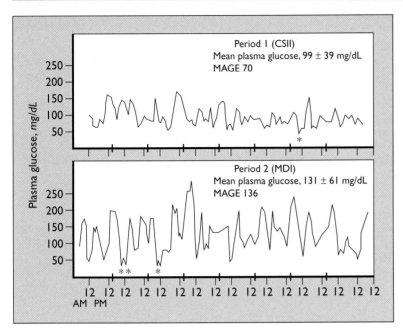

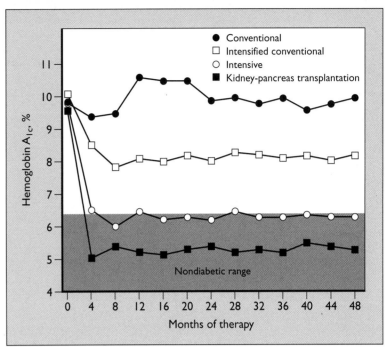

FIGURE 5-9. Glycemia in type 1 diabetes treated with physiologic insulin replacement using a multiple daily injection (MDI) regimen or continuous subcutaneous insulin infusion (CSII) with an external pump. In this study, a patient with type 1 diabetes performed multiple (15) self-glucose monitoring tests in a single day as an outpatient. Other than the frequent glucose checks, the accuracy of which were confirmed by simultaneous laboratory assay, the patient maintained a normal outpatient schedule, including self-selected meals and sedentary office work. During one 24-hour period (see bottom section of Fig. 5-8), the patient used a continuous subcutaneous insulin infusion with an external insulin pump and gave himself multiple daily injections with insulin placebo. During a second 24-hour period (see middle section of Fig. 5-8), the patient reversed therapy, using insulin placebo in the pump and active insulin in the injections. Although the glucose profile is somewhat less labile with CSII than with MDI, both therapies achieved blood glucose levels that are close to or within the normal range for much of the day. MAGE—mean amplitude of glycemic excursions. *Asterisk* indicates clinical hypoglycemia. (*Adapted from* Nathan *et al.* [17].)

FIGURE 5-10. Comparison of long-term glycemia, as measured by hemoglobin A_{1c} (HbA$_{1c}$), for different treatments of type 1 diabetes. Patients were nonrandomly assigned to one of three groups: conventional therapy, intensified conventional therapy, or intensive therapy with continuous subcutaneous insulin infusion (CSII) or multiple daily injection (MDI) (n = 18, 22, and 21, respectively). *Conventional therapy* was defined in 1980 to 1984 as 1 or 2 daily insulin injections without frequent self-monitoring of glucose levels or dose adjustment. The injections usually consisted of a combination of intermediate-acting and rapid-acting insulin before breakfast and dinner. *Intensified conventional therapy* is similar to conventional therapy but with the addition of twice-daily glucose monitoring and adjustment of the pre-breakfast and pre-dinner doses based on monitoring results. The fourth group represents patients with end-stage renal disease after receiving a simultaneous kidney-pancreas transplantation (n = 34).

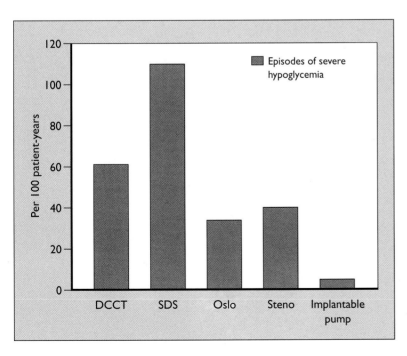

FIGURE 5-11. Frequency of severe hypoglycemia with intensive therapy of diabetes mellitus. As in the Diabetes Control and Complications Trial (DCCT), *severe hypoglycemia* is defined as any episode of chemical hypoglycemia (usually with plasma glucose <60 mg/dL) requiring help from another person to treat. Severe hypoglycemia includes a spectrum of hypoglycemia, ranging from only minimal confusion to episodes of loss of consciousness or seizures. If the patient is able to swallow, 15 g of a rapidly absorbable simple sugar should be given in the form of 4 oz of orange juice, soda, or sugar candy. If unable to swallow, intramuscular glucagon, usually 1 mg, or intravenous dextrose, 12.5–50 mL of 50% dextrose, is administered. The DCCT [2], SDS (Stockholm Diabetes Study) [18], Oslo Study [5], and Steno Studies [4] studied patients with type 1 diabetes and used either multiple daily injections or external insulin pump therapy. The only intensive therapy for patients with type 1 diabetes with demonstrably lower rates of severe hypoglycemia has used implantable pumps delivering insulin intravenously or intraperitoneally [19].

Long-term Complications: Pathophysiology and Results of Intensive Therapy

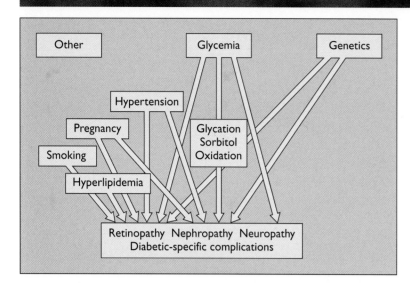

FIGURE 5-12. Pathogenesis of complications. The specific mechanism or mechanisms that cause the microvascular and neurologic complications of diabetes remain unidentified. Several obvious contributing factors, however, have been noted in epidemiologic studies, animal models, and interventional studies. Whereas no single mechanism is likely to explain the myriad complications, glycemia appears to be an underlying cause for all of them, as demonstrated in interventional studies such as the Diabetes Control and Complications Trial [2]. It is probable that different clinical stages of specific complications, eg, nonproliferative and proliferative retinopathy, have different causes. Genetic susceptibility to retinopathy and neuropathy is suggested by familial clustering [20]. Hypertension and pregnancy are well known to accelerate the development of retinopathy and nephropathy. In addition, interventional studies using anti-hypertensive agents, and especially angiotensin-converting enzyme inhibitors, have demonstrated attenuation of the otherwise inexorable progression of nephropathy [21–23].

LONG-TERM COMPLICATIONS OF TYPE 1 DIABETES AND THE RISK OF DEVELOPING CLINICAL MANIFESTATIONS OF SPECIFIED COMPLICATIONS

Cataract: 25% to 30% lifetime risk with 3% to 5% requiring cataract extraction

Glaucoma (open angle): 10% risk after 30 years

Retinopathy: 90% develop some degree over lifetime; 40% to 50% require laser and 3% to 5% blind after 30 years' duration

Adhesive capsulitis: frozen shoulder, prevalence 10%

Coronary artery disease: major cause of mortality

Gastroparesis: 1% to 5% develop symptoms—lifetime risk

Carpal tunnel syndrome: 30% with electrophysiologic evidence, 9% with symptoms (prevalence)

Nephropathy: 35% develop end-stage renal disease over lifetime

Trigger finger, DuPuytren's contractures: 10% prevalence

Autonomic neuropathy (prevalence): bladder, 1% to 5% with dysfunction; impotence, 10% to 40%; diarrhea, 1%

Peripheral vascular disease

Peripheral neuropathy: 54% lifetime risk; 2% to 3% foot ulcers/y

FIGURE 5-13. Long-term complications of type 1 diabetes and the risks of developing clinical manifestations of specified complications. Data for some complications are sparse. The estimates provided reflect the era before the Diabetes Control and Complications Trial. Intensive therapy of type 1 diabetes is anticipated to reduce the lifelong development of retinopathy, nephropathy, and neuropathy by 50% to 80%. The overall effect of diabetic complications results in a substantial 15-year reduction in life span, predominantly owing to the development of nephropathy and cardiovascular disease.

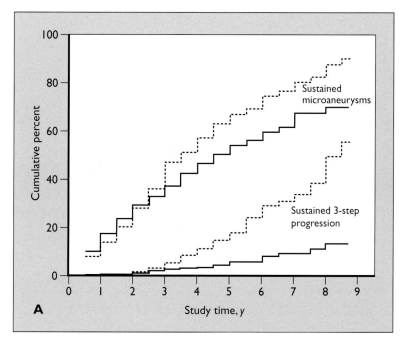

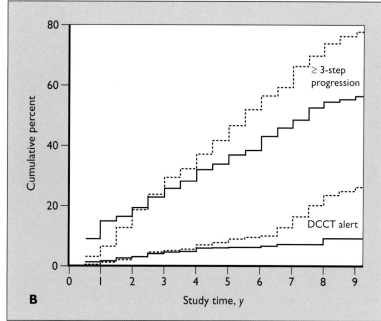

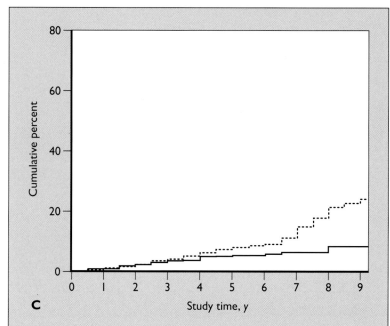

FIGURE 5-14. In the Diabetes Control and Complications Trial (DCCT), retinopathy measured in 18,000 sets of photographs with seven-field stereoscopic fundus photography performed every 6 months. The development and progression of retinopathy at virtually every stage were decreased by intensive therapy. **A,** The primary prevention cohort had 1 to 5 years' duration of diabetes and no retinopathy at baseline. In the primary cohort, the development of *sustained microaneurysms*, defined as one or more microaneurysms detected at two consecutive 6-month examinations, and of sustained three-step or greater progression according to the Early Treatment of Diabetic Retinopathy Study (ETDRS) scale, were decreased by 27% and 76% (*P*<0.002), respectively. **B,** The secondary intervention cohort was defined as having 1 to 15 years' duration of diabetes and at least one microaneurysm in either eye at baseline. In the secondary intervention cohort, intensive therapy was highly effective at reducing the progression to more severe levels of retinopathy, including a 34% reduction in three-step or greater progression (*P*<0.001) and a 47% reduction in severe nonproliferative retinopathy (*P*<0.02) (DCCT alert). **C,** The development of even more severe retinopathy, defined as neovascularization either on the disc or elsewhere, was reduced by 48% (*P*<0.02). (*Adapted from* DCCT Research Group [24].)

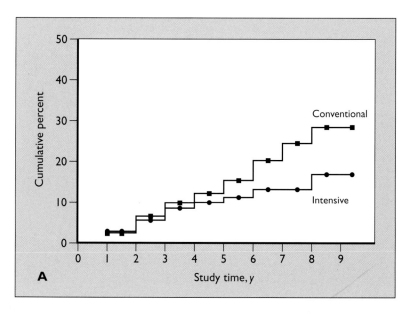

FIGURE 5-15. Nephropathy. Nephropathy in patients with type 1 diabetes progresses through several stages, usually over 15 to 25 years. The development of microalbuminuria, defined as between 20 and 40 mg of albumin excretion per 24 hours, is the first detectable stage, progressing to clinical albuminuria (>300 mg albumin excretion per 24 h), usually over more than a decade. Albumin excretion progresses to the level consistent with nephrotic syndrome followed by decreasing glomerular filtration rate and culminating in end-stage renal disease. Hypertension uniformly accompanies the development of nephropathy. Treatment of hypertension, especially with angiotensin-converting enzyme (ACE) inhibitors, and use of ACE inhibitors during the microalbuminuric stage, even in the absence of hypertension, have been shown to attenuate the progression rate of nephropathy.

The Diabetes Control and Complications Trial (DCCT) demonstrated a uniformly beneficial effect of intensive therapy on the development of microalbuminuria (40 mg/24 h). **A,** In patients with primary prevention, a 34% risk reduction (*P*=0.04).

(Continued on next page)

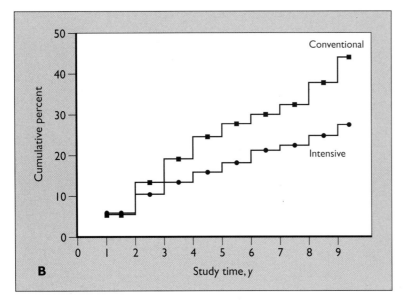

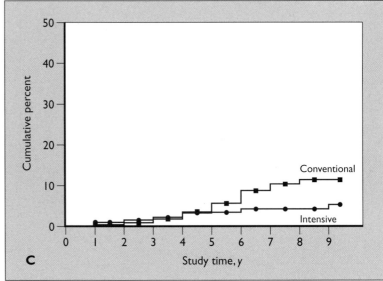

FIGURE 5-15. (*Continued*) **B,** In patients with secondary intervention, a 43% reduction (*P*<0.0001). **C,** A 56% reduction in the development of more advanced stages of nephropathy, such as clinical albuminuria (*P*<0.01). (*Adapted from* DCCT Research Group [25].)

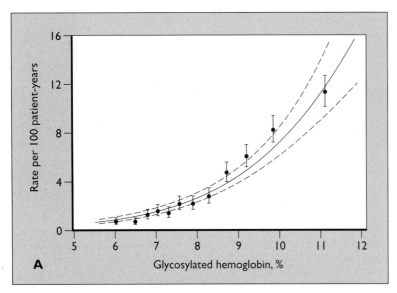

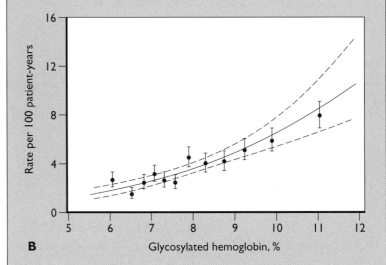

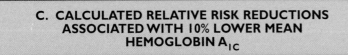

Complication	Risk Reduction, %*
Retinopathy	
Onset	35
Sustained progression	39
Severe nonproliferative	37
Nephropathy	
Microalbuminuria (≥40 mg/24 h)	25
Microalbuminuria (≥100 mg/24 h)	39
Albuminuria (≥300 mg/24 h)	34
Neuropathy	30

C. CALCULATED RELATIVE RISK REDUCTIONS ASSOCIATED WITH 10% LOWER MEAN HEMOGLOBIN A$_{1c}$

Calculated reduction in risk for every 10% lowering of hemoglobin A$_{1c}$.

FIGURE 5-16. Glycemia and complications. The Diabetes Control and Complications Trial (DCCT) performed primary analyses comparing the effects of intensive and conventional therapy on long-term complications. In addition, the DCCT performed secondary analyses examining the relationship of glycemia (mean of all hemoglobin A$_{1c}$ [HbA$_{1c}$] values for each subject during the trial) and the development or progression of complications, independent of treatment assignment. These analyses provide an assessment of the expected risk for different complications based on HbA$_{1c}$ achieved. **A,** Rate of retinopathy progression in combined treatment groups. **B,** Rate of development of microalbuminuria (>40 mg/24 h) in combined treatment groups. In addition, the risk reduction for a specified decrease in HbA$_{1c}$ can be calculated (**C**). (*Adapted from* DCCT Research Group [9].)

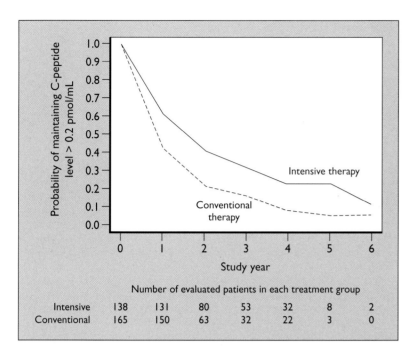

FIGURE 5-17. Preservation of endogenous insulin secretion with intensive therapy. In the Diabetes Control and Complications Trial (DCCT), patients with less than 5 years' duration of diabetes could have a modest degree of residual insulin secretion (C-peptide level 0.2–0.5 pmol/mL 90 min after a standardized meal). Of the patients, 303 fulfilled this criteria; 138 were randomly assigned to intensive therapy and 165 to conventional therapy. During the DCCT, repeated tests of endogenous insulin secretion were performed. As shown, intensive therapy was more likely to preserve endogenous secretion of insulin than was conventional therapy, extending the residual secretion by at least 2 years. Compared with patients having intensive treatment without residual insulin secretion, those having intensive treatment with residual insulin secretion maintained lower hemoglobin A_{1c} levels with less exogenous insulin and had less frequent severe hypoglycemia and a lower risk of retinopathy progression. Thus, preservation of endogenous insulin secretion is clinically important, facilitating the safe implementation of intensive therapy. Intensive therapy should be initiated as early as possible in the course of type 1 diabetes. (*Adapted from* DCCT Research Group [26].)

New Approaches to Therapy

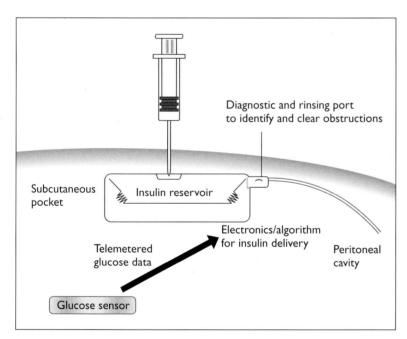

FIGURE 5-18. Implantable pump. The first step in creating an artificial pancreas was the development of a totally enclosed implantable pump. Ideally, the pump should deliver insulin reliably and in physiologic patterns to achieve normoglycemia. In addition, the requirement for rapid changes in insulin levels precludes subcutaneous delivery. Either intravenous or intraperitoneal delivery can achieve rapid changes and avoid peripheral hyperinsulinemia. Intraperitoneal delivery has a slight advantage in delivering insulin directly to the liver.

Several implantable pumps have been developed and tested extensively. The pumps share many characteristics. They hold enough insulin for 4 to 8 weeks and are filled subcutaneously through a port. The pumps are implanted in either a subclavian pocket or in the lower abdomen, with a catheter tunneled either into the subclavian vein or peritoneal cavity. The catheters become obstructed, on average, every 4 to 9 months, and usually can be cleared through a flushing procedure, although occasionally catheter replacement is necessary. All pumps operate by telemetry and can be programmed to provide many different insulin profiles. The pumps are capable of achieving glycemic control similar to conventional intensive therapy but with a lower risk of severe hypoglycemia. A functional and practical glucose sensor has yet to be developed.

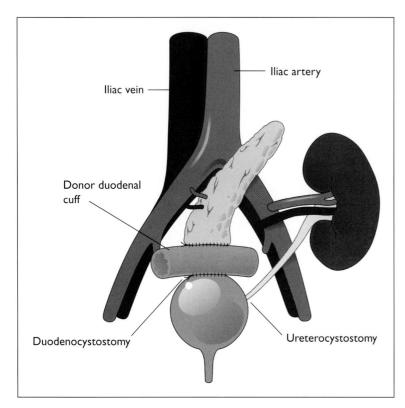

FIGURE 5-19. Whole-organ transplantation. Pancreatic allografts have become increasingly successful as a form of hormone replacement therapy. When successful, they obviate the need for exogenous insulin, "diabetes diets,"

frequent self-monitoring, and the panoply of other day-to-day chores and lifestyle adjustments that are a part of the management of type 1 diabetes. Whereas most pancreas transplantations are performed in type 1 diabetes with cadaveric organs and simultaneously with kidney transplantation (to treat end-stage renal disease), some centers perform isolated pancreas transplantations, partial pancreatic transplantations from living donors, and, rarely, transplantation in type 2 diabetes. The current consensus is that simultaneous kidney-pancreas transplantation is most acceptable because the risks of immunosuppression and surgery are subsumed by renal transplantation. Moreover, pancreas transplantation survival is superior in the setting of a combined kidney-pancreas transplantation compared with an isolated pancreas transplantation. However, patients who come to kidney transplantation always have a high burden of well-established, long-term complications, including decreased vision from retinopathy and peripheral and cardiovascular disease, and neuropathy. As such, these patients are less likely to benefit from the putative improvement in long-term complications that might be expected from transplantation at an earlier stage of the disease. The balance, therefore, is between the acute risk of surgery and recognized complications of long-term immunosuppression and the putative benefit of pancreas transplantation at an earlier age, before the development of complications. Current recommendations suggest that patients with type 1 diabetes undergoing kidney transplantation, and those rare patients with very brittle diabetes that interferes substantially with their day-to-day existence because of repeated hypoglycemia and ketoacidosis, be considered as candidates for pancreas transplantation.

The most common procedure is shown. It includes anastomosis of the pancreas attached to the duodenal cuff to the bladder for exocrine drainage, and anastomosis of the pancreatic blood supply into the iliac vessels, resulting in systemic rather than mesenteric insulin delivery. More physiologic approaches also are being used, including enteric drainage of the exocrine pancreas and mesenteric vessel anastomoses to provide more direct insulin delivery to the liver.

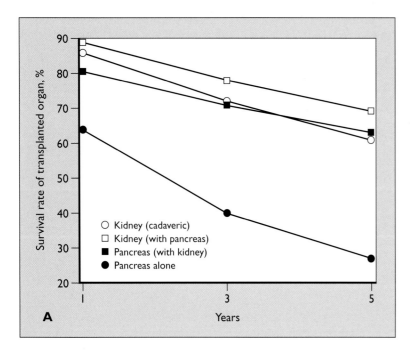

FIGURE 5-20. Transplantation results. Increasingly successful technical results of pancreas transplantation have made it a viable choice of therapy, especially in the setting of a kidney transplantation (*see* Fig. 5-19). **A,** The metabolic results of pancreas transplantation, *ie,* pancreas transplantation "survival" defined as normal glycemia (fasting glucose or hemoglobin A_{1c} results) without any exogenous insulin or other hypoglycemic agents, are beginning to parallel the results of kidney transplantation.

(*Continued on next page*)

B. OUTCOMES OF WHOLE-ORGAN PANCREATIC TRANSPLANTATION

	Simultaneous with Kidney	After Kidney	Solitary
Patient survival, %			
1 y	93	97	90
3 y	86	88	85
5 y	82	83	77
Pancreas graft survival, %			
1 y	81	73	64
3 y	71	42	40
5 y	63	34	27
Kidney graft survival, %	86		
Effect on diabetic complications			
Retinopathy	None		
Neuropathy	Reduces peripheral and autonomic		
Nephropathy			
Native kidney			Reverses lesions after >5 y
Transplanted kidney	May prevent development	Prevents progression	
Quality of life	Improves (compared with solitary kidney transplantation)		

FIGURE 5-20. (*Continued*) The complications of pancreas transplantation are relatively frequent and must be considered before recommending the procedure to patients. No controlled clinical trials have been performed. However, studies of retinopathy, nephropathy, and neuropathy have been performed that compare patients who have had kidney transplantation alone or failed pancreas transplantation with patients who have had successful pancreas transplantations. These studies have demonstrated improvements in outcome that generally support the role of pancreas transplantation in ameliorating long-term complications (**B**). All data based on published or registry data for 1988 to 1996 [27–39]. Of all pancreas transplantations in patients with diabetes, 87% have been performed as simultaneous kidney-pancreas procedures. Approximately 8% have been done as pancreas after kidney transplantation and 5% as solitary pancreas transplantations. Results from pancreas transplantation performed before 1986 generally were less successful, whereas results from the most recently performed pancreas transplantations reveal better short-term pancreas survival. (*Adapted from* UNOS [27].)

POTENTIAL ADVANTAGES AND DISADVANTAGES OF WHOLE-ORGAN VERSUS ISLET TRANSPLANTATION

	Whole Organ	Isolated Islets
Surgery	Major surgery required; must drain exocrine secretions	Can be infused in minor procedure
Postoperative complications	Frequent	None
Transplantation tissue		
Source	Human allograft	Human or other species
Number	Single donor	Islets harvested from multiple donors
Immunosuppression	Major	May be minimal for immunoprotected (encapsulated or masked antigenic sites)
Current efficacy (restoration of normoglycemia at 1 y with no exogenous insulin)	80%–90% success rate	80%

FIGURE 5-21. Islet transplantation. Many of the drawbacks of whole-organ transplantation, including major abdominal surgery, requirement for long-term immunosuppression, and postoperative complications are potentially eliminated with the use of isolated islets. Masking of antigenic sites or immunoprotection with encapsulation may not only reduce the need for immunosuppression but may allow the use of islets from other species. Limited data from Edmonton, Canada have demonstrated approximately 80% insulin independence following islet transplantation. The Edmonton protocol includes islet isolation and preparation without culture, steroid-free immunosuppression with tacrolimus and sirolimus, and transhepatic infusion of isolates from donor pancreas into the portal vein with the goal of 10,000 islet equivalents per kilogram of body weight of the recipient [40].

References

1. Dolger H: Clinical evaluation of vascular damage in diabetes mellitus. *JAMA* 1947, 134:1289–1291.

2. DCCT Research Group: The effect of intensive diabetes treatment on the development and progression of long-term complications in insulin-dependent diabetes mellitus: The Diabetes Control and Complications Trial. *N Engl J Med* 1993, 329:978–986.

3. The Kroc Collaborative Study Group: Blood glucose control and the evolution of diabetic retinopathy and albuminuria. *N Engl J Med* 1994, 311:365–372.

4. Feldt-Rasmussen B, Mathiesen ER, Deckert T: Effect of two years of strict metabolic control on progression of incipient nephropathy in insulin-dependent diabetes. *Lancet* 1986, 2(8519):1300–1304.

5. Binchmann-Hansen O, Dahl-Jorgensen K, Hanssen KR, Sandvik L: The response of diabetic retinopathy to 41 months of multiple insulin injections, insulin pumps, and conventional insulin therapy. *Arch Ophthalmol* 1988, 106:1242–1246.

6. Reichard P, Nilsson B-Y, Rosenqvist U: The effect of long-term insulin treatment on the development of microvascular complications of diabetes mellitus. *N Engl J Med* 1993, 329:304–309.

7. Nathan DM: The modern management of insulin-dependent diabetes mellitus. *Med Clin NA* 1988, 72:1365–1378.

8. Nathan DM, Singer DE, Hurxthal K, Goodson JD: The clinical information value of the glycosylated hemoglobin assay. *N Engl J Med* 1984, 310:341–346.

9. DCCT Research Group: The absence of a glycemic threshold for the development of long-term complications. *Diabetes* 1996, 45:1289–1298.

10. Cryer PE, Fisher JN, Shamoon H: Hypoglycemia. *Diabetes Care* 1994, 17:734–751.

11. Fanelli C, Epifano L, Rambotti AM, *et al.*: Meticulous prevention of hypoglycemia normalizes the glycemic thresholds and magnitude of most of neuroendocrine responses to, symptoms of, and cognitive function during hypoglycemia in intensively treated patients with short-term IDDM. *Diabetes* 1993, 42:1683–1689.

12. Saleh TY, Cryer PE: Alanine and terbutaline in the prevention of nocturnal hypoglycemia in IDDM. *Diabetes Care* 1997, 20:1231–1236.

13. Zinman B, Tildesley H, Chiasson J-L, *et al.*: Insulin lispro in CSII. *Diabetes* 1997, 46:440–443.

14. Nathan DM: Long-term complications of diabetes mellitus. *N Engl J Med* 1993, 328:676–685.

15. Galloway JA, Spradlin CT, Howey DC, Dupre J: Intrasubject differences in pharmacokinetic and pharmacodynamic responses: the immutable problem of present-day treatment? In *Diabetes*. Edited by Serrano-Rios M, Lefebvre PJ. New York: Elsevier Science; 1985.

16. Molnar GD, Taylor WF, Langworthy AL: Plasma immunoreactive insulin patterns in insulin-treated diabetics. Studies during continuous blood glucose monitoring *Mayo Clin Proc* 1972, 47:709–719.

17. Nathan DM, Lou P, Avruch J: Intensive conventional and insulin pump therapies in type 1 diabetes. A crossover study. *Ann Intern Med* 1982, 97:31–36.

18. Reichard P, Pihl M: Mortality and treatment side effects during long-term intensified conventional insulin treatment in the Stockholm Diabetes Intervention Study. *Diabetes* 1994, 43:313–317.

19. Dunn FL, Nathan DM, Scavini M, Selam J-L: Long-term therapy of IDDM with an implantable insulin pump. *Diabetes Care* 1997, 20:59–63.

20. DCCT Research Group: Clustering of long-term complications in families with diabetes in the Diabetes Control and Complications Trial. *Diabetes* 1997, 46:1829–1839.

21. Parving HH, Smidt UM, Friisberg B, *et al.*: A prospective study of glomerular filtration rate and arterial blood pressure in insulin-dependent diabetics with nephropathy. *Diabetologia* 1981, 20:457–461.

22. Klein BEK, Moss SE, Klein R: Effect of pregnancy on progression of diabetic retinopathy. *Diabetes Care* 1990, 13:34–40.

23. Lewis EJ: The effect of angiotensin-converting-enzyme inhibition on diabetic nephropathy. *N Engl J Med* 1993, 329:1456–1462.

24. Progression of retinopathy with intensive versus conventional treatment in the Diabetes Control and Complications Trial. Diabetes Control and Complications Trial Research Group. *Ophthalmology* 1995, 102:647–661.

25. Effect of intensive therapy on the development and progression of diabetic nephropathy in the Diabetes Control and Complications (DCCT) Research Group. *Kidney Int* 1995, 47:1703–1720.

26. DCCT Research Group. Effect of intensive therapy on residual β cell function in patients with type 1 diabetes in the Diabetes Control and Complications Trial. *Ann Int Med* 1998, 128:517–523.

27. UNOS. 1997 Annual Report: U.S. Scientific Registry of Transplant Recipients and The Organ Procurement and Transplantation Network. Bethesda, MD: Department of Health and Human Services, ISBN 1-886651-25-6.

28. Gruessner RW, Sutherland DER: Simultaneous kidney and segmental pancreas transplants from living related donors: the first two successful cases. *Transplantation* 1996, 61:1265–1268.

29. Stegall M, Wachs M, Kam I: Successful pancreas transplantation in adult-onset diabetes mellitus. *Diabetes* 1997, 46(Suppl 1):64A.

30. American Diabetes Association: Pancreas transplantation for patients with diabetes mellitus. *Diabetes Care* 1998, 21(Suppl 1):S79.

31. Sutherland DER, Gruessner RWG: Current status of pancreas transplantation for the treatment of type 1 diabetes mellitus. *Clin Diabetes* 1997, 15:152–156.

32. Ramsay RC, Goetz FC, Sutherland DER, *et al.*: Progression of diabetic retinopathy after pancreas transplantation for insulin-dependent diabetes mellitus. *N Engl J Med* 1988, 318:208–214.

33. Navarro X, Sutherland DER, Kennedy WR: Long-term effects of pancreatic transplantation on diabetic neuropathy. *Ann Neurol* 1997, 42:727–736.

34. Navarro X, Kennedy WR, Sutherland DER: Autonomic neuropathy and survival in diabetes mellitus: effects of pancreas transplantation. *Diabetologia* 1991, 34(Suppl 1): S108–S112.

35. Fioretto P, Steffes MW, Sutherland DER, *et al.*: Reversal of lesions of diabetic nephropathy after pancreas transplantation. *N Engl J Med* 1998, 339:69–75.

36. Bohman SO, Tyden G, Wilczek, *et al.*: Prevention of kidney graft diabetic nephropathy by pancreas transplantation in man. *Diabetes* 1985, 34:306–308.

37. Bilous RW, Mauer SM, Sutherland DER, *et al.*: The effects of pancreas transplantation on the glomerular structure of renal allografts in patients with insulin-dependent diabetes. *N Engl J Med* 1989, 321:80–85.

38. Nathan DM Fogel HA, Norman D, *et al.*: Long-term metabolic and quality of life results with pancreatic/renal transplantation in IDDM. *Transplantation* 1991, 52:85–91.

39. Milde FK, Hart LK, Zehr PS: Quality of life of pancreatic transplant recipients. *Diabetes Care* 1992, 15:1459–1463.

40. Shapiro AM, Lakey JR, Ryan EA, *et al.*: Islet transplantation in seven patients with type 1 diabetes mellitus using a glucocorticoid-free immunosuppressive regimen. *N Engl J Med* 2000, 343(4):230–238.

PATHOGENESIS OF TYPE 2 DIABETES

John E. Gerich and Niyaz Gosmanov

6

Type 2 diabetes (formerly maturity-onset or non–insulin-dependent diabetes mellitus) is among the most common chronic diseases, affecting about 6% of the United States population (approximately 16 million people) [1]. Phenotypically, about 95% of people with diabetes mellitus have type 2 diabetes [2]. This disorder, however, is extremely heterogeneous (Fig. 6-1). Approximately 10% of patients have late-onset type 1 diabetes; about another 5% develop diabetes as a result of rare monogenic defects in either insulin secretion or insulin action. The remaining patients have "garden variety" type 2 diabetes. The number of people with type 2 diabetes worldwide is expected to increase from 135 million to over 300 million by 2025, with most of this increase occurring in developing countries. The prevalence of type 2 diabetes in the United States has increased rapidly over the past 50 years (Fig. 6-2) and is highest in minority populations, including blacks, Hispanics, and especially Native Americans. In the Pima Indians of Arizona, 50% of adults older than age 35 years have the disease [3]. In all populations, the prevalence increases with age; in whites, the prevalence reaches 20% by the age of 80 years [2] (Fig. 6-3).

The pathogenesis of type 2 diabetes involves the interaction of genetic and environmental (acquired) factors which adversely affect insulin secretion (pancreatic β-cell function) and tissue responses to insulin (insulin sensitivity) (Fig. 6-4). Both impaired β-cell function and insulin resistance are present before the onset of type 2 diabetes and are predictive of its subsequent development [4–7]. Type 2 diabetes is a polygenic disorder [8]; the additive effects of an as yet unknown number of genetic polymorphisms (risk factors) are required for development of the disorder, although they may not be sufficient necessarily in the absence of environmental (acquired) risk factors (Fig. 6-5). Although searches for candidate genes based on various proteins involved in mediating insulin action have failed to find diabetic genes in this category [8], these genetic factors likely will be elucidated as the Human Genome Project progresses. To date, only two polymorphisms have been identified. One involves an amino acid polymorphism (pro12 ala) in the peroxisome proliferator receptor gamma, which is expressed in insulin target tissues and pancreatic β cells and is involved in modulating effects of insulin [9]. The other involves the gene encoding calpain-10, a cysteine protease that modulates insulin secretion and insulin effects in muscle and adipose tissue [10].

The importance of inheritable factors is underscored by the fact that a person with either both parents or a monozygotic twin with type 2 diabetes has up to an 80% lifetime risk of developing this disorder [11]. Having a single parent or sibling with type 2 diabetes carries a risk of about 30%, which represents a twofold to fourfold increase above that of the general population [12,13]. Impaired β-cell function is the earliest detectable defect in people with normal glucose tolerance who are genetically predisposed to develop type 2 diabetes [6,7,14], eg, first-degree relatives of individuals with type 2 diabetes (Fig. 6-8) [15]. The strongest evidence for this comes from studies of monozygotic twins where one

twin has type 2 diabetes while the other has normal glucose tolerance [16]. The twin with normal glucose tolerance has about an 80% chance of developing type 2 diabetes and thus can be considered to be a true genetically prediabetic individual. All four studies of such twin pairs have found that the twin with normal glucose tolerance had impaired β-cell function [16–19]; the only study that simultaneously assessed insulin sensitivity found it to be normal [16].

Environmental (acquired) factors, however, are also critical for developing diabetes, since without these, genetic factors may be insufficient to cause type 2 diabetes. The most important factors are those that influence insulin sensitivity: obesity (especially visceral obesity), physical inactivity, high-fat–low-fiber diets, smoking, and low birth weight (Fig. 6-6) [13,20–25]. Intervention trials have consistently demonstrated that the risk for developing type 2 diabetes can be reduced by up to 60% by caloric restriction, diet modification, and increased physical activity [26–30]. Although most (>90%) patients with classic type 2 diabetes are obese (and therefore insulin resistant), most insulin-resistant obese individuals are not diabetic. What distinguishes obese individuals with and without diabetes is the ability to compensate for insulin resistance with increased insulin secretion (Fig. 6-7) [31].

There are numerous examples in the literature where type 2 diabetes can occur solely as a result of impaired insulin secretion in the absence of insulin resistance [32–40]. Most of the insulin resistance found in people with type 2 diabetes can be ascribed to environmental (acquired) factors such as obesity, physical inactivity, high-fat diets, and glucose and lipid toxicity [41]. After binding to its receptor, insulin triggers a complex series of events (Fig. 6-10). The insulin resistance of obesity is associated with reduced numbers of insulin receptors, reduced insulin receptor kinase activity, and reduced activation of insulin signaling proteins and glucose transport [42]. Quantitatively similar defects have been found in obese individuals with type 2 diabetes compared to obese individuals without type 2 diabetes [42]. Several factors may be involved in the insulin resistance associated with obesity: altered release from adipose tissue of free fatty acids [43], tumor necrosis factor-α [44], resistin [45], leptin [46], adipsin [47], and adiponectin [48], as well as accumulation of lipid in insulin target organs [49, 50] (Fig. 6-11).

People destined to develop type 2 diabetes initially have impaired glucose tolerance (IGT), a state characterized by isolated postprandial hyperglycemia (Figs. 6-12—6-14). In type 2 diabetes, the basic metabolic derangements are the same except that progressive deterioration in β-cell function and a modest decrease in insulin sensitivity now result in overproduction of glucose by the liver and kidney in the postabsorptive state (ie, fasting hyperglycemia) and impaired splanchnic glucose sequestration (glycogen formation) in the postprandial state [51,52]. Fasting hyperglycemia is directly related to rates of glucose production (Fig. 6-15). Because of the mass action effect of hyperglycemia and prevailing insulin levels, glucose utilization rates are still in an absolute sense normal in type 2 diabetes, although the distribution of tissue uptake and metabolic fates may be altered (Fig. 6-16) [52].

Poorly controlled diabetes leads to microvascular complications (retinopathy, nephropathy, and neuropathy) and macrovascular complications (premature atherosclerosis). Interventional clinical trials (such as the Diabetes Control and Complications Trial, the UKPDS, the Kumamoto Study, and the Stockholm Diabetes Intervention Study) [53–55] have shown that microvascular complications can be prevented if HbA_{1c} levels are maintained below 7.0% (upper limit of normal, 6.0%) (Fig. 6-7), whereas it appears that lower HbA_{1c} levels are needed to prevent macrovascular complications [56–58]. Improved insulin preparations and new oral agents that specifically target either impaired insulin secretion and insulin resistance are now available that can achieve this degree of glycemic control (Fig. 6-18). Furthermore, lifestyle changes (weight loss, exercise) and drugs that reduce insulin resistance can reverse IGT and prevent its progression to type 2 diabetes. Because of the progressive deterioration in insulin secretion, most patients initially successfully managed on one oral agent will need additional drugs, and up to 50% may ultimately need some form of insulin therapy to maintain adequate glycemic control [59–70].

Epidemiology

HETEROGENEITY OF PHENOTYPIC TYPE 2 DIABETES

Subtype	Patients, %
I. LADA [71]	≈10
II. MODY [72]	≈3
MODY 1: HNF-4α	
MODY 2: Glucokinase	
MODY 3: HNF-1α	
MODY 4: PDX-1 (IPF-1)	
MODY 5: HNF-1β	
MODY 6: Neuro D1/BETA 2	
III. Maternally inherited diabetes and deafness	<1
(Mutations in mitochondrial DNA$_t$RNA)	
IV. Insulin receptor defects	<1
Leprechanism	
Type A insulin resistance and acanthosis nigricans	
Rabson-Mendenhall syndrome	
V. Type 2 diabetes	≈85

FIGURE 6-1. Heterogeneity of phenotypic type 2 diabetes. Patients with late-onset autoimmune diabetes (LADA) [71] experience onset of disease after age 30 years, are generally lean, have islet cell or glutamic acid decarboxylase antibodies, and usually progress to insulin dependence in less than 5 years. Patients with maturity-onset diabetes of youth (MODY) [72] generally experience onset of disease between 15 and 30 years of age, can be either obese or lean, and have a strong family history of diabetes consistent with an autosomal dominant inheritance resulting in impaired insulin release but little or no insulin resistance. Five monogenetic mutations have been identified and more are expected. HNF—hepatic nuclear factor; IPF—insulin-promoting factor; neuro D1/BETA 2—1/β cell box transactivator 2; PDX—pancreatic development factor.

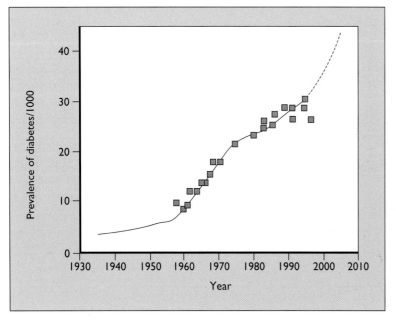

FIGURE 6-2. Increasing prevalence of diabetes in the United States. The prevalence of diagnosed diabetes in the United States has risen steadily since 1930 and is expected to continue to increase rapidly in the early part of the 21st century. About 90% of cases of diagnosed diabetes are of type 2 diabetes. It is estimated that at any given time, at least one third of persons with type 2 diabetes are undiagnosed. (*Adapted from* [1].)

PREVALENCE OF TYPE 2 DIABETES AND IMPAIRED GLUCOSE TOLERANCE

Age, y	Diabetes		IGT	
	Men, %	Women, %	Men, %	Women, %
20–39	1.6	1.7	—	—
30–49	6.8	6.1	12.6	11.2
50–59	12.9	12.4	13.3	15.3
60–74	20.2	17.8	19.2	21.9
>75	21.1	17.5	—	—

FIGURE 6-3. Prevalence of type 2 diabetes and impaired glucose tolerance (IGT). (*Data from* Harris *et al.* [2].)

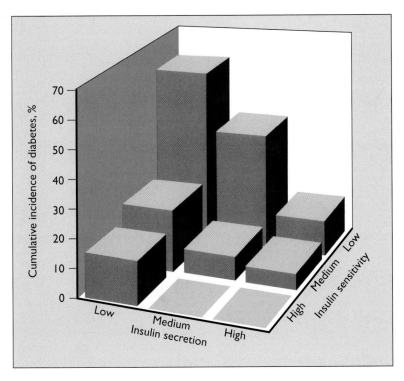

FIGURE 6-4. Incidence of diabetes among Pima Indians. The relative impact of variations in β-cell function and insulin sensitivity on the subsequent development of diabetes among 262 Pima Indians is shown. The acute insulin secretory response to intravenous glucose and insulin action at baseline was measured in patients who initially had normal glucose tolerance. Patients were divided into tertiles of insulin secretion and insulin sensitivity and were followed for an average of 7 years. The observations, however, do not take into consideration whether the β-cell function was appropriate for the degree of insulin resistance; they merely illustrate the fact that both factors influence the risk for developing type 2 diabetes. (*Adapted from* Pratley and Weyer [7].)

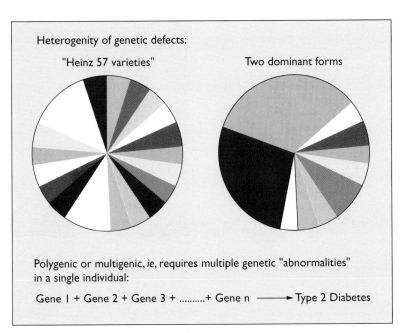

FIGURE 6-5. Two major features of the genetics of type 2 diabetes in the general population. First, this disease is a genetically heterogeneous disorder. At present, however, it is not clear how many forms of diabetes exist, whether there are one or two predominant forms, or whether each form represents only a small percentage of the total population. For most patients, the disease is polygenic: some abnormality or sequence polymorphism is present in several genes, each contributing a small amount to the overall pathogenesis. Although there is no definitive information on the number of genes involved in each form, most investigators believe that at least three genes, and perhaps as many as 10 or 20, may contribute to the final phenotype. Most likely, these are "normal" genetic variants or sequence polymorphisms, which slightly alter insulin action or insulin secretion [73].

Environmental Factors

RELATIVE RISKS FOR DEVELOPING TYPE 2 DIABETES

Obesity, BMI, kg/m^2	Relative Risk
< 23	1
23–25	3
25–30	8
30–35	20
< 35	40
Physical Activity, *h/wk*	
> 7	1.0
4–7	1.1
2–4	1.2
0.5–2	1.5
<0.5	1.8
Healthy Diet, *quintiles based on fat/fiber content*	
5	1.00
4	1.15
3	1.30
2	1.50
1	2.00

FIGURE 6-6. Relative risks for developing type 2 diabetes. A physically inactive individual (less than 30 min/wk of exercise) who consumes an unhealthy diet (level 1) and is modestly overweight (body mass index [BMI] 25–30) would have a 30-fold increased (1.8 × 2.0 × 8) risk of developing type 2 diabetes compared to the general population, which would translate to a lifetime risk of nearly 100%. (*Adapted from* Choi and Shi [21].)

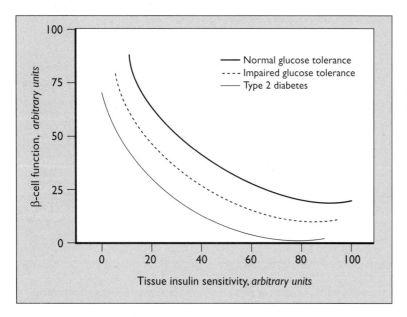

FIGURE 6-7. Reciprocal relationship between β-cell function and tissue insulin sensitivity. A hyperbolic function relates β-cell function to tissue insulin sensitivity such that when insulin decreases, β-cell function increases to maintain normal glucose homeostasis. Patients who develop impaired glucose tolerance (IGT) or type 2 diabetes have an inadequate β-cell compensation for insulin resistance in that for any degree of reduced tissue insulin sensitivity, the β-cell response is below normal [5–7,74].

Genetic Factors

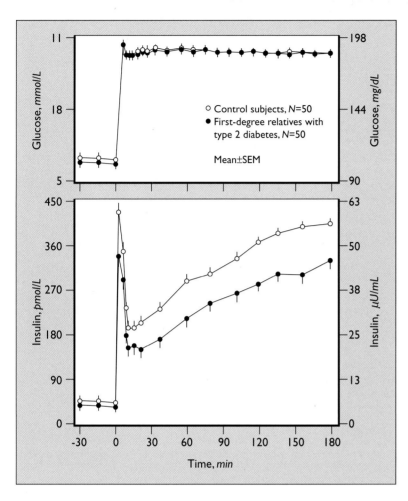

FIGURE 6-8. Plasma glucose (*top*) and insulin (*bottom*) concentrations in hyperglycemic clamp experiments. In response to an acute elevation of blood glucose concentrations, insulin is secreted in a biphasic manner; a first phase lasting approximately 10 minutes followed by a gradually increasing second phase. The first phase of insulin release has been linked to insulin granules located near the β-cell membrane (rapidly releasable pool). Second phase insulin release depends in part on mobilizing insulin granules from a storage pool to the rapidly releasable pool as well as increased synthesis of insulin. In this study [15], subjects with normal glucose tolerance but a first-degree relative with type 2 diabetes were studied using a hyperglycemic clamp to assess their β-cell function and insulin sensitivity relative to a group of subjects with normal glucose tolerance but no family history of diabetes. Subjects were matched for age, gender, and obesity to exclude environmental (acquired) risk factors. It was demonstrated that individuals with a first-degree relative with type 2 diabetes had reduced early (first phase) and late (second phase) insulin release and were not insulin resistant. (*Adapted from* Pimenta *et al.* [15].)

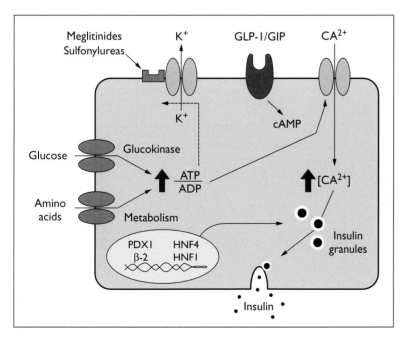

FIGURE 6-9. Nutrient sensing and insulin secretion by the pancreatic β cell. The β cell takes up glucose and amino acids via specific transporters on the cell membrane, such as the GLUT2 glucose transporter. This isoform of transporter is expressed only by the β cell and the liver and has a Km in the physiologic range. Once inside the cell, glucose is phosphorylated by a specialized form of hexokinase called glucokinase. The subsequent metabolism of glucose results in a change in the adenosine triphosphate (ATP):adenosine diphosphate (ADP) ratio in the cell, which in turn causes activation of the ATP-sensitive potassium channel. This results in depolarization of the cell, an influx of calcium, and subsequent release of insulin from secretory granules. The sulfonylurea receptor can also activate the ATP-sensitive potassium channel, mimicking the effect of glucose. Other secretagogues, such as glucagon-like peptide-1 (GLP-1), bypass this system by changing cellular cyclic adenosine monophosphate (cAMP) levels. The level of expression of the several molecules involved in glucose sensing, including the GLUT2 glucose transporter, and the development of the β cell, are controlled by several nuclear transcription factors. The best studied of these are HNF-1α, HNF-1β, HNF-4α, and PDX-1 (IPF-1). Maturity-onset diabetes of youth can result from genetic defects in any of these transcription factors or a genetic defect in glucokinase. In type 2 diabetes, the exact site of the defect in glucose sensing is unknown, but studies in animal models of disease have suggested that this may be the result of a down-regulation of the GLUT2 glucose transporter [75].

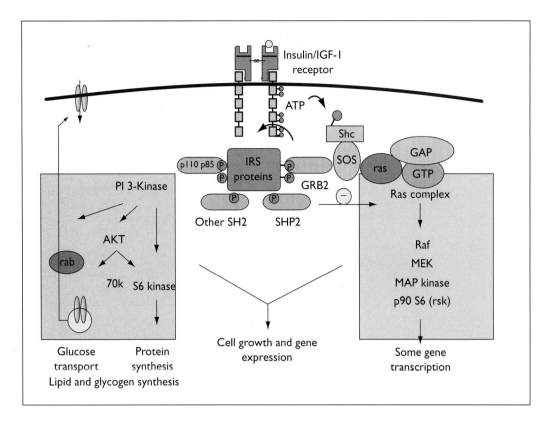

FIGURE 6-10. The insulin signaling network. The full network is complex and can be divided into five levels: 1) activation of the insulin receptor tyrosine kinase and closely linked events; 2) phosphorylation of a family of substrate proteins; 3) interaction of the receptor and its substrates with several intermediate signaling molecules via SH2 (src homology 2) and other recognition domains; 4) activation of serine and lipid kinases, resulting in a broad range of phosphorylation-dephosphorylation events; and 5) regulation of the final biological effectors of insulin action, such as glucose transport, lipid synthesis, gene expression, and mitogenesis. The SH2 proteins link the insulin receptor substrate (IRS) proteins to a series of cascading reactions involving serine/threonine kinases and phosphatases such as the mitogen-activated protein (MAP) kinases, S6 kinases, and protein phosphatase-1A. These serine kinases act on enzymes such as glycogen synthase, transcription factors, and other proteins to produce many of the final biological effects of the hormone. In adipose tissue and muscle, insulin stimulation also increases glucose uptake by promoting translocation of an intracellular pool of glucose transporters to the plasma membrane. Exactly how this action is linked to the phosphorylation cascade is unknown, but several studies suggest that this important action of insulin, as well as most metabolic effects, is downstream of the enzyme phosphatidylinositol 3-kinase (PI 3-kinase). Other effects of insulin, such as stimulation of glycogen and lipid synthesis, occur through additional intracellular effects to stimulate the enzymes involved in these reactions. ATP—adenosine triphosphate; GAP—GTPase-activating protein; GRB2—growth-factor receptor binding protein 2; GTP—guanosine triphosphate; IGF—insulin-like growth factor; MEK—MAP-Erk kinase; SOS—son-of-seven less protein.

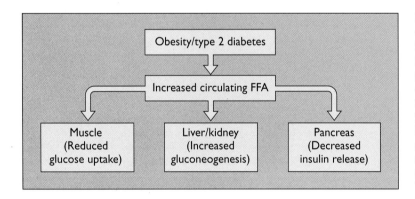

FIGURE 6-11. Insulin resistance and obesity. The insulin resistance associated with type 2 diabetes largely can be explained by obesity, since comparably obese individuals with and without type 2 diabetes have quantitatively similar reductions in insulin-receptor binding, insulin-receptor tyrosine kinase activity, and muscle glucose transport [42,76]. Most of these abnormalities in patients with type 2 diabetes can be normalized by weight loss [77]. Current evidence indicates that the most important factor involved in the insulin resistance of obesity in humans is the increased circulating levels of plasma free fatty acids (FFA) [43]. Experimental elevation of FFA in normal humans decreases muscle glucose uptake and increases endogenous glucose production and in animal models impairs insulin secretion [78,79]. All of these actions would promote hyperglycemia by altering rates of the balance between entry and removal of glucose from the circulation. The mechanisms for the effects of FFA are twofold: substrate competition [80] and impaired insulin signaling [81]. Acetylated products of FFA metabolism decrease glucose oxidation via inhibition of pyruvate dehydrogenase and activate serine/threonine kinases possibly through increases in protein kinase C (theta), leading to reduced activity of insulin receptor substrate (IRS) proteins. The main effect of the latter appears to be a reduction in glucose transport [82–84].

STAGES IN THE DEVELOPMENT OF TYPE 2 DIABETES

	Impaired β-Cell Function	Insulin Resistance	Glucose Tolerance
Stage 1	Demonstrable upon testing (+)	Absent	Normal
Stage 2	Demonstrable upon testing (++)	Present (variable)	Normal
Stage 3	Clearly abnormal (+++)	Worse than above	IGT*
Stage 4	More abnormal (++++)	Worse than above	IGT + IFG†
Stage 5	Markedly abnormal (+++++)	Worse than above	Type 2 diabetes‡

*Fasting plasma glucose generally normal < 110 mg/dL (6.1 mM) but 2 hr postprandial > 140 mg/dL (7.8 mM) < 200 mg/dL (11.1 mM).

†Fasting plasma glucose >110 mg/dL (6.1 mM) but less than 126 mg/dL (7.0 mM) and 2 hr postprandial.

‡Fasting plasma glucose > 126 mg/dL (7.0 mM) and/or 2 hr postprandial > 200 mg/dL (11.1 mM).

FIGURE 6-12. Stages in development of type 2 diabetes. Longitudinal and cross-sectional studies indicate that individuals destined to develop type 2 diabetes pass through five stages. The first stage begins at birth, when glucose homeostasis is normal but individuals are at risk for type 2 diabetes because of genetic polymorphisms predisposing them to become obese and limiting the ability of pancreatic β cells to compensate for insulin resistance. During stage 2, decreases in insulin sensitivity emerge as a result of a genetic predisposition and unhealthy lifestyle, which is initially compensated for by an increase in β-cell function so that glucose tolerance remains normal. During stage 3, β-cell function and insulin sensitivity both deteriorate so that when challenged, as during a glucose tolerance test or a standardized meal, postprandial glucose tolerance becomes abnormal. At this point, β-cell function is clearly abnormal but sufficient to maintain normal fasting plasma glucose concentrations. In stage 4, as a result of further deterioration in β-cell functioning and worsening of insulin sensitivity (probably a result of postprandial hyperglycemia), fasting plasma glucose concentrations increase due to an increase in basal endogenous glucose production. Finally, in stage 5, as a result of further deterioration in β-cell function (due to genetic and environmental factors such as glucose and lipotoxicity), both fasting and postprandial glucose levels reach diabetic levels. IFG—impaired fasting glucose; IGT—impaired glucose tolerance.

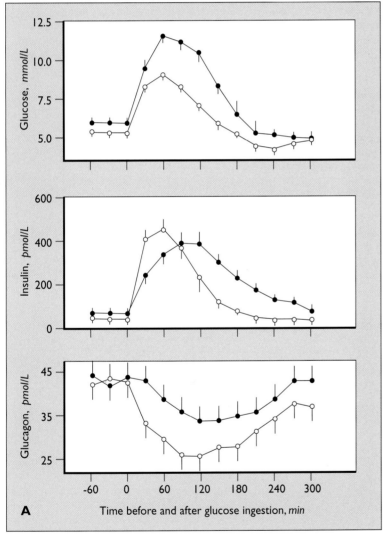

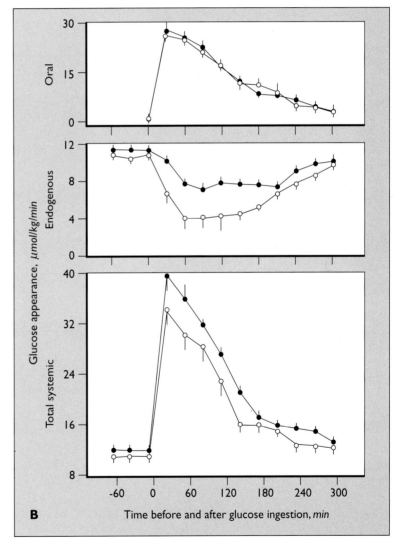

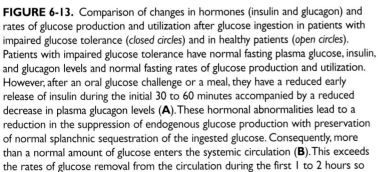

FIGURE 6-13. Comparison of changes in hormones (insulin and glucagon) and rates of glucose production and utilization after glucose ingestion in patients with impaired glucose tolerance (*closed circles*) and in healthy patients (*open circles*). Patients with impaired glucose tolerance have normal fasting plasma glucose, insulin, and glucagon levels and normal fasting rates of glucose production and utilization. However, after an oral glucose challenge or a meal, they have a reduced early release of insulin during the initial 30 to 60 minutes accompanied by a reduced decrease in plasma glucagon levels (**A**). These hormonal abnormalities lead to a reduction in the suppression of endogenous glucose production with preservation of normal splanchnic sequestration of the ingested glucose. Consequently, more than a normal amount of glucose enters the systemic circulation (**B**). This exceeds the rates of glucose removal from the circulation during the first 1 to 2 hours so

that plasma glucose levels increase more than normal. The hyperglycemia eventually leads to delayed and greater than normal plasma insulin levels which, along with the hyperglycemia, cause glucose utilization to exceed glucose production so that plasma glucose eventually returns to normal fasting levels [85,86]. During the 4- to 6-hour postprandial period, a greater than normal amount of glucose entered the circulation and plasma glucose levels started at a normal level and returned to a normal level; therefore, it is obvious that a greater than normal amount of glucose had been removed from circulation. Although tissue glucose utilization is not reduced in patients with impaired glucose tolerance (IGT), it is less than would have been found in patients with normal glucose tolerance whose plasma glucose and insulin levels matched those of patients with IGT, indicating that patients with IGT are insulin resistant [87]. (*Adapted from* Mitrakou *et al.* [86].)

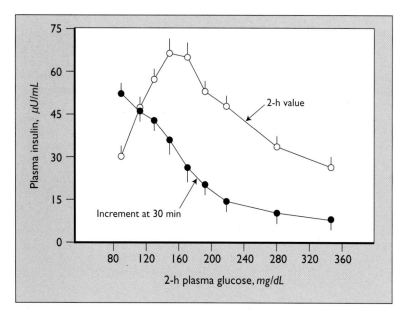

FIGURE 6-14. Comparison of early and late plasma insulin responses during oral glucose tolerance tests. The decrease in early (30 min) postprandial insulin secretion has been correlated with the reduced suppression of endogenous glucose production [86], and decreases progressively as glucose tolerance deteriorates [87]. In contrast, 2-hour insulin levels increase initially and only decrease after 2-hour plasma glucose levels reach diabetic values [88]. The latter phenomenon had been erroneously interpreted to imply that insulin resistance occurs earlier than impaired insulin secretion in the evolution of type 2 diabetes [89], whereas it is now evident that this results from the hyperglycemia due to delayed early insulin release [6,7,88,90].

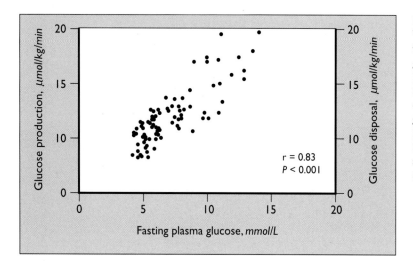

FIGURE 6-15. Glucose production and disposal in the postabsorptive state. With further deterioration in β-cell function, plasma glucose levels in the fasting state increase as a result of impaired suppression of hepatic and renal glucose release by insulin [52]. This is largely due to increased gluconeogenesis [91–94]. As shown in this figure, glucose removal from the circulation also increases as fasting blood glucose levels increase, illustrating that the primary cause of fasting hyperglycemia is overproduction of glucose, not reduced glucose utilization. The increased glucose production results from impaired β-cell function as well as insulin resistance, mediated in part indirectly by increased plasma free fatty acids, increased availability of gluconeogenic substrates, and lack of appropriate suppression of glucagon secretion. (*Adapted from* Dinneen *et al.* [52].)

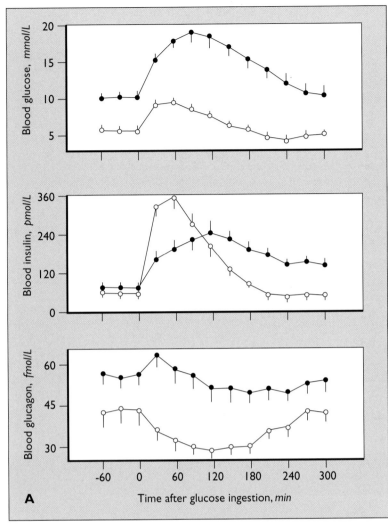

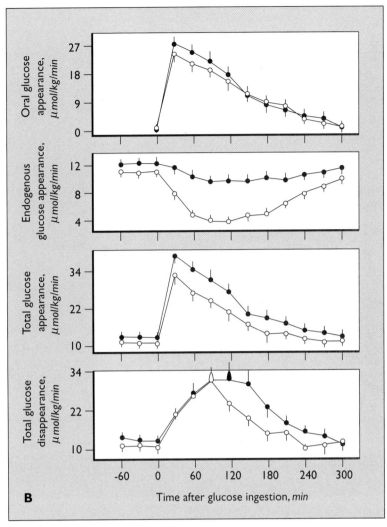

FIGURE 6-16. Comparison of postprandial changes in plasma insulin and glucagon levels (**A**) and rates of glucose appearance and removal from plasma (**B**) in patients with type 2 diabetes and healthy patients. The postprandial abnormalities in patients with type 2 diabetes (*closed circles*) are quite similar to those of people with impaired glucose tolerance (*open circles*), except that they are more exaggerated. The only major difference is that with excessive glycosuria, uptake of glucose in liver is diminished [51,52,95,96]. (*Adapted from Mitrakou et al.* [51].)

Control, Complications, and Treatment

UKPDS: EFFECTS OF INTENSIVE TREATMENT OF TYPE 2 DIABETES

Reduced HbA_{1c} by 11% with intensive therapy (7.9% vs. 7.0%)
This leads to
  12% decrease in any diabetes-related endpoint
  25% decrease in microvascular endpoints
  21% decrease in retinopathy at 12 years
  33% decrease in microalbuminuria at 12 years
  24% decrease in cataract
  16% decrease in myocardial infarction (ns)
  5% decrease in stroke (ns)

FIGURE 6-17. Effects of intensive treatment of type 2 diabetes. Results of the United Kingdom Prospective Diabetes Study (UKPDS) showed an unequivocal effect of intensive insulin therapy on long-term complications of diabetes and mortality [97,98]. HbA_{1c}—glycated hemoglobin.

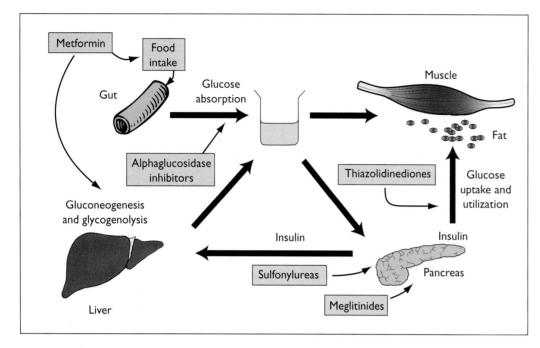

whereas thiazolidinediones (TZDs) are thought to work primarily on adipose tissue and muscle to reduce free fatty acid release and increase glucose uptake, respectively [64]. The exact mechanism of action of these agents on a molecular level is still poorly understood. Metformin may act on gluconeogenic and mitochondrial enzymes, whereas TZDs acting on peroxisome proliferator gamma receptors may alter adipose tissue metabolism (eg, decreased free fatty acids, tumor necrosis factor-α, and resistin release), which then has secondary effects on muscle and liver metabolism [101,102]. In contrast, the mechanism of action of alphaglucosidase inhibitors is well established [103]. By inhibiting the digestion of dietary starches, they slow the postprandial absorption of glucose. Recently, so-called designer insulins produced by modification of their molecular structure have led to preparations with improved pharmacokinetics. Lispro and aspart insulins are absorbed more rapidly than regular insulin and have a shorter half-life, so that injection of these agents immediately prior to meal ingestion more closely mimics the normal physiologic profile than that of regular human insulin which, for optimal benefit, must be injected 30 minutes prior to meal ingestion [66,104–106]. Glargine insulin is a peakless insulin preparation that lasts, on average, 24 hours and has distinct advantages over NPH insulin, which peaks at 6 to 8 hours and lasts only 14 hours [66,67,107,108].

FIGURE 6-18. Sites of action of drugs used to treat type 2 diabetes. Various oral agents are now available for the treatment of type 2 diabetes. These agents differ in their modes of action, efficacy, pharmacokinetics, and side effects. Sulfonylureas and meglitinides are insulin secretagogues that act directly on the pancreatic β cells via inhibiting adenosine triphosphate (ATP)-sensitive potassium channels [59]. Metformin, a biguanide, and thiazolidinediones are classified as insulin sensitizers [63,99]. Metformin appears to act preferentially to inhibit glucose production and to reduce appetite [100],

References

1. *Diabetes in America*, edn 2. Edited by Harris M, Cowie C, Stern M, et al. Bethesda: National Institutes of Health; 1995.

2. Harris M, Flegal K, Cowie C, et al.: Prevalence of diabetes, impaired fasting glucose, and impaired glucose tolerance in U.S. adults. The Third National Health and Nutrition Examination Survey, 1988–1994. *Diabetes Care* 1998, 21:518–524.

3. Bogardus C, Lillioja S, Bennett P: Pathogenesis of NIDDM in Pima Indians. *Diabetes Care* 1991, 14:685–690.

4. Weyer C, Tataranni PA, Bogardus C, et al.: Insulin resistance and insulin secretory dysfunction are independent predictors of worsening of glucose tolerance during each stage of type 2 diabetes development. *Diabetes Care* 2000, 24:89–94.

5. Weyer C, Bogardus C, Mott D, et al.: The natural history of insulin secretory dysfunction and insulin resistance in the pathogenesis of type 2 diabetes mellitus. *J Clin Invest* 1999, 104:787–794.

6. Kahn S: The importance of β-cell failure in the development and progression of type 2 diabetes. *J Clin Endocrinol Metab* 2001, 86:4047–4058.

7. Pratley R, Weyer C: The role of impaired early insulin secretion in the pathogenesis of type II diabetes mellitus. *Diabetologia* 2001, 44:929–945.

8. Hamman R: Genetic and environmental determinants of noninsulin-dependent diabetes mellitus (NIDDM). *Diabetes Metab Rev* 1992, 8:287–338.

9. Stefan N, Fritsche A, Haring H, et al.: Effect of experimental elevation of free fatty acids on insulin secretion and insulin sensitivity in healthy carriers of the Pro12Ala polymorphism of the peroxisome proliferator-activated receptor-gamma2 gene. *Diabetes* 2001, 50:1143–1148.

10. Horikawa Y, Oda N, Cox N, et al.: Genetic variation in the gene encoding calpain-10 is associated with type 2 diabetes mellitus. *Nat Genet* 2000, 26:163–175.

11. Gloyn A: The genetics of diabetes: a progress report. *Practical Diabetes Int* 2001, 18:246–250.

12. Shaw J, Purdie D, Neil H, et al.: The relative risks of hyperglycemia, obesity and dyslipidemia in relatives of patients with type II diabetes mellitus. *Diabetologia* 1999, 42:24–27.

13. Shatten B, Smith G, Kuller L, et al.: Risk factors for the development of type 2 diabetes among men enrolled in the usual care group of the multiple risk factor intervention trial. *Diabetes* 1993, 16:1331–1338.

14. Gerich J, Van Haeften T: Insulin resistance versus impaired insulin secretion as the genetic basis for type 2 diabetes. *Curr Opin Endo Diab* 1998, 5:144–148.

15. Pimenta W, Kortytkowski M, Mitrakou A, et al.: Pancreatic beta-cell dysfunction as the primary genetic lesion in NIDDM. *JAMA* 1995, 273:1855–1861.

16. Vaag A, Alford F, Beck-Nielsen H: Intracellular glucose and fat metabolism in identical twins discordant for non–insulin-dependent diabetes mellitus (NIDDM): acquired versus genetic metabolic defects. *Diabetic Med* 1996, 13:806–815.

17. Cerasi E, Luft R: Insulin response to glucose infusion in diabetic and nondiabetic monozygotic twin pairs: genetic control of insulin response. *Acta Endocrinol* 1967, 55:330–345.

18. Barnett A, Spiliopoulos A, Pyke D, et al.: Metabolic studies in unaffected co-twins of noninsulin-dependent diabetics. *Br Med J* 1981, 282:1656–1658.

19. Pyke D, Taylor K: Glucose tolerance and serum insulin in unaffected identical twins of diabetics. *Br Med J* 1967, 4:21–22.

20. Hu F, Manson J, Stampfer M, et al.: Diet, lifestyle, and the risk of type 2 diabetes mellitus in women. *N Engl J Med* 2001, 345:790–797.

21. Choi B, Shi F: Risk factors for diabetes mellitus by age and sex: results of the national population health survey. *Diabetologia* 2001, 44:1221–1231.

22. Marshall J, Hoag S, Shetterly S, et al.: Dietary fat predicts conversion of impaired glucose tolerance to NIDDM. *Diabetes Care* 1994, 17:50–56.

23. Wei M, Schweitner H, Blair S: The association between physical activity, physical fitness and type 2 diabetes mellitus. *Compr Ther* 2000, 26:176–182.

24. Wannamethee S, Shaper A, Perry I: Smoking as a modifiable risk factor for type 2 diabetes in middle-aged men. *Diabetes Care* 2001, 24:1590–1595.

25. Rich-Edwards J, Colditz G, Stampfer M, et al.: Birthweight and the risk for type 2 diabetes mellitus in adult women. *Ann Intern Med* 1999, 130:278–284.

26. Eriksson J, Lindstrom J, Tuomilehto J: Potential for prevention of type 2 diabetes. *Br Med Bull* 2001, 60:183–199.

27. Knowler W, Barrett-Connor E, Fowler S, et al.: Reduction in the incidence of type 2 diabetes with lifestyle intervention or metformin. *N Engl J Med* 2002, 346:393–403.

28. Tuomilehto J, Lindström J, Eriksson J, et al.: Prevention of type 2 diabetes mellitus by changes in lifestyle among subjects with impaired glucose tolerance. *N Engl J Med* 2001, 344:1343–1350.

29. Pan XR, Li GW, Hu YH, et al.: Effects of diet and exercise in preventing NIDDM in people with impaired glucose tolerance: The Da Qing IGT and Diabetes Study. *Diabetes Care* 1997, 20:537–544.

30. Erikkson K, Lindgarde F: Prevention of type 2 (noninsulin-dependent) diabetes mellitus by diet and exercise. *Diabetologia* 1991, 34:891–898.

31. Porte D, Jr., Kahn S: Beta-cell dysfunction and failure in type 2 diabetes: potential mechanisms. *Diabetes* 2001, 50(Suppl 1):S160–S163.

32. Carey D, Jenkins A, Campbell L, et al.: Abdominal fat and insulin resistance in normal and overweight women: direct measurements reveal a strong relationship in subjects at both low and high risk of NIDDM. *Diabetes* 1996, 45:633–638.

33. Banerji M, Chaiken R, Gordon D, et al.: Does intra-abdominal adipose tissue in black men determine whether NIDDM is insulin-resistant or insulin-sensitive? *Diabetes* 1995, 44:141–146.

34. Byrne M, Sturgis J, Sobel R, et al.: Elevated plasma glucose 2 h postchallenge predicts defects in beta-cell function. *Am J Physiol* 1996, 270:E572–E579.

35. Nesher R, Casa Della L, Litvin Y, et al.: Insulin deficiency and insulin resistance in type II (noninsulin-dependent) diabetes: quantitative contributions of pancreatic and peripheral responses to glucose homeostasis. *Eur J Clin Invest* 1987, 17:266–274.

36. Campbell P, Mandarino L, Gerich J: Quantification of the relative impairment in actions of insulin on hepatic glucose production and peripheral glucose uptake in non–insulin-dependent diabetes mellitus. *Metabolism* 1988, 37:15–21.

37. Kalant N, Leibovici D, Fukushima N, et al.: Insulin responsiveness of superficial forearm tissues in type 2 (noninsulin-dependent) diabetes. *Diabetologia* 1982, 22:239–244.

38. Bonora E, Bonadonna R, DelPrato S, et al.: In vivo glucose metabolism in obese and type II diabetic subjects with or without hypertension. *Diabetes* 1993, 42:764–772.

39. Nosadini R, Solini A, Velussi M, et al.: Impaired insulin-induced glucose uptake by extrahepatic tissue is hallmark of NIDDM patients who have or will develop hypertension and microalbuminuria. *Diabetes* 1994, 43:491–499.

40. Groop L, Ekstrand A, Forsblom C, et al.: Insulin resistance, hypertension and microalbuminuria in patients with type 2 (non–insulin-dependent) diabetes mellitus. *Diabetologia* 1993, 36:642–647.

41. Gerich J: The genetic basis of type 2 diabetes mellitus: Impaired insulin secretion versus impaired insulin sensitivity. *Endocr Rev* 1998, 19:491–503.

42. Dohm GL, Tapscott E, Pories W, et al.: An in vitro human muscle preparation suitable for metabolic studies. Decreased insulin stimulation of glucose transport in muscle from morbidly obese and diabetic subjects. *J Clin Invest* 1988, 82:486–494.

43. Boden G: Role of fatty acids in the pathogenesis of insulin resistance and NIDDM. *Diabetes* 1997, 46:3–10.

44. Hotamisligil G, Spiegelman B: Tumor necrosis factor-α: a key component of the obesity-diabetes link. *Diabetes* 1994, 43:1271–1278.

45. Steppan C, Bailey S, Bhat S, et al.: The hormone resistin links obesity to diabetes. *Nature* 2001, 409:307–312.

46. Ahima R, Flier J: Leptin. *Annu Rev Physiol* 2000, 62:413–437.

47. Ahima R, Flier J: Adipose tissue as an endocrine organ. *Trends Endocrinol Metab* 2000, 11:327–332.

48. Saltiel A, Kahn C: Insulin signalling and the regulation of glucose and lipid metabolism. *Nature* 2001, 414:799–806.

49. Kelley D, Goodposter B: Skeletal muscle triglyceride: an aspect of regional adiposity and insulin resistance. *Diabetes Care* 2001, 24:933–941.

50. Virkamaki A, Korsheninnikova E, Seppala-Lindroos A, et al.: Intramyocellular lipid is associated with resistance to in vivo insulin actions on glucose uptake, antipolysis, and early insulin signaling pathways in human skeletal muscle. *Diabetes* 2001, 50:2337–2343.

51. Mitrakou A, Kelley D, Veneman T, et al.: Contribution of abnormal muscle and liver glucose metabolism in postprandial hyperglycemia in noninsulin-dependent diabetes mellitus. *Diabetes* 1990, 39:1381–1390.

52. Dinneen S, Gerich J, Rizza R: Carbohydrate metabolism in noninsulin-dependent diabetes mellitus. *N Engl J Med* 1992, 327:707–713.

53. DCCT Research Group: The effect of intensive treatment of diabetes on the development and progression of long-term complications in insulin dependent diabetes mellitus. *N Engl J Med* 1993, 329:977–986.

54. UK Prospective Diabetes Study (UKPDS) Group: Effect of intensive blood-glucose control with metformin on complications in overweight patients with type 2 diabetes (UKPDS 34). *Lancet* 1998, 352:854–865.

55. Reichard P, Pihl M, Rosenqvist U, et al.: Complications in IDDM are caused by elevated blood glucose level: The Stockholm Diabetes Intervention Study (SDIS) at 10-year follow up. *Diabetologia* 1996, 39:1483–1488.

56. Stratton I, Adler A, Neil HA, et al.: Association of glycaemia with macrovascular and microvascular complications of type 2 diabetes (UKPDS 35): prospective observational study. *Br Med J* 2000, 321:405–412.

57. Gerstein H, Pais P, Pogue J, et al.: Relationship of glucose and insulin levels to the risk of myocardial infarction: a case-control study. *J Am Coll Cardiol* 1999, 33:612–619.

58. Khaw K-T, Wareham N, Luben R, et al.: Glycated haemoglobin, diabetes, and mortality in men in Norfolk cohort of European Prospective Investigation of Cancer and Nutrition (EPIC-Norfolk). *Br Med J* 2001, 322:15–18.

59. Lebovitz H: Insulin secretagogues: old and new. *Diab Rev* 1999, 7:139–153.

60. Langtry H, Balfour J: Glimepiride. A review of its use in the management of type 2 diabetes mellitus. *Drugs* 1998, 55:563–584.

61. Dunn C, Faulds D: Nateglinide. *Drugs* 2000, 60:607–615.

62. Lee Y, Hirose H, Ohneda M, et al.: Beta-cell lipotoxicity in the pathogenesis of non–insulin-dependent diabetes mellitus of obese rats: impairment in adipocyte–beta-cell relationships. *Proc Natl Acad Sci USA* 1994, 91:10878–10882.

63. Mudaliar S, Henry R: New oral therapies for type 2 diabetes mellitus: the glitazones or insulin sensitizers. *Annu Rev Med* 2001, 52:239–257.

64. Inzucchi S, Maggs D, Spollett G, et al.: Efficacy and metabolic effects of metformin and troglitazone in type II diabetes mellitus. *N Engl J Med* 1998, 338:867–872.

65. Campbell L, Baker D, Campbell RK: Miglitol: assessment of its role in the treatment of patients with diabetes mellitus. *Ann Pharmacother* 2000, 34:1291–1301.

66. Bolli G, Di Marchi R, Park G, et al.: Insulin analogues and their potential in the management of diabetes mellitus. *Diabetologia* 1999, 42:1151–1167.

67. Lepore M, Pampanelli S, Fanelli C, et al.: Pharmacokinetics and pharmacodynamics of subcutaneous injection of long-acting human insulin analog glargine, NPH insulin, and ultralente human insulin and continuous subcutaneous infusion of insulin lispro. *Diabetes* 2000, 49:2142–2148.

68. Abraira C, Henderson W, Colwell J, et al.: Response to intensive therapy steps and glipizide dose in combination with insulin in type 2 diabetes. Diabetes Care 1998, 21:574–579.

69. Turner R, Cull C, Frighi V, et al.: Glycemic control with diet, sulfonylurea, metformin, or insulin in patients with type 2 diabetes mellitus. Progressive requirement for multiple therapies (UKPDS 49). JAMA 1999, 281:2005–2012.

70. Siegel E, Mayer G, Nauck M, et al.: [Factitious hypoglycemia caused by taking a sulfonylurea drug] [German]. Dtsch Med Wochenschr 1987, 112:1575–1579.

71. Wroblewski M, Gottsater A, Lindgarde F, et al.: Gender, autoantibodies, and obesity in newly diagnosed diabetic patients aged 40–75 years. Diabetes Care 1998, 21:250–255.

72. Bell G, Polonsky K: Diabetes mellitus and genetically programmed defects in β-cell function. Nature 2001, 414:788–791.

73. Kahn C: Insulin action, diabetogenes, and the cause of type II diabetes. Diabetes 1994, 43:1066–1084.

74. Kahn S: The importance of the β-cell in the pathogenesis of type 2 diabetes mellitus. Am J Med 2000, 108(Suppl 6A):2S–8S.

75. Thorens B, Wu Y, Leahy J, et al.: The loss of GLUT2 expression by glucose-unresponsive beta cells of db/db mice is reversible and is induced by the diabetic environment. J Clin Invest 1992, 90:77–85.

76. Caro J, Sinha M, Raju SM, et al.: Insulin receptor kinase in human skeletal muscle from obese subjects with and without noninsulin-dependent diabetes. J Clin Invest 1987, 79:1330–1337.

77. Bak J, Moller N, Schmitz O, et al.: In vivo action and muscle glycogen synthase activity in type II (noninsulin-dependent) diabetes mellitus: effects of diet treatment. Diabetologia 1992, 35:777–784.

78. McGarry J, Dobbins R: Fatty acids, lipotoxicity and insulin secretion. Diabetologia 1999, 42:128–138.

79. Unger R, Zhou Y: Lipotoxicity of beta cells in obesity and in other causes of fatty acid spillover. Diabetes 2001, 50(Suppl 1):S118–S121.

80. Randle P, Priestman D, Mistry S, et al.: Glucose fatty acid interactions and the regulation of glucose disposal. J Cell Biochem 1994, 55S:1–11.

81. Shulman G: Cellular mechanisms of insulin resistance. J Clin Invest 2000, 106:171–176.

82. Garvey W, Huecksteadt T, Matthaei S, et al.: Role of glucose transporters in the cellular insulin resistance of type II noninsulin-dependent diabetes mellitus. J Clin Invest 1988, 81:1528–1536.

83. Kelley D, Mintun M, Watkins S, et al.: The effect of non–insulin-dependent diabetes mellitus and obesity on glucose transport and phosphorylation in skeletal muscle. J Clin Invest 1996, 97:2705–2713.

84. Cline G, Petersen K, Krssak M, et al.: Impaired glucose transport as a cause of decreased insulin-stimulated muscle glycogen synthesis in type 2 diabetes. N Engl J Med 1999, 341:240–246.

85. Gerich J: Metabolic abnormalities in impaired glucose tolerance. Metabolism 1997, 46:40–43.

86. Mitrakou A, Kelley D, Mokan M, et al.: Role of reduced suppression of glucose production and diminished early insulin release in impaired glucose tolerance. N Engl J Med 1992, 326:22–29.

87. Van Haeften T, Pimenta W, Mitrakou A, et al.: Relative contributions of β-cell function and tissue insulin sensitivity to fasting and postglucose-load glycemia. Metabolism 2000, 49:1318–1325.

88. Gerich J, Van Haeften T: Insulin resistance versus impaired insulin secretion as the genetic basis for type 2 diabetes. Curr Opin Endo Diab 1998, 5:144–148.

89. DeFronzo R: The triumvirate: B-cell, muscle, and liver: a collusion responsible for NIDDM. Diabetes 1988, 37:667–687.

90. Calles-Escandon J, Robbins D: Loss of early phase of insulin release in humans impairs glucose tolerance and blunts thermic effect of glucose. Diabetes 1987, 36:1167–1172.

91. Meyer C, Stumvoll M, Nadkarni V, et al.: Abnormal renal and hepatic glucose metabolism in type 2 diabetes mellitus. J Clin Invest 1998, 102:619–624.

92. Consoli A, Nurjhan N, Capani F, et al.: Predominant role of gluconeogenesis in increased hepatic glucose production in NIDDM. Diabetes 1989, 38:550–561.

93. Magnusson I, Rothman D, Katz L, et al.: Increased rate of gluconeogenesis in type II diabetes. A 13C nuclear magnetic resonance study. J Clin Invest 1992, 90:1323–1327.

94. Nurjhan N, Consoli A, Gerich J: Increased lipolysis and its consequences on gluconeogenesis in noninsulin-dependent diabetes mellitus. J Clin Invest 1992, 89:169–175.

95. Kelley D, Mokan M, Veneman T: Impaired postprandial glucose utilization in non–insulin-dependent diabetes mellitus. Metabolism 1994, 43:1549–1557.

96. Roden M, Petersen K, Shulman G: Nuclear magnetic resonance studies of hepatic glucose metabolism in humans. Recent Prog Horm Res 2001, 56:219–237.

97. Intensive blood-glucose control with sulphonylureas or insulin compared with conventional treatment and risk of complications in patients with type 2 diabetes (UKPDS 33). UK Prospective Diabetes Study (UKPDS) Group. Lancet 1998, 352:837–853.

98. Turner R: The U.K. Prospective Diabetes Study. A review. Diabetes Care 1998, 21(Suppl 3):C35–C38.

99. Cusi K, DeFronzo R: Metformin: a review of its metabolic effects. Diab Rev 1998, 6:89–131.

100. Stumvoll M, Nurjhan N, Perriello G, et al.: Metabolic effects of metformin in non–insulin-dependent diabetes mellitus. N Engl J Med 1995, 333:550–554.

101. Gerich J: Oral hypoglycemic agents. N Engl J Med 1989, 321:1231–1245.

102. Inzucchi S: Oral antihyperglycemic therapy for type 2 diabetes: scientific review. JAMA 2002, 287:360–372.

103. Göke B, Herrmann-Rinke C: The evolving role of α-glucosidase inhibitors. Diabetes Metab Rev 1998, 14:S31–S38.

104. Mudaliar S, Lindberg F, Joyce M, et al.: Insulin aspart (B28 Asp-Insulin): a fast-acting analog of human insulin. Absorption kinetics and action profile compared with regular human insulin in healthy nondiabetic subjects. Diabetes Care 1999, 22:1501–1506.

105. Dimitriadis G, Gerich J: Importance of timing preprandial subcutaneous insulin administration in the management of diabetes mellitus. Diabetes Care 1983, 6:374–377.

106. Hedman C, Lindstrom T, Arnqvist H: Direct comparison of insulin lispro and aspart shows small differences in plasma insulin profiles after subcutaneous injection in type 1 diabetes. Diabetes Care 2001, 24:1120–1121.

107. Ratner R, Hirsch I, Neifing J, et al.: Less hypoglycemia with insulin glargine in intensive insulin therapy for type 1 diabetes. Diabetes Care 2000, 23:639–643.

108. Rosenstock J, Schwartz S, Clark C, et al.: Basal insulin therapy in type 2 diabetes. Diabetes Care 2001, 24:631–636.

MANAGEMENT AND PREVENTION OF DIABETIC COMPLICATIONS

Sunder R. Mudaliar and Robert R. Henry

7

Type 2 diabetes is a chronic disease characterized by insulin resistance, impaired insulin secretion, and hyperglycemia. The long-term complications of diabetic retinopathy, nephropathy, neuropathy, and accelerated atherosclerosis lead to significant morbidity in the form of preventable blindness, end-stage renal disease, limb amputations, and premature cardiovascular disease [1]. Diabetics suffer from the morbidity of their microvascular complications, and most of them ultimately die from the complications of macrovascular coronary artery disease.

A pathophysiologic hallmark of type 2 diabetes is insulin resistance, which has both genetic and acquired components [2]. Glucose intolerance and hyperglycemia supervene only when the pancreatic β cell is unable to maintain compensatory hyperinsulinemia to overcome tissue resistance to insulin action [3]. In addition to having hyperglycemia and insulin resistance, nearly 80% of diabetics are obese and have a host of other metabolic abnormalities, including dyslipidemia (increased small dense low-density lipoprotein cholesterol, decreased high-density lipoprotein cholesterol, and raised triglyceride levels), hypertension, and abnormalities of coagulation and the fibrinolytic system. This cluster of metabolic abnormalities, which has been termed the insulin resistance syndrome [4] or the cardiovascular dysmetabolic syndrome, is associated with a higher incidence of cardiovascular morbidity and mortality [5].

The major cause of tissue damage in diabetes is vascular disease in the micro- and macrovasculature [6,7]. Four major molecular mechanisms have been implicated in glucose-mediated vascular damage. These include increased polyol pathway flux, increased flux through the hexosamine pathway, increased formation of diacylglycerol with subsequent activation of specific protein kinase C isoforms, and accelerated nonenzymatic formation of advanced glycation end products. Recent evidence seems to suggest that each of the above mechanisms is triggered by a single hyperglycemia-induced process of overproduction of superoxide by the mitochondrial electron transport chain [7]. The net result of the above changes induced by hyperglycemia in diabetes is overproduction of potentially damaging reactive oxygen species and upregulation of cytokines and tissue growth factors. In insulin-resistant patients with type 2 diabetes, in addition to hyperglycemia, insulin resistance also plays a major role in the induction of macrovascular abnormalities and atherosclerotic cardiovascular disease [4,5].

The development of diabetic complications is no longer inevitable. Results from the United Kingdom Prospective Diabetes Study (UKPDS) clearly demonstrate that tight glucose and blood pressure control in patients with type 2 diabetes prevents the development of and delays the progression of microvascular complications and possibly macrovascular disease [8–10]. In addition, results from the UKPDS and other studies have also shown that treatment of concomitant risk factors like lipids and blood pressure and the use of aspirin have favorable effects on cardiovascular complications in patients with type 2 diabetes [11]. However, the ultimate goal in the management of diabetes is the prevention of diabetes. Recent results from the Diabetes Prevention Program have shown that with intensive lifestyle modification, it is possible to delay or prevent the onset of type 2 diabetes in high-risk individuals [12].

Complications of Diabetes

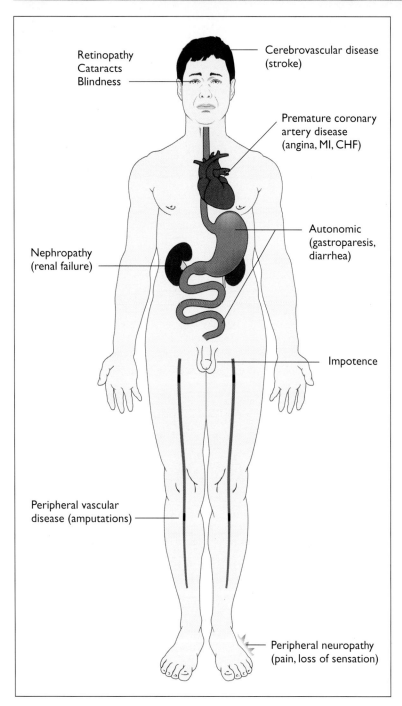

Retinopathy
Cataracts
Blindness

Cerebrovascular disease
(stroke)

Premature coronary
artery disease
(angina, MI, CHF)

Autonomic
(gastroparesis,
diarrhea)

Nephropathy
(renal failure)

Impotence

Peripheral vascular
disease (amputations)

Peripheral neuropathy
(pain, loss of sensation)

FIGURE 7-1. Clinical manifestations of diabetes. The complications of diabetes are protean and encompass nearly all organ systems. Diabetes currently is the leading cause of adult-onset blindness in the United States, and it accounts for more than one third of new cases of end-stage renal disease (ESRD). Accelerated lower extremity arterial disease in diabetics with neuropathy is responsible for 50% of all nontraumatic amputations, and the death rate for cardiovascular disease in diabetics is at least 2.5 times that in nondiabetic patients [1]. Heart disease appears earlier in type 2 diabetes and is more often fatal. Throughout their lives, diabetics suffer from the microvascular complications of blindness, ESRD, and neuropathy, and, sooner rather than later, most diabetics ultimately die from the complications of macrovascular cardiovascular disease. CHF—congestive heart failure; MI—myocardial infarction.

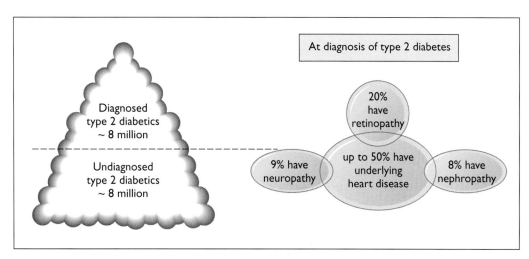

At diagnosis of type 2 diabetes

Diagnosed
type 2 diabetics
~ 8 million

Undiagnosed
type 2 diabetics
~ 8 million

20%
have
retinopathy

9% have
neuropathy

up to 50% have
underlying
heart disease

8% have
nephropathy

FIGURE 7-2. The epidemiology of diabetes and its complications. Diabetes mellitus is an important clinical and public health problem in the United States. Nearly 8 million adults have been diagnosed with diabetes, 90% to 95% of whom have type 2 diabetes. In addition, it is estimated that a further 8 million persons who meet the diagnostic criteria for diabetes remain undiagnosed. It has been estimated that among patients in the United States, type 2 diabetes may have been present for up to 12 years before clinical diagnosis. During this period of undiagnosed and untreated diabetes, micro- and macrovascular disease progress. By the time of diagnosis, 20% of patients have retinopathy, 8% have nephropathy, 9% have neuropathy, and up to 50% have cardiovascular disease [1,5,13].

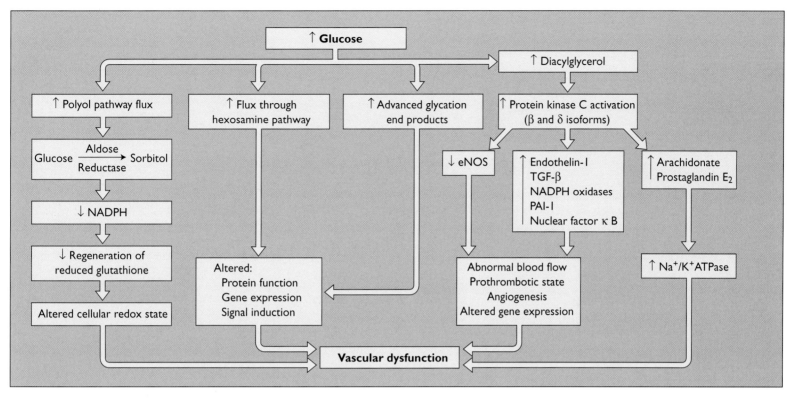

FIGURE 7-3. Possible cellular and molecular mechanisms of vascular disease in diabetes. Hyperglycemia in diabetes causes damage to many tissues, including the retina, kidney, nerves, heart, brain, and skin. A major cause of tissue damage is vascular disease affecting both the micro- and macrovasculature. Hyperglycemia-induced mechanisms that induce vascular damage include increased polyol pathway flux, increased flux through the hexosamine pathway, increased formation of diacylglycerol and the subsequent activation of specific protein kinase C isoforms, and accelerated nonenzymatic formation of advanced glycation end products (AGEs). Each of these mechanisms contributes to vascular dysfunction through a number of mechanisms, including the production of vasodilatory prostaglandins, overproduction of potentially damaging reactive oxygen species, and upregulation of cytokines and growth factors. eNOS—endothelial nitric oxide synthase; TGF-β—transforming growth factor-β. (*Adapted from* King *et al.* [6] and Brownlee [7].)

Diabetic Retinopathy

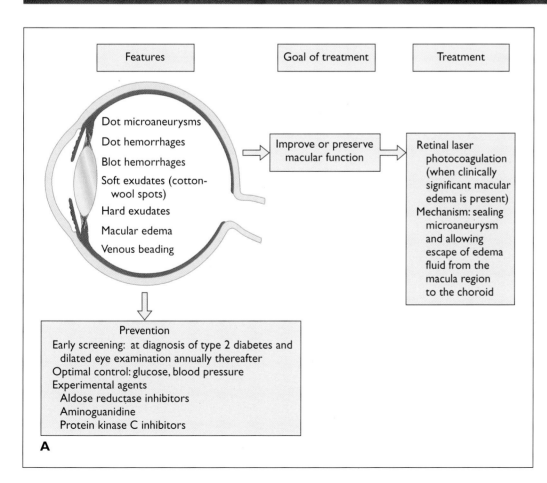

A

FIGURE 7-4. Clinical features and management. Diabetes is the leading cause of new blindness in adults. Retinopathy is present in a considerable proportion of type 2 diabetics at the time of diagnosis. After 15 or more years of disease, the risk of any retinopathy is about 78%, with about one third of patients having macular edema and about one sixth of patients having proliferative retinopathy [14]. Diabetic retinopathy may be classified as nonproliferative diabetic retinopathy (NPDR) or proliferative diabetic retinopathy (PDR). **A,** Nonproliferative diabetic retinopathy. This condition is characterized by structural abnormalities of the retinal vessels (primarily capillaries, but also venules and arterioles), varying degrees of retinal nonperfusion, retinal edema, lipid exudates, and intraretinal hemorrhage. Nonproliferative diabetic retinopathy may be mild, moderate, or severe.

(*Continued on next page*)

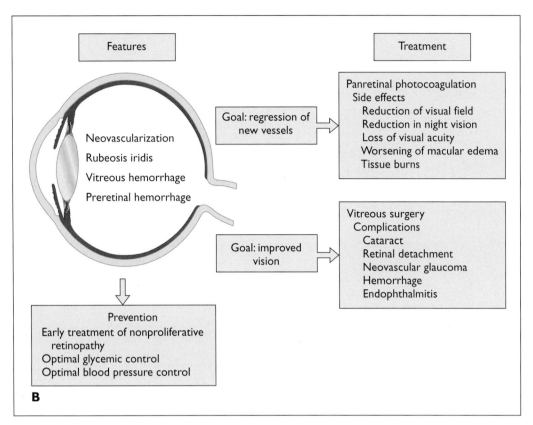

FIGURE 7-4. (*Continued*) **B**, Proliferative diabetic retinopathy. The presence of extensive areas of hemorrhages, microaneurysms, venous beading, or intraretinal microvascular abnormalities (tortuous dilated vessels adjacent to nonperfused areas of the retina) predicts the progression to proliferative retinopathy. For patients with mild, moderate, or severe NPDR, the risk of developing PDR is 5%, 12% to 24%, and 50%, respectively [14].

All patients with type 2 diabetes should have a dilated eye examination at the time of diagnosis and annually or more often thereafter [15]. Prevention of retinopathy is best accomplished by maintaining near-normal glycemia. Once NPDR develops, intensive attempts should be made to optimize glucose and blood pressure control, and clinically significant macular edema (*ie*, retinal edema that threatens the fovea) should be treated with focal or grid photocoagulation, which reduces the risk of moderate visual loss by about 50%. Panretinal photocoagulation may be beneficial in PDR, along with measures to optimize glucose and blood pressure control [14]. The United Kingdom Prospective Diabetes Study has confirmed that intensive blood glucose and blood pressure control reduces the risk of retinopathy progression [8–10].

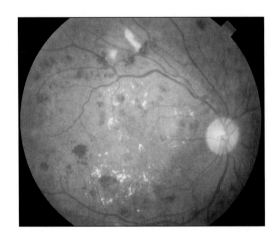

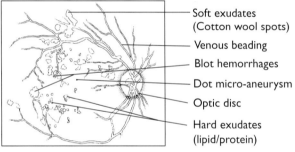

FIGURE 7-5. (See Color Plate) Nonproliferative diabetic retinopathy (NPDR). The characteristic features of NPDR include dot aneurysms (hypercellular, saccular outpouchings of the capillary wall), blot hemorrhages resulting from vascular occlusion, cotton-wool spots (retinal nerve fiber infarcts due to ischemia), hard exudates (lipid and protein exudates due to excessive vascular permeability), and venous beading (abnormal appearance of retinal veins with localized swellings and constrictions resembling sausage links). (*Courtesy of* Dr. M. Goldbaum, UCSD/VA San Diego Health Care System, San Diego, CA.)

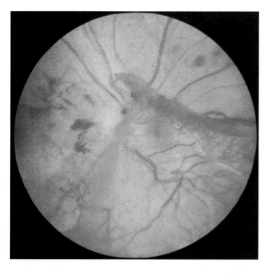
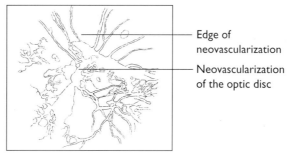

Edge of
neovascularization

Neovascularization
of the optic disc

FIGURE 7-6. (See Color Plate) Classic features of proliferative diabetic retinopathy (PDR). The development of neovascularization is pathognomonic of this stage. The presence of new vessels on the optic nerve head or on more than one fourth of the disc area, together with preretinal or vitreous hemorrhages, is indicative of high-risk proliferative retinopathy and is an absolute indication for panretinal photocoagulation, if technically possible. (*Courtesy of* Dr. M. Goldbaum, UCSD/VA San Diego Health Care System, San Diego, CA.)

Diabetic Nephropathy

URINARY ALBUMIN EXCRETION RATE

	Urinary AER, 24-h Collection, *mg*	Timed Collection, *µg/min*	Spot Collection, *µg/mg* Creatinine
Normal	<30	<20	<30
Microalbuminuria	30–299	20–199	30–299
Macroalbuminuria (Overt nephropathy)	≥300	≥200	≥300

FIGURE 7-7. Urinary albumin excretion rate (AER). The incidence of end-stage renal disease (ESRD) in type 2 diabetes ranges from 4% to 20%. Because type 2 diabetes is 10 times or more prevalent than type 1 diabetes, the incidence of ESRD is approximately the same in both types of diabetes [1]. The cost of treatment for ESRD in diabetes exceeds $2 billion annually [16].

A nondiabetic patient with normal kidneys excretes less than 30 mg of albumin/24 hours (20 µg/min) into the urine, and in a spot urine collection has an albumin:creatinine ratio of less than 30 (µg of albumin/mg of creatinine). Microalbuminuria is present at diagnosis in 3% to 30% of patients with type 2 diabetes. Without specific interventions, 20% to 40% of patients with type 2 diabetes with

microalbuminuria progress to overt nephropathy. However, 20 years after the onset of overt nephropathy, only about 20% have progressed to ESRD [17]. There is substantial evidence that the onset of microalbuminuria and progression of nephropathy correlate closely with poor glycemic control and, more importantly, that improved glycemic control and blood pressure control reduce the onset and progression of microalbuminuria and nephropathy [8–10,18]. Screening for microalbuminuria should be performed at the time of diagnosis and annually thereafter by a random/spot urine albumin and creatinine measurement. (This test has good correlation with 24-hour albumin measurements.) Because the urine albumin excretion rate (UAER) is variable, two of three specimens collected within a 3- to 6-month period should be abnormal before a patient is considered to have crossed a diagnostic threshold. Exercise within the preceding 24 hours, fever, heart failure, marked hyperglycemia, and marked hypertension may elevate UAER over borderline values [17].

STAGES OF DIABETIC NEPHROPATHY IN TYPE 2 DIABETES

Asymptomatic	Renal Insufficiency	End-stage Renal Disease
Normal GFR/creatinine	Decreasing GFR	Uremia
Hypertension	Increasing creatinine	Greatly increased creatinine
Microalbuminuria (30–300 mg/d)	Proteinuria >500 mg/d	Greatly decreased GFR (<15 ml/min)

FIGURE 7-8. Stages of diabetic nephropathy in type 2 diabetes. The natural history of nephropathy in type 2 diabetes is not as clear as it is in type 1 diabetes, for which five stages of nephropathy have been described: 1) an early stage of increased glomerular filtration, progressing through 2) a stage of early glomerular lesions with glomerular basement thickening and mesangial matrix expansion, and on to 3) incipient diabetic nephropathy with microalbuminuria (urinary albumin 30 to 300 mg/day). Ultimately, 4) clinical nephropathy with overt proteinuria over 500 mg/day and declining glomerular filtration rate (GFR) develops and culminates in 5) end-stage renal disease. The early stages of nephropathy have not yet been well documented in type 2 diabetes. (*Data from* Friedman [19].)

MEASURES TO PREVENT OR RETARD DIABETIC NEPHROPATHY

Optimal glycemic control: HbA$_{1c}$ <7% (caution in the elderly)

Adequate blood pressure control: BP <130/80 (caution in those with autonomic neuropathy)

ACE inhibitors (when microalbuminuria is present with urinary albumin 30–300 mg/day)

Dietary protein restriction (when overt nephropathy is present with urinary protein >500 mg/day or when there is a strong family history of nephropathy)

Experimental

Aminoguanidine (inhibits AGE formation)

Protein kinase C inhibitors

FIGURE 7-9. Measures to prevent or retard diabetic nephropathy. In the United Kingdom Prospective Diabetes Study, both tight glycemic control (with a median HbA$_{1c}$ of <7%) and blood pressure (BP) control (with a mean blood pressure of 144/82) was associated with reductions in the progression of microalbuminuria [8–10]. More recently, in the MICRO-HOPE study [20], 3577 subjects with type 2 diabetes were randomized to either placebo or 10 mg daily of ramipril, an angiotensin-converting enzyme (ACE) inhibitor. The study was stopped 6 months early (after 4.5 years) because ramipril had consistent benefits not only in reducing the risk of overt nephropathy by 16%, but was also associated with significant reductions in the risk of myocardial infarction, stroke, cardiovascular mortality, and all-cause mortality by about 30%. AGE—advanced glycation end products.

Diabetic Neuropathy

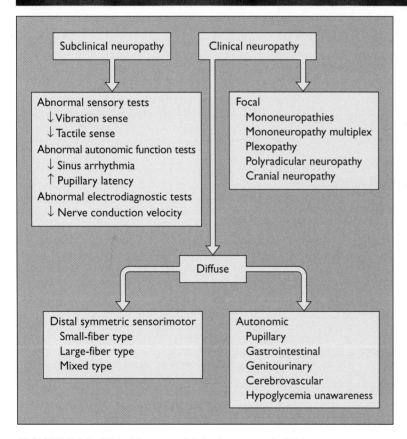

FIGURE 7-10. Clinical features of diabetic neuropathy. Diabetic neuropathy is one of the most common complications of diabetes. Its clinical manifestations cause much suffering among diabetic patients. Acute hyperglycemia decreases nerve function, and chronic hyperglycemia is characterized by progressive loss of nerve fibers, a loss that can be assessed noninvasively by several tests of nerve function, including quantitative sensory tests, autonomic function tests, and electrophysiologic testing [21].

CLINICAL FEATURES OF DISTAL SENSORIMOTOR DIABETIC NEUROPATHY

Large Fiber Type	Small Fiber Type
Unsteady gait	Pain predominates
Absent reflexes	Variable reflexes
Decreased vibration/position sense	Variable position/vibration sense
Charcot's joints possible	Variable presence of Charcot's joints
Mimics posterior column lesions	Ultimately leads to sensory loss

FIGURE 7-11. Distal sensorimotor diabetic neuropathy.

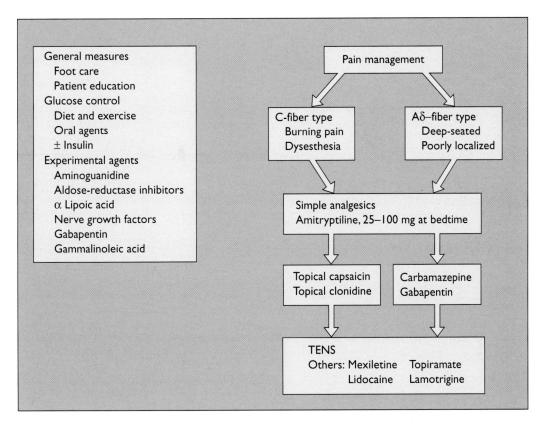

FIGURE 7-12. Management of peripheral diabetic neuropathy. The pathophysiologic mechanisms underlying decreased nerve function and nerve fiber loss in diabetics still are not fully understood but may include formation of sorbitol by aldose reductase and the formation of advanced glycation end products (AGEs) [21]. Like other diabetic complications, the progression of neuropathy is related to glycemic control. Chronic sensory neuropathy with moderate or severe sensory loss involving large-fiber sensation (touch, vibration, and joint position sense) or small-fiber sensation (pain and temperature sense) is associated with a high risk of ulceration.

Current approaches to prevention and treatment of diabetic neuropathy include measures to optimize glucose control, various symptomatic measures for pain control, and use of aldose reductase inhibitors, which appear to slow the progression of neuropathy rather than provide symptomatic relief [22]. TENS—transcutaneous electrical nerve stimulation.

Diabetic Foot Disease

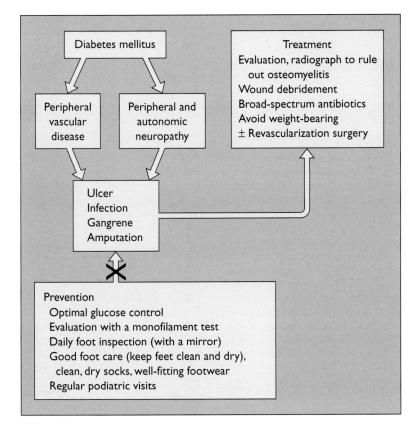

FIGURE 7-13. Clinical features and management of diabetic foot disease. Diabetic foot lesions are a major cause of hospitalization, with approximately 20% of all diabetics entering the hospital because of foot problems. Nearly 55,000 lower extremity amputations are performed each year on diabetic patients, accounting for 50% of all nontraumatic amputations [23]. Diabetic foot lesions are the result of a combination of peripheral and autonomic neuropathy and peripheral vascular disease (ischemia). The cascade of events begins with foot ulcers, infection, and gangrene, and ultimately results in amputation. Management of diabetic foot ulcers should be aggressive, and should include detailed evaluation of the ulcer and the foot, radiography to exclude osteomyelitis, broad-spectrum antibiotics, wound debridement (if indicated), and avoidance of weight bearing. Topical application of antibacterial agents and platelet-derived growth factors may be useful adjunctive measures. Preventive measures include optimal glycemic control, daily foot inspections (with the aid of a mirror), good foot care (keeping feet clean and dry), wearing clean socks and appropriate, well-fitting shoes, and regular podiatric visits. Good patient education and a team approach are the keys to the prevention and treatment of diabetic foot disease.

Diabetics are particularly prone to foot deformities and the development of cocked-up toes, which results in pressure at the tips of the toes and under the first metatarsal head, leading to ulceration and infection. The ideal treatment is prophylactic surgery to straighten the toes. If this is not feasible, special shoes with a cushioned insole to protect the toes and metatarsal head should be worn.

All diabetics should have the protective sensory function in their feet evaluated with a 10-g Semmestel-Weinstein monofilament. If a patient cannot consistently feel a 10-g monofilament, protective sensory function has been lost, and the patient is at high risk of developing foot ulcers [24].

Diabetic Male Sexual Dysfunction

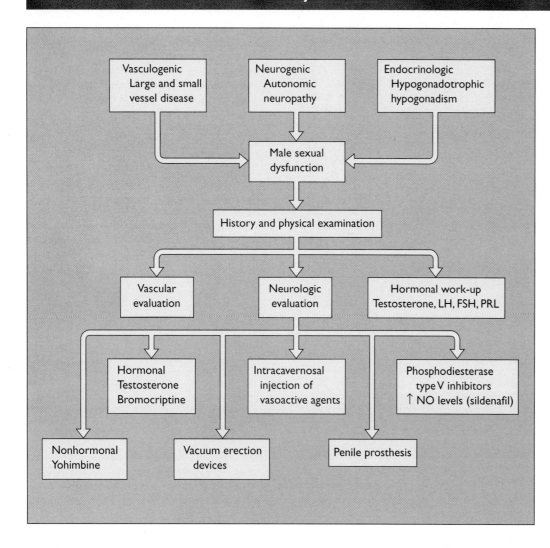

FIGURE 7-14. Evaluation and management of diabetic male sexual dysfunction. The prevalence of erectile dysfunction in diabetic men ranges from 35% to 75%, significantly higher than that in the general population [25]. Its onset is insidious, and it may occur early in the disease. The major underlying abnormalities are vascular (cavernosal artery insufficiency, corporal veno-occlusive dysfunction) and neurologic (autonomic neuropathy). The role of hormonal abnormalities is controversial. All diabetic men with erectile dysfunction require a detailed endocrinologic work-up (luteinizing hormone [LH], follicle-stimulating hormone [FSH], prolactin [PRL], and testosterone levels) and, in select cases, vascular evaluation (intracavernosal injection test, visual sexual stimulation, and penile duplex ultrasonography) and neurologic evaluation (nocturnal penile tumescence test, cavernosal electrical activity potential, somatosensory evoked potentials, and sacral latency test). Treatment options include nonhormonal α-2-adrenergic blocking agents (yohimbine); hormonal therapy, if indicated (testosterone replacement in hypogonadism, bromocriptine/surgery for prolactinomas, discontinuation of medications causing hyperprolactinemia); vacuum erection devices; intracavernosal injection of vasoactive agents; penile prostheses (in selected cases); and the phosphodiesterase V inhibitor sildenafil, which acts by increasing nitric oxide levels.

Cardiovascular Disease in Diabetes

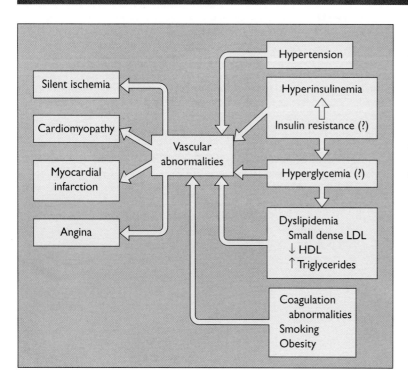

FIGURE 7-15. Pathogenesis and clinical features of heart disease in diabetes. The risk for cardiovascular disease in patients with diabetes is two to five times that in nondiabetic persons [26]. At the time of diagnosis of type 2 diabetes, more than 50% of patients have preexisting coronary artery disease (CAD) [13]. Numerous risk factors contribute to macrovascular dysfunction in type 2 diabetes. Some appear related to the insulin resistance and hyperinsulinemia that are characteristic of the early stages of type 2 diabetes before the onset of pancreatic β-cell exhaustion and overt hyperglycemia. These include the various components of the cardiovascular dysmetabolic syndrome (ie, hypertension, central obesity, dyslipidemia, glucose intolerance, and coagulation abnormalities) [5]. Heart disease in diabetics may result in silent myocardial ischemia or manifest as angina, myocardial infarction, or congestive heart failure (diabetic cardiomyopathy). HDL—high-density lipoprotein; LDL—low-density lipoprotein.

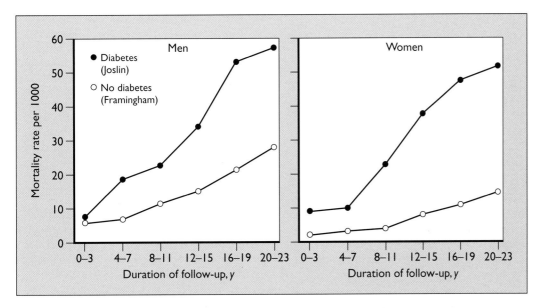

FIGURE 7-16. Cardiovascular disease is the major cause of mortality in patients with type 2 diabetes. Comparison of data from the Joslin Study and the Framingham Study shows that the mortality rate due to coronary artery disease (CAD) is doubled in men with diabetes and nearly quadrupled in women with diabetes, as compared to the nondiabetic population [27]. Moreover, within the diabetic population, glucose control is an important predictor of CAD mortality and all CAD events [28].

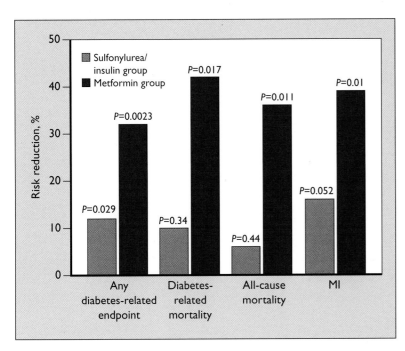

FIGURE 7-17. Cardiovascular/mortality risk reduction with intensive therapy in diabetic patients. In the United Kingdom Prospective Diabetes Study (UKPDS), 5102 patients with newly diagnosed type 2 diabetes were followed for an average of 10 years in order to determine whether intensive glucose lowering reduces cardiovascular and microvascular complications and also to determine the benefits and disadvantages of sulfonylureas, metformin, and insulin [8,9]. The UKPDS results demonstrated that although microvascular complications are decreased by nearly 25% by lowering HbA_{1c} to a median of 7% (compared to 7.9% in the conventional group), there was no significant effect on cardiovascular complications, with only a nonsignificant 16% reduction in the risk of combined fatal/nonfatal myocardial infarction (MI). However, an epidemiologic analysis showed a continuous association between the risk of cardiovascular complications and glycemia, such that for every percentage point decrease in HbA_{1c} (eg, 9% to 8%), there was a 25% reduction in diabetes-related deaths, a 7% reduction in all-cause mortality, and an 18% reduction in fatal/nonfatal MI.

In the subgroup of obese diabetic patients treated with metformin, intensive glucose lowering with a median HbA_{1c} of 7.4% (compared to 8.0% in the conventional group) was associated with significantly decreased risks of diabetes-related deaths, all-cause mortality, and MI [9]. But in a surprise outcome, for those obese diabetic patients in this substudy who had metformin added to existing sulfonylurea treatment, there was an unexpected significant increase in all-cause and diabetes-related mortality, and no beneficial effects on cardiovascular or microvascular outcomes.

In the UKPDS, reassuringly, tight blood pressure control (144/82 vs 154/87 mm Hg) was associated with significant reductions in virtually all cardiovascular and microvascular outcomes [10].

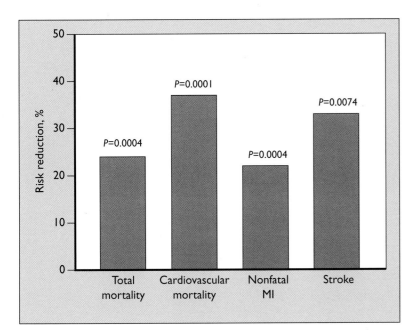

FIGURE 7-18. Cardiovascular/mortality risk reduction with ramipril therapy in diabetic patients. In contrast to the United Kingdom Prospective Diabetes Study, which studied patients with newly diagnosed diabetes, the recently concluded MICRO-HOPE study randomized 3577 patients with long-standing type 2 diabetes (12 years' duration) to treatment with either placebo or ramipril (an angiotensin-converting enzyme inhibitor) [20]. The study was stopped 6 months early (after 4.5 years) because 10 mg of ramipril daily significantly lowered the risk of all the measured cardiovascular outcomes, including fatal and nonfatal myocardial infarction (MI), stroke, nephropathy, and also all-cause and cardiovascular mortality, by 22% to 37%. The cardiovascular benefit in this study was greater than that attributable to the small decrease in blood pressure seen and also additive to those of baseline therapeutic agents, which included aspirin, lipid-lowering agents, and other blood pressure–lowering drugs.

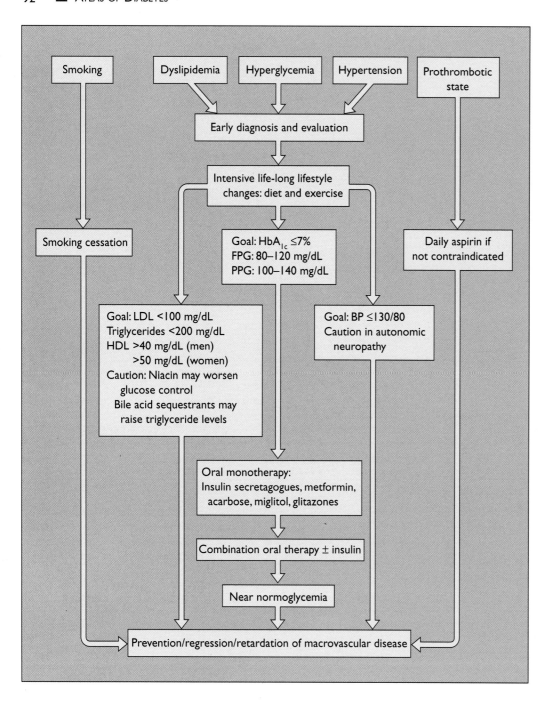

FIGURE 7-19. A multifactorial approach to management of cardiovascular disease in diabetes. Multiple risk factors contribute to accelerated atherosclerosis and premature coronary artery disease (CAD) in diabetes. The cornerstone of prevention is aggressive intervention to identify and favorably modify established risk factors, including hyperglycemia, hyperlipidemia, and hypertension. Because of the extremely high risk of macrovascular disease in diabetes, the National Cholesterol Education Program has recently designated diabetes as a CAD-risk equivalent and hence in patients with diabetes, the target low-density lipoprotein (LDL) cholesterol should be <100 mg/dL; the target high-density lipoprotein (HDL) cholesterol goal should be >40 mg/dL in men and >50 mg/dl in women; and the triglyceride goal should be <200 mg/dL [29]. Unless contraindicated, all eligible diabetic patients should be on daily aspirin. The importance of lifestyle changes and strict adherence to dietary and exercise recommendations should be emphasized at all times. BP—blood pressure; FPG—fasting plasma glucose; PPG—postprandial plasma glucose.

Economic Implications of Diabetic Complications

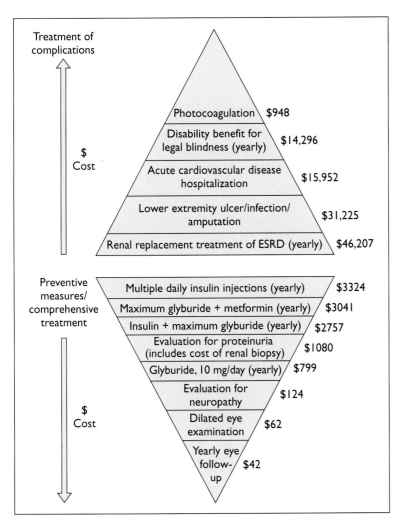

FIGURE 7-20. Cost of diabetic complications: prevention versus treatment, in 1997 US dollars. The annual expense of treating diabetes and its complications in the United States (most of which is for treatment of type 2 diabetes) is estimated at about $100 billion [16]. Not only is type 2 diabetes costly, but it also causes excessive morbidity and mortality. Analysis of data has shown that prevention of this disease not only is preferable to treatment but also is more cost-effective. This figure compares the cost of comprehensive treatment of diabetes with medications and preventive measures with the monumental costs of treating disease complications such as retinopathy, nephropathy, neuropathy, foot disease, and cardiovascular disease. It has been estimated that comprehensive treatment of type 2 diabetes with HbA_{1c} values maintained at 7.2% will reduce the cumulative incidence of blindness by 72%, end-stage renal disease (ESRD) by 87%, and lower extremity amputation by 67%. Lifetime cardiovascular disease risk is increased by 3% due to increased life expectancy, which is increased by 1.39 years. The estimated incremental cost per quality-adjusted life year gained is $16,002. This efficiency of treating type 2 diabetes is similar to that for screening and treating hypertension and is in the range of interventions considered cost-effective. Treatment is more cost-effective for those with earlier onset of diabetes, minorities, and those with higher HbA_{1c} under standard care. (*Data from* Eastman *et al.* [30].)

Future Directions: Prevention of Type 2 Diabetes

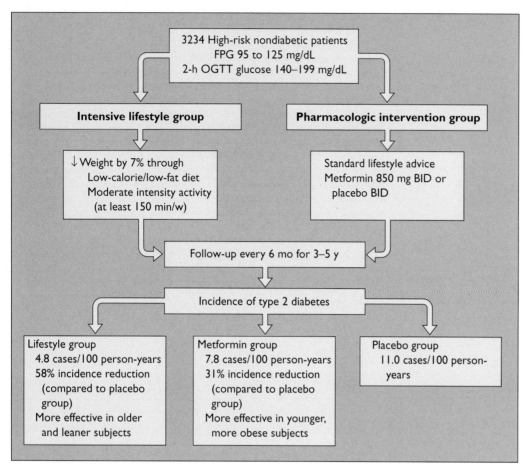

diabetic complications [8–11]. However, even with early intervention and intensive treatment, there are high costs and significant morbidity. Ultimately, preventing or delaying the onset of diabetes may be more cost-effective [12]. Impaired glucose tolerance (IGT) (fasting plasma glucose [FPG]: 110–125 mg/dL, or 2-hour post-oral glucose tolerance test [OGTT] glucose 140–199 mg/dL) has been shown to be a strong risk factor for development of type 2 diabetes and a possible risk factor for CAD. There are data to suggest that at this stage of IGT, patients are at high risk for diabetes and CAD, but have not yet developed end-organ disease. The Diabetes Prevention Program (DPP) supported by the National Institutes of Health was designed to determine if it is possible to prevent or delay the progression to type 2 diabetes through lifestyle changes or pharmacologic intervention in high-risk patients with IGT [12]. The DPP study randomized 3234 high-risk subjects with IGT to either an intensive lifestyle intervention arm or pharmacologic/placebo treatment with standard lifestyle advice. The study was stopped a year early (average follow-up, 2.8 years) because of a significant reduction in the incidence of diabetes in the lifestyle arm of the study. Subjects randomized to a low-calorie and low-fat diet combined with moderate intensity physical activity lost an average of 5.6 kg and had a 58% reduction in the incidence of diabetes over 2.8 years. On the other hand, pharmacologic treatment with metformin 850 mg BID resulted in only a 31% reduction in the incidence of diabetes compared to placebo.

Currently, studies are in progress to determine if other pharmacologic agents like ramipril (an angiotensin-converting enzyme inhibitor) and rosiglitazone (a thiazolidinedione antidiabetic agent) are also effective in reducing the incidence of type 2 diabetes in high-risk individuals.

FIGURE 7-21. Prevention of type 2 diabetes. It is now clear that type 2 diabetes is not a milder form of diabetes. Its complications can be the same as or more severe than those in type 1 diabetes. Moreover, these complications occur early during the natural course of the disease, even before clinical onset. At the time of diagnosis of type 2 diabetes, 20% of patients have retinopathy, 8% have nephropathy, 9% have neuropathy [5], and up to 50% have underlying coronary artery disease (CAD) [26]. Results from several large randomized studies including the United Kingdom Prospective Diabetes Study have confirmed that treatment of hyperglycemia, hypertension, and hyperlipidemia may prevent or retard the progression of

References

1. Harris MI: Summary. In *Diabetes in America.* NIH Publication No. 95-1468. Edited by Harris MI, Cowie CC, Stern MP, *et al.* Washington, DC: US Government Printing Office; 1995:1–14.

2. De Fronzo RA: Lilly Lecture 1987: The triumvirate: β cell, muscle, liver. A collusion responsible for NIDDM. *Diabetes* 1988, 37:667–687.

3. Pratley RE, Weyer C: The role of impaired early insulin secretion in the pathogenesis of Type II diabetes mellitus. *Diabetologia* 2001, 44(8):929–945.

4. Reaven GM: Role of insulin resistance in human disease. *Diabetes* 1988, 37:1596–1607.

5. Fagan TC, Deedwania PC: The cardiovascular dysmetabolic syndrome. *Am J Med* 1998, 105(1A):77S–82S.

6. King GL, Brownlee M: The cellular and molecular mechanisms of diabetic complications. *Endocrinol Metab Clin North Am* 1996, 25:255–270.

7. Brownlee M: Biochemistry and molecular cell biology of diabetic complications. *Nature* 2001, 414:813–820.

8. United Kingdom Prospective Diabetes Study Group: Intensive blood-glucose control with sulfonylurea or insulin compared with conventional treatment and risk of complications in patients with type 2 diabetes (UKPDS 33). *Lancet* 1998, 352(9131):837–853.

9. United Kingdom Prospective Diabetes Study Group: Effect of intensive blood-glucose control with metformin on complications in overweight patients with type 2 diabetes (UKPDS 34). *Lancet* 1998, 352(9131):854–865.

10. United Kingdom Prospective Diabetes Study Group: Tight blood pressure control and risk of macrovascular and microvascular complications in type 2 diabetes: UKPDS 38. *Br Med J* 1998, 7160:703–713.

11. Reaven GM: Multiple CHD risk factors in type 2 diabetes: beyond hyperglycemia. *Diabetes, Obesity and Metabolism* 2002, 4(Suppl 1):S13–S18.

12. Diabetes Prevention Program Research Group: Reduction in the incidence of type 2 diabetes with lifestyle intervention or metformin. *N Engl J Med* 2002, 346(6):393–403.

13. Garber AJ: Vascular disease and lipids in diabetes. *Med Clin North Am* 1998, 82:931–948.

14. Aiello LP, Cavallerano J, Bursell S: Diabetic eye disease. *Endocrinol Metab Clin North Am* 1996, 25:271–291.

15. American Diabetes Association: Position statement: Diabetic retinopathy. *Diabetes Care* 2002, 25:S90–S93.

16. American Diabetes Association: Direct and Indirect Costs of Diabetes in the United States in 1992. Alexandria, VA: American Diabetes Association, 1993.

17. American Diabetes Association: Position statement: Diabetic nephropathy. *Diabetes Care* 2002, 25:S85–S89.

18. Marks JB, Raskin P: Nephropathy and hypertension in diabetes. *Med Clin North Am* 1998, 82:877–907.

19. Friedman E: Renal syndromes in diabetes. *Endocrinol Metab Clin North Am* 1996, 25:293–324.

20. Heart Outcomes Prevention Evaluation Study Investigators: Effects of ramipril on cardiovascular and microvascular outcomes in people with diabetes mellitus: results of the HOPE study and MICRO-HOPE substudy. *Lancet* 2000, 355(9200):253–259.

21. Harati Y: Diabetes and the nervous system. *Endocrinol Metab Clin North Am* 1996, 25:325–359.

22. Boulton AJM, Malik RA: Diabetic neuropathy. *Med Clin North Am* 1998, 82:909–929.

23. Levin ME: Foot lesions in patients with diabetes mellitus. *Endocrinol Metab Clin North Am* 1996, 25:447–462.

24. American Diabetes Association: Position statement: foot care in diabetes. *Diabetes Care* 2002, 25(Suppl):S69–S70.

25. Hakim LS, Goldstein I: Diabetic sexual function. *Endocrinol Metab Clin North Am* 1996, 25:379–400.

26. Zimmet PZ, Alberti KGMM: The changing face of macrovascular disease in NIDDM: An epidemic in progress. *Lancet* 1997, 350(SI):1–4.

27. Krowelski AS, Warram JH, Valsania P, et al.: Evolving natural history of coronary artery disease in diabetes mellitus. *Am J Med* 1991, 90(Suppl 2A):56S–61S.

28. Kuusisito J, Mykannen L, Pyorala K, et al.: NIDDM and its metabolic control predict coronary artery disease in elderly subjects. *Diabetes* 1994, 43:960–967.

29. American Diabetes Association: Position statement: management of dyslipidemia in adults with diabetes mellitus. *Diabetes Care* 2002, 25:S74–S77.

30. Eastman RC, Javitt JC, Herman WH, et al.: Model of complications in NIDDM: Analysis of the health benefits and cost-effectiveness of treating NIDDM with the goal of normoglycemia. *Diabetes Care* 1997, 20:735–744.

INSULIN RESISTANCE

Ele Ferrannini

8

At the whole-body level, hormone response is the compounded result of secretory rate and cellular sensitivity. For many hormones, action is modulated through hormonal feedback (*eg,* corticotropin-releasing hormone [CRH] and adrenocorticotropic hormone [ACTH] for cortisol, gonadotrophin-releasing hormone and gonadotrophins for sex steroids). With this design, sensitivity is provided by the specific hormone receptors on target tissues as well as on the companion gland of the feedback loop. In the case of insulin, there is no major pituitary or hypothalamic relay; target tissues control secretion directly by determining the level of positive and negative stimuli. Thus, the circulating concentrations of substrates (mostly glucose, but also amino acids, free fatty acids [FFA], and ketone bodies), which result from insulin action on intermediary metabolism in different tissues, feed signals back to the β cell. Sensitivity gating is provided by insulin receptors on target tissues (and on the β cell itself). Possibly as a consequence of the peculiar system design, insulin resistance is a relatively common phenomenon in physiology as well as pathophysiology.

Insulin exerts multiple actions on many cell types, but the primary servoregulated signal for insulin release is the plasma glucose concentration. According to this construct, insulin resistance is a reduced sensitivity of glucose uptake to insulin stimulation sensed by the β cell through elevated plasma glucose levels. Consequently, insulin resistance is defined as defective glucose disposal in the face of raised glucose and insulin concentrations.

Insulin sensitivity is set not only by the number and affinity of the insulin receptors but also by the functional state of the intracellular signaling pathways that transduce insulin binding to the various effectors (*eg,* glucose transport, phosphorylation and oxidation, glycogen synthesis, lipolysis, and ion exchange). Therefore, a massive reduction in the number of insulin receptors (or the presence of high titers of circulating anti-insulin or anti–insulin-receptor autoantibodies) is associated with a form of insulin resistance that is generalized and extreme (*ie,* all pathways are involved). These are, however, rare cases. More commonly, cellular resistance of the glucose pathway is caused by a malfunction of the signal transduction machinery. The various insulin effectors are, at least in part, independent of one another. As a consequence, cellular insulin resistance can be of any degree and usually is incomplete, or pathway specific. In addition, resistance in the glucose pathway reinforces the insulin signal to other pathways (*eg,* protein turnover) via stimulation of β cell activity. To the extent that they have preserved their sensitivity, other pathways are overly stimulated by the compensatory hyperinsulinemia. The pathophysiologic implication of this phenomenon is that, in insulin-resistant states, any abnormality that is found to be associated with defective glucose metabolism (*eg,* dyslipidemia, higher blood pressure, platelet hypercoagulation, or prothrombotic changes) theoretically can be the result of either the insulin resistance itself or the chronic effects of the attendant hyperinsulinemia. This is the origin of the insulin resistance syndrome.

Definition and Measurement

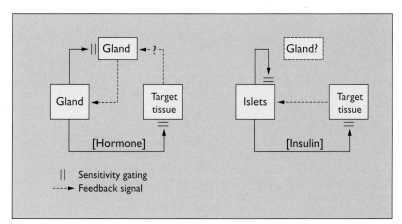

FIGURE 8-1. General organization of an endocrine system and peculiarity of the insulin system. For many protein and non-protein hormones, action is modulated by at least one, often two, hierarchical hormonal feedback paths (eg, corticotropin-releasing hormone and adrenocorticotropic hormone for cortisol, gonadotrophin-releasing hormone and gonadotrophins for sex steroids). Sensitivity is provided by the circulating hormone concentrations ([hormone]) acting upon specific hormone receptors located on target tissues as well as on the companion gland of the feedback loop. In the case of insulin, there is no major pituitary or hypothalamic relay; target tissues control secretion directly by determining the level of positive and negative stimuli. Thus, the circulating concentrations of substrates (mostly glucose, but also amino acids, free fatty acids, and ketone bodies), which result from insulin action on intermediary metabolism in different tissues, feed signals back to the β cell. Sensitivity gating is provided by insulin receptors on target tissues; some degree of autoregulation is given by insulin receptors on the β cell itself.

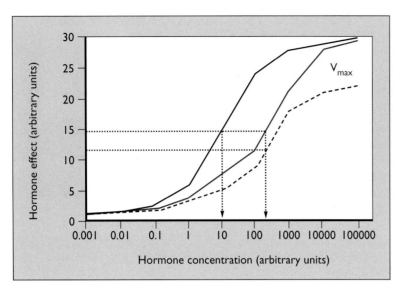

FIGURE 8-2. Shape and parameters of the dose-response curve for a hormone. In general, the relationship between concentration and action of a hormone is sigmoidal (*black line*): the response is sluggish in the low concentration range, then rises in an approximately linear manner, and then tapers off to saturation. Mathematically, this kind of dose-response relationship can be approximated by a Michaelis-Menten equation, in which the maximal effect is termed V_{max}, the hormone concentration at which the effect is half-maximal is termed K_m, and sensitivity is expressed by the ratio V_{max}/K_m. The figure exemplifies two types of abnormal response: reduced sensitivity, characterized by a 20-fold increase in K_m (*blue line*), and the same reduction in sensitivity coupled with an impaired maximal response (*dotted line*).

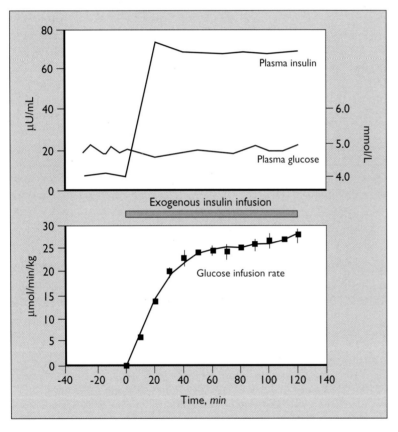

FIGURE 8-3. Euglycemic hyperinsulinemic insulin clamping. Euglycemic hyperinsulinemic insulin clamping is regarded as the gold standard for the measurement of insulin sensitivity in vivo [1,2]. Exogenous insulin is infused in a primed-constant format to raise plasma insulin concentrations to any desired level (in this figure, the postprandial range). As peripherally infused insulin is cleared rapidly from the plasma (at the rate of 0.6 to 1.4 L/min in nonobese healthy subjects [3]), a stable hyperinsulinemic plateau is reached within 20 minutes. Exogenous glucose is infused simultaneously to prevent insulin-induced hypoglycemia; the glucose infusion rate is adjusted every 5 to 10 minutes under the guidance of on-line plasma glucose measurements. During the second hour of a 2-hour clamp study, endogenous glucose release generally is suppressed, and the glucose infusion rate equals the total amount of glucose taken up by all tissues in the body. The *black squares* in the *lower panel* of the figure represent mean (± SEM) values of whole-body insulin-mediated glucose uptake (normalized for body weight) in 30 nondiabetic patients of a range of ages and body weights.

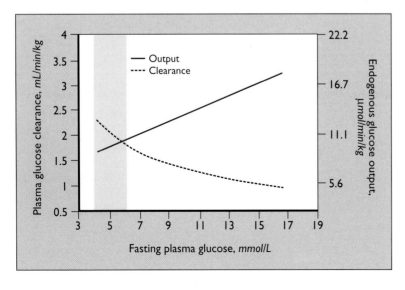

FIGURE 8-4. Glucose turnover in the fasting state. The use of a glucose isotope, either stable or radioactively labeled, allows one to measure the rate at which glucose is produced endogenously and cleared from the plasma in the fasting state. Following a prolonged primed-constant intravenous infusion, the tracer reaches isotopic equilibrium (*ie*, constant specific activity) throughout the body glucose space. Under these circumstances, the ratio of the tracer infusion rate to its steady-state plasma concentration measures whole-body glucose clearance (expressed in mL/min/kg of body weight). Endogenous glucose output (mostly from the liver) then is calculated as the product of glucose clearance by the fasting plasma glucose concentration and expressed in μmol/min per kg of body weight. The graph shows how glucose clearance and endogenous glucose output vary across a range of fasting plasma glucose concentrations, encompassing the normal (*shaded area*) and diabetic state. Whereas glucose clearance is reduced already for minor degrees of fasting hyperglycemia (<7 mmol/L), endogenous glucose output increases in approximate proportion to the severity of hyperglycemia [4].

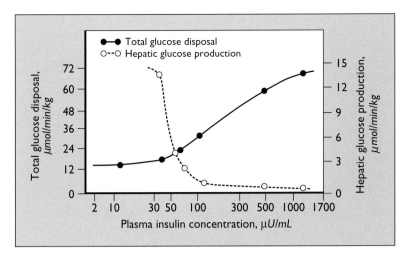

FIGURE 8-5. Insulin dose-response curves for stimulation of whole-body glucose uptake and inhibition of endogenous glucose production in healthy subjects. Curves were constructed by combining the insulin clamp technique at five insulin levels encompassing the physiologic and pharmacologic concentration range with tracer glucose infusion. The effect of insulin on endogenous (hepatic) glucose release is already maximal at plasma insulin concentrations that are submaximal for stimulation of glucose uptake [5]. Thus, under physiologic conditions, the earliest and most effective action of insulin to limit postprandial hyperglycemia is to suppress release of endogenous glucose into the systemic circulation.

Insulin Action

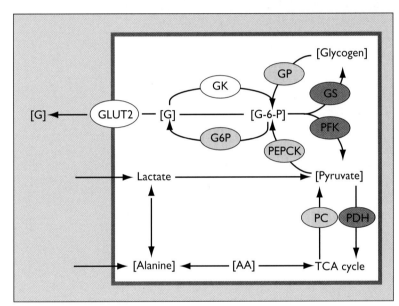

FIGURE 8-6. Hepatic glucose production. Simplified scheme of the main intracellular pathways of glucose production in the liver, glycogenolysis and gluconeogenesis (*thick lines*). *Shaded ovals* indicate key insulin-sensitive enzymes in the pathway. Substrate concentrations are in brackets; insulin-sensitive enzymes are inscribed in circles, shaded to indicate stimulatory action or gray to indicate inhibitory action. Whereas glycogen breakdown directly increases the intracellular concentrations of glucose-6-phosphate (G-6-P), uptake of lactate, alanine, and other gluconeogenic amino acids provides 3-carbon precursors for de novo G-6-P synthesis. G—free glucose; GP—glycogen phosphorylase; GS—glycogen synthase; G6P—glucose-6-phosphatase; GK—glucokinase; PFK—phosphofructokinase; PEPCK—phospho-enolpyruvate-carboxykinase; PC—pyruvate carboxylase; PDH—pyruvate dehydrogenase; AA—amino acids; GLUT2—isoform 2 (non–insulin-sensitive) of the glucose transporter; TCA—tricarboxylic acid cycle.

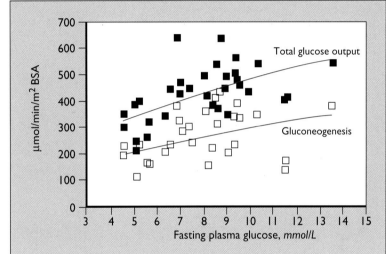

FIGURE 8-7. Contribution of gluconeogenesis to fasting plasma glucose concentration. Total endogenous glucose output (measured by the tracer dilution technique) and gluconeogenesis (determined by the deuterated water technique [6]) were simultaneously measured in fasting nondiabetic subjects and patients with type 2 diabetes mellitus. As expected (*see* Fig. 8-4), endogenous glucose output (*filled squares, solid line*) is related directly to the degree of hyperglycemia over a range of fasting plasma glucose concentrations. Gluconeogenesis (*empty squares, blue line*) makes up roughly one half of total glucose output in nondiabetic subjects, and is increased in diabetic patients, thereby contributing substantially to their fasting hyperglycemia [7]. BSA—body surface area.

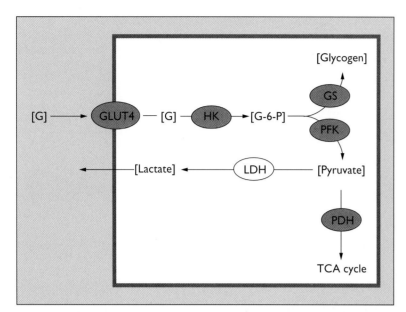

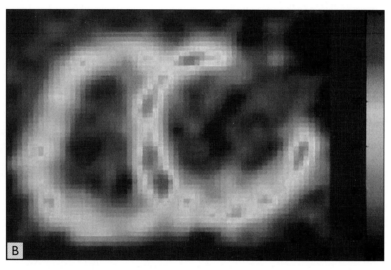

FIGURE 8-8. Peripheral glucose disposal. Simplified scheme of glycogen synthesis and glucose oxidation, the main pathways of intracellular glucose disposition in insulin target tissues. *Shaded ovals* indicate key insulin-sensitive enzymes in the pathway. G—free glucose; G-6-P—glucose-6-phosphate; GLUT4—isoform 4 (insulin-sensitive) of the glucose transporter; HK—hexokinase II; GS—glycogen synthase; PFK—phosphofructokinase; PDH—pyruvate dehydrogenase; LDH—lactic dehydrogenase; TCA—tricarboxylic acid cycle.

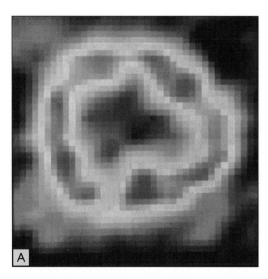

FIGURE 8-9. (See Color Plate) Insulin action in the heart. Myocardial muscle is insulin-sensitive. Whereas free fatty acids (FFA) represent the dominant fuel for cardiac muscle in the fasting state, an increase in circulating insulin concentrations inhibits lipolysis, thereby restraining FFA availability and promoting glucose uptake. By using ^{18}F-deoxyglucose (FDG), an analog of glucose (which is transported and phosphorylated in the same manner as D-glucose but not further metabolized) labeled with a short-lived radioactive isotope of fluorine (^{18}F), positron-emitting tomography (PET) detects a signal that is proportional to the rate of myocardial glucose uptake. The figure shows FDG images of human heart muscle during a euglycemic insulin clamp study like the one illustrated in Figure 8-3. The colors (with red being the most intense) indicate regions with different rates of glucose utilization. **A**, The left ventricle of a normal patient. **B**, The ventricular walls of a patient who suffered from an anterior myocardial infarction 6 months before the PET study. A "cold" area of missing glucose uptake is clearly visible at the upper right corner (the anterior wall of the left ventricle). Also evident is a diffuse decrease in insulin-mediated glucose uptake (insulin resistance) throughout the left ventricular wall, involving myocardial regions distant from the infarcted area and normally perfused (perfusion scan not shown) [8].

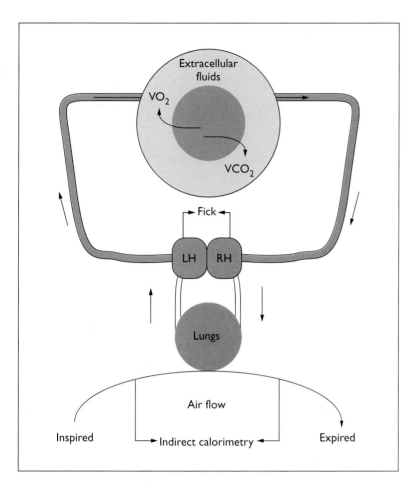

FIGURE 8-10. Measuring intracellular glucose disposition and energy expenditure in vivo via indirect calorimetry. The schematic illustrates the correspondence between indirect calorimetry (in which oxygen consumption = [O_2 in expired air - O_2 in inspired air] × air flow; carbon dioxide production = [CO_2 in expired air - CO_2 in inspired air] × air flow) and the Fick principle (by which oxygen consumption = (arterial blood O_2 - central venous blood O_2) × cardiac output; carbon dioxide production = (arterial blood CO_2 - venous blood CO_2) × cardiac output). With the use of calorimetric equations, net rates of oxidation of lipids and carbohydrates and of energy expenditure can be quantified at the whole-body as well as the organ level starting from gas-exchange data. LH—left heart; RH—right heart; VO_2—oxygen consumption; VCO_2—carbon dioxide production.

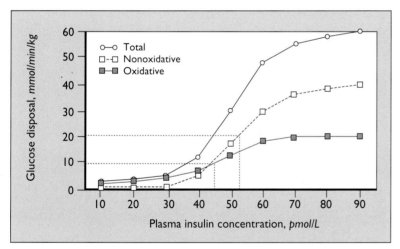

FIGURE 8-11. Dose-response curve for action of insulin on glucose oxidation and nonoxidative glucose disposal in the healthy subject. Indirect calorimetry can be combined with the insulin clamp technique to estimate glucose oxidation at various plasma insulin plateaus. Nonoxidative glucose disposal, consisting primarily of glycogen synthesis, is then obtained as the difference between total glucose uptake and net glucose oxidation. The figure presents data from healthy subjects studied over a range of plasma insulin levels; the dotted lines identify the K_m values for oxidative glucose disposal and glycogen synthesis. Glucose oxidation has a high sensitivity and low capacity; glycogen synthesis has lower sensitivity but higher capacity. Thus, under physiologic conditions, mild hyperinsulinemia stimulates glucose oxidation, whereas stronger insulinization promotes glucose storage into glycogen. Clamp studies combined with regional calorimetry have demonstrated that skeletal muscle is the insulin target tissue responsible for most (50% to 70%) insulin-mediated glucose uptake and storage in vivo [9].

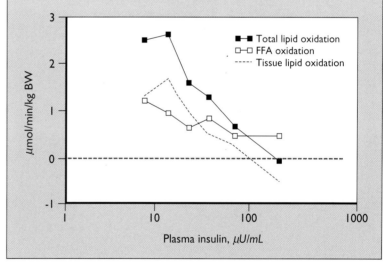

FIGURE 8-12. Dose-response curves for insulin action on lipid metabolism. Indirect calorimetry also yields estimates for total net lipid oxidation. The oxidation of circulating free fatty acid (FFA) can be measured by collecting labeled CO_2 in the expired air during the constant infusion of carbon-labeled palmitate. Tissue lipid oxidation is then defined as the difference between total lipid and FFA oxidation. In the clamp studies in normal subjects summarized in the figure, low insulin doses effectively inhibited both total lipid and FFA oxidation; high physiologic insulin doses (or chronic hyperinsulinemia) did not affect FFA oxidation any further, but caused net lipid synthesis (ie, negative values of lipid oxidation). BW—body weight. (*Data from* Groop *et al.* [10].)

Insulin Resistance

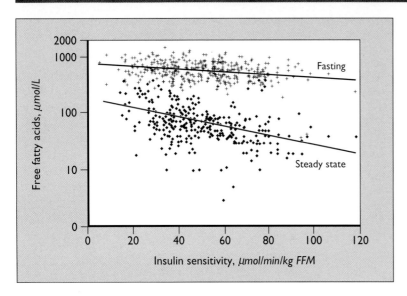

FIGURE 8-13. Relation between free fatty acid (FFA) concentrations and insulin sensitivity. In each of 450 nondiabetic subjects, plasma FFA concentrations measured in the fasting state and again at the end of a euglycemic insulin clamp (*see* Fig. 8-3) are plotted against the individual level of insulin sensitivity. The distance between the two regression lines measures the suppressive effect of insulin on lipolysis (*ie*, inhibition of tissue hormone-sensitive lipase). Lipolysis is resistant to insulin inhibition (in the fasting state as well as during insulinization) in subjects who are resistant to the effect of insulin on glucose uptake [11]. Thus, insulin sensitivity in lipolysis and glucose pathways is a coupled phenomenon. FFM—fat-free mass.

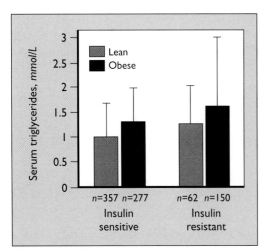

FIGURE 8-14. Insulin sensitivity and serum triglycerides. If the effect of insulin on lipolysis is deficient, both the peripheral tissues and the liver are exposed to an excess of circulating free fatty acids (FFA). In peripheral tissues, FFA impede insulin-mediated glucose uptake (by substrate competition, according to Randle [12]); in the liver, FFA are incorporated into triglycerides at an increased rate. In accordance with the latter observation, serum triglyceride concentrations are higher in insulin-resistant individuals (*ie*, subjects in the lowest quartile of the distribution of insulin sensitivity) than in more insulin-sensitive subjects, whether they are obese or lean. The figure plots median and interquartile range for four groups: insulin-sensitive lean subjects; insulin-sensitive obese subjects; insulin-resistant lean subjects; and insulin-resistant obese subjects. (*Data from* the European Group for the Study of Insulin Resistance database [11]).

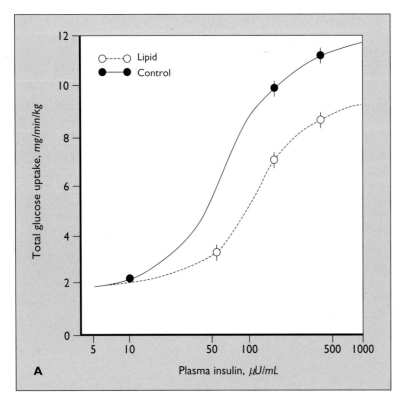

FIGURE 8-15. Experimental proof of substrate competition. Dose-response curves for total glucose uptake (**A**) and its main components,

(*Continued on next page*)

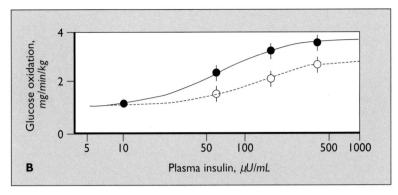

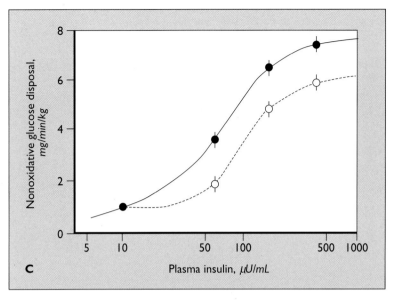

FIGURE 8-15. (*Continued*) glucose oxidation (**B**), and nonoxidative glucose disposal (**C**) (equivalent to glycogen synthesis), in healthy volunteers under control conditions (*solid lines*), and during the simultaneous infusion of Intralipid (KabiVitrum, Franklin, OH), a triglyceride emulsion (*dotted lines*). Provision of exogenous fatty substrates acutely impairs both total glucose uptake and its main components (glucose oxidation and glycogen synthesis), as predicated by substrate competition.

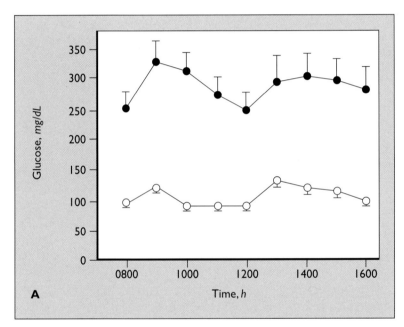

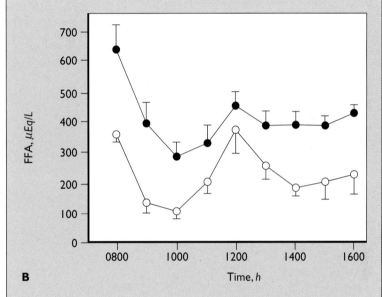

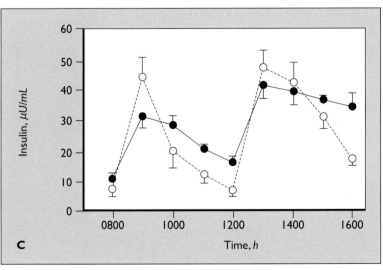

FIGURE 8-16. Day-long metabolic profile in type 2 diabetes. Plasma glucose (**A**), free fatty acids (FFA) (**B**), and insulin (**C**) concentrations in response to breakfast and lunch were measured in nondiabetic patients (*open circles*) and in type 2 diabetic patients (*closed circles*). Whereas average insulin levels were comparable in the two groups, both plasma glucose and FFA were markedly elevated in the diabetic patients [12]. Thus, patients with type 2 diabetes are resistant to insulin action on glucose disposal (*ie,* higher plasma glucose concentrations) as well as lipolysis (*ie,* higher plasma FFA levels) throughout the day. Consequently, insulin target tissues are exposed to chronically elevated FFA and may become laden with triglyceride deposits. (*Adapted from* Golay *et al.* [13].)

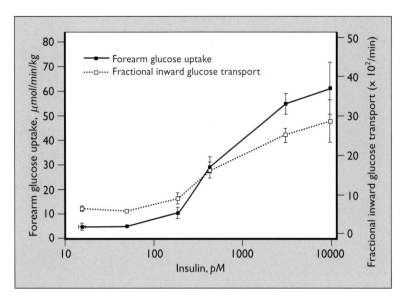

FIGURE 8-17. Glucose transport in vivo. In the human forearm, glucose transport can be measured under in vivo conditions by a triple-tracer method [14]. By this technique, the washout curves of three intra-arterially injected tracers (mannitol, to trace extracellular kinetics; 3-ortho-methylglucose, to trace glucose transport; and labeled glucose, to monitor intracellular glucose metabolism) are measured in a deep forearm vein that drains mostly muscle tissue. A compartmental model then is used on these data to calculate fractional inward glucose transport across the plasma membrane of skeletal muscle. The dose-response curve for glucose transport in the human forearm tissues was measured in healthy subjects by the triple tracer technique during graded hyperinsulinemia created by the insulin clamp technique. The graph also shows the parallelism between inward glucose transport and total glucose uptake in forearm tissues.

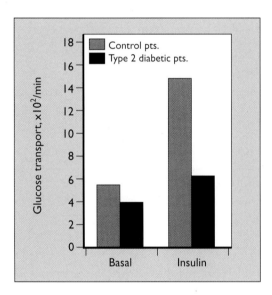

FIGURE 8-18. Defective glucose transport in type 2 diabetes. Inward glucose transport was measured by the triple-tracer technique in the basal state (overnight fast) and during euglycemic hyperinsulinemia in matched groups of patients with type 2 diabetes and nondiabetic controls. Diabetes is associated with a marked defect in the ability of insulin to stimulate glucose transport in skeletal muscle tissues [15].

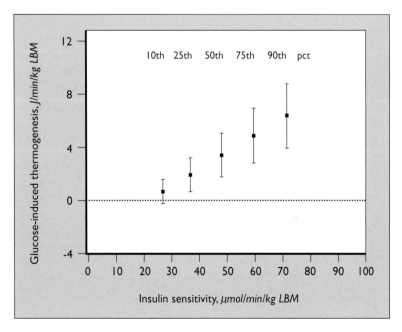

FIGURE 8-19. Insulin resistance and thermogenesis. One of the actions of insulin in vivo is to stimulate energy expenditure (ie, thermogenesis). Glucose-induced thermogenesis (GIT) is the change in energy expenditure observed during euglycemic hyperinsulinemia, as measured by indirect calorimetry during an insulin clamp in this case. The figure shows point estimates (± SEM) of GIT at different percentiles (pct) of insulin sensitivity in 322 nondiabetic subjects after statistical adjustment by gender, age, and body mass index. Insulin-resistant subjects show a defect in glucose-induced thermogenesis that is proportional to the degree of insulin resistance [16]. LBM—lean body mass.

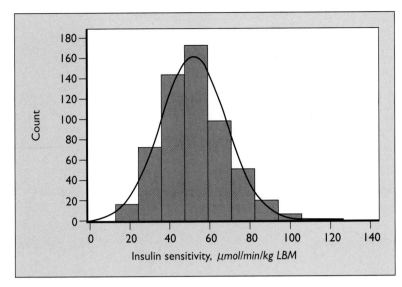

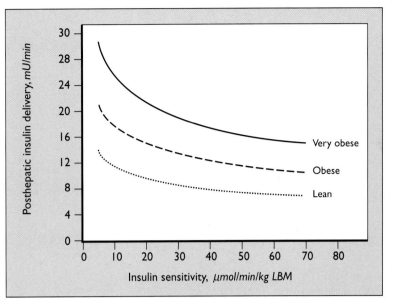

FIGURE 8-20. Insulin sensitivity in the general population. The graph shows the frequency distribution plot of insulin sensitivity (as measured by the euglycemic insulin clamp) in a cohort of 580 nondiabetic, nonobese (body mass index ≤25 kg/m²) white patients of both sexes. The distribution is significantly different from the normal distribution. The graft is skewed to the left as a result of an excess of insulin-resistant individuals (data from the European Group for the Study of Insulin Resistance [17]). There is, however, no evidence to suggest a bimodal or multimodal distribution of this trait. In general terms, this distribution is compatible with a model in which genetic drive is influenced by powerful environmental factors. LBM—lean body mass.

FIGURE 8-21. Relation between insulin sensitivity and insulin secretion. In a cohort of 1200 nondiabetic white patients of both sexes, the relationship between insulin sensitivity (by the insulin clamp technique) and insulin secretion (estimated from the clamping data as the posthepatic insulin delivery rate) is highly curvilinear (hyperbolic), such that in insulin-resistant individuals small changes in insulin sensitivity are associated with large (compensatory) changes in insulin secretion. The plot also shows the impact of obesity as an independent factor that greatly amplifies insulin secretion at any given level of insulin resistance. Thus, any degree of insulin hypersecretion (and, therefore, of hyperinsulinemia) can be described as the sum of a component that is secondary (compensatory) to insulin resistance and a part that is primary. The primary component is particularly common in obese individuals. (*Data from* Ferrannini *et al.* [18].)

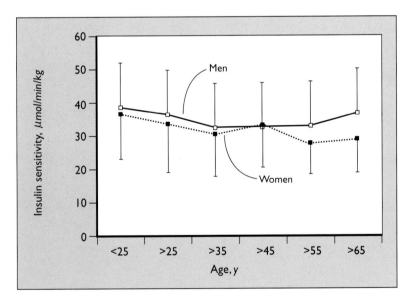

FIGURE 8-22. Impact of age on insulin sensitivity. In nondiabetic, otherwise healthy patients, aging has a marginal effect on insulin resistance [15]. Thus, the aging population tends to be insulin resistant because it is enriched with individuals with impaired glucose tolerance, essential hypertension, or obesity rather than as a result of senescence itself.

Insulin Resistance Syndrome

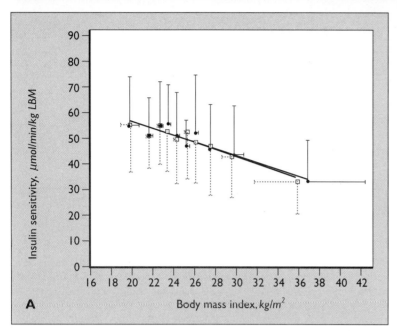

A

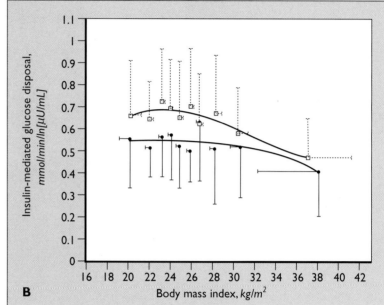

B

FIGURE 8-23. Insulin resistance and obesity. The dependence of insulin sensitivity on obesity (expressed as the body mass index [BMI]) is expressed in two ways in this figure. When total insulin-mediated glucose uptake is normalized by lean body mass (LBM) (**A**), insulin sensitivity declines linearly with body mass equally in men (*dotted lines*) and women (*solid bars*). However, when insulin-mediated glucose disposal is expressed in absolute terms (**B**) (in mmol/min, corrected for the steady-state plasma insulin concentration achieved during the clamp), the negative impact of obesity is seen only in very obese individuals (BMI >32 kg/m²). Thus, in the obese person, each unit mass of lean tissue (mostly skeletal muscle) is resistant to the action of insulin in direct proportion to the excess body fat. However, the expanded body mass of the moderately obese person compensates for the reduced insulin sensitivity and contributes to the maintenance of glucose tolerance [18].

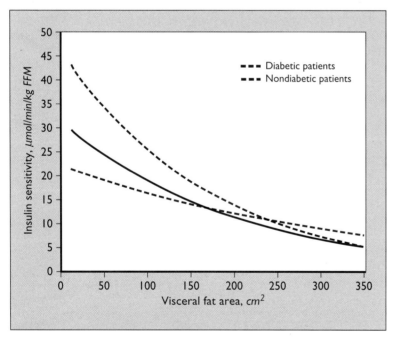

FIGURE 8-24. Fat as a determinant of insulin action. Adipose mass is not the sole link between obesity and insulin resistance. Excessive deposition of fat in the abdominal visceral area and within skeletal muscle cells is a potent determinant of insulin action. This graph shows the reciprocal association between insulin sensitivity (on the euglycemic insulin clamp) and intra-abdominal fat accumulation (measured as the visceral fat area by MRI) in adult humans. The *solid line* is the predicted relationship after adjustment by sex, age, and body mass index in 70 patients (*P* < 0.001). The *dotted lines* are the separate relationships in nondiabetic patients and diabetic patients. Note that the impact of visceral fat accumulation on insulin sensitivity is stronger in nondiabetic, insulin-sensitive subjects than in insulin-resistant diabetic patients (*P* < 0.02). FFM—fat-free mass.

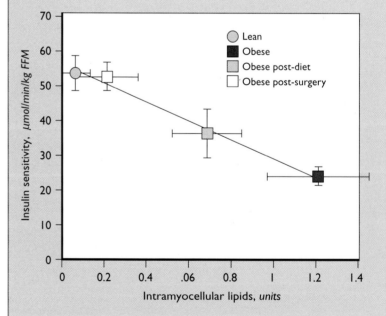

FIGURE 8-25. Reciprocal association between insulin sensitivity and intra-myocellular lipid accumulation (estimated by histochemistry on biopsy specimens of vastus lateralis muscle) in lean patients, morbidly obese patients, and morbidly obese patients following weight reduction by hypocaloric diet or surgery (biliopancreatic diversion). FFM—fat-free mass. (*Adapted from* Greco *et al.* [19].)

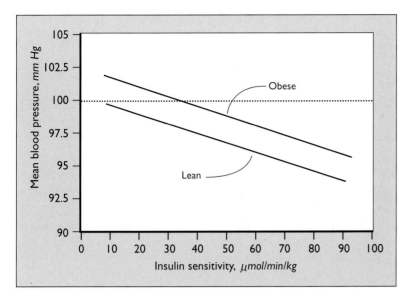

FIGURE 8-26. Insulin resistance and blood pressure. Patients with essential hypertension are, as a group, insulin resistant. This is not a special feature of essential hypertension, however, but the extension of a physiologic link to the disease domain. In fact, insulin resistance is associated with higher blood pressure levels in the normotensive population. The graph shows the significant inverse relationship between mean blood pressure and insulin sensitivity (as measured by the clamping technique) in 450 nondiabetic subjects in the European Group for the Study of Insulin Resistance cohort. The regression lines are adjusted by gender and age, and are drawn across the observed range of insulin sensitivity. The lower line (*lean*) is the predicted dependence in a subject with a body mass index of 25 kg/m², whereas the upper line (*obese*) is the function for an individual with a body mass index of 35 kg/m². The dotted line is an arbitrary threshold for clinical hypertension. Obesity and insulin resistance work together to raise arterial blood pressure [20].

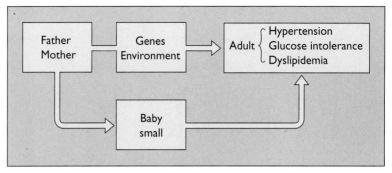

FIGURE 8-27. Insulin resistance and intrauterine development. Low birthweight has been found to be associated with the emergence in adulthood of hypertension, impaired glucose tolerance, and dyslipidemia, all states of impaired insulin action. Therefore, in addition to genes and environmental factors, insulin sensitivity may be modulated by changes that occur during intrauterine development. Thus, intrauterine growth retardation, possibly caused by maternal insulin resistance, may exert negative effects on the development of β cells, insulin sensing in target tissues, and the vasculature.

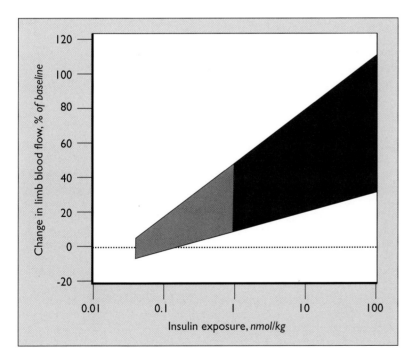

FIGURE 8-28. Hemodynamic actions of insulin: I. Insulin induces dilatation of peripheral (forearm, leg, or calf) vasculature as a function of exposure (dose of insulin × length of exposure, expressed as total nmol/kg of body weight). The lightly shaded area represents the physiologic insulin exposure, over which the average vasodilatory response is in the range 15% to 30%. This represents a compilation of a number of published studies. (*Adapted from* Yki-Järvinen and Utriainen [21]).

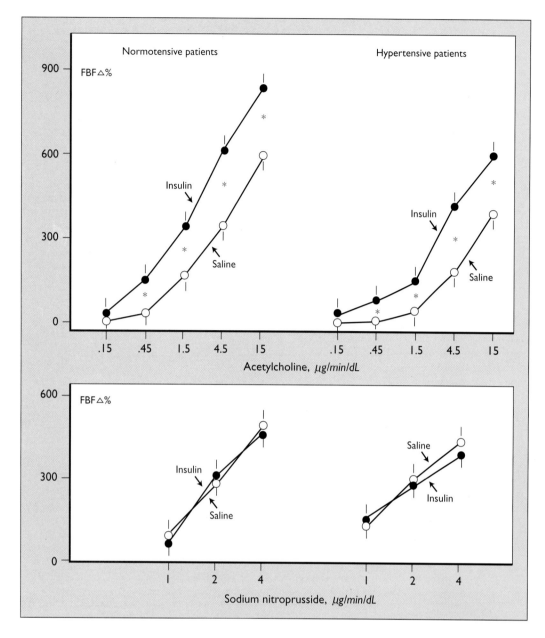

FIGURE 8-29. Hemodynamic actions of insulin: II. When infused locally (*ie,* through the brachial artery) at physiologic doses, insulin potentiates acetylcholine-induced (*top*), but not nitroprusside-induced (*bottom*), vasodilatation in humans [22], both in normotensive patients (*left*) and in patients with essential hypertension (*right*). These data suggest that insulin vasodilatation is an endothelium-dependent phenomenon. In addition, the potentiating effect of insulin was similar in healthy patients and hypertensive patients (who were resistant to the effect of insulin on glucose uptake), suggesting that the actions of insulin on the vasculature and glucose metabolism are largely independent of each other. *Asterisks* indicate mean values that are significantly different between insulin and saline infusion. FBF—forearm blood flow.

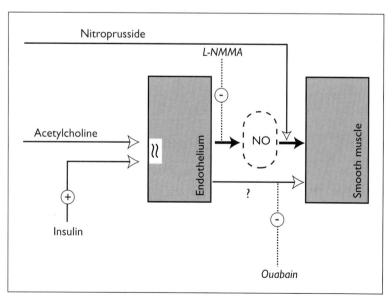

FIGURE 8-30. Hemodynamic actions of insulin: III. Insulin receptors are present on endothelial as well as on smooth muscle cells; thus, both types of cells are potential targets for insulin action. Insulin-induced vasodilatation [23] and insulin potentiation of acetylcholine-induced vasodilatation can both be blocked by L-monomethyl-arginine (L-NMMA), a competitive inhibitor of nitric oxide (NO) synthase [22], indicating that a likely mechanism for this effect of insulin is NO release from the endothelium. Direct provision of NO with nitroprusside bypasses the endothelial step. Furthermore, both insulin-induced vasodilatation [24] and insulin potentiation of acetylcholine-induced vasodilatation [22] can be blocked by ouabain, an inhibitor of sodium-potassium ATPase, suggesting that cell membrane hyperpolarization is an alternative mechanism for this action of insulin. Insulin-induced hyperpolarization can be exerted directly on the smooth muscle cell or involve the release of an unidentified hyperpolarizing factor from the endothelium.

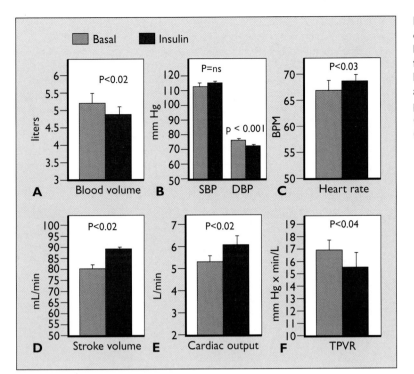

FIGURE 8-31. Hemodynamic actions of insulin: IV. Vasodilatation is not the only vascular action of insulin. Following physiologic hyperinsulinemia established by insulin clamping, blood volume is reduced (**A**); diastolic blood pressure (DBP) falls slightly, whereas systolic blood pressure (SBP) increases somewhat (**B**); heart rate goes up (**C**); stroke volume and cardiac output increase (**D** and **E**); and total peripheral vascular resistances (TPVR) decrease (**F**). This hemodynamic picture is compatible with a direct effect of insulin to reduce vascular resistance (vasodilatation) and a simultaneous effect of insulin to stimulate adrenergic activity (enhanced cardiac contractility). BPM—beats per minute.

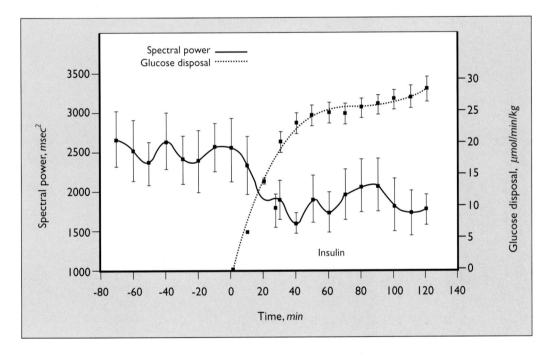

FIGURE 8-32. Hemodynamic actions of insulin: V. Spectral analysis of heart rate variability provides information on the autonomic nervous control of cardiac function. Total spectral power reflects parasympathetic and adrenergic inputs related to baroreflex control of heart rate; these inputs are mediated through the central nervous system. During a standard euglycemic insulin clamp, insulin causes a prompt and marked decline in total spectral power, which is temporally and quantitatively unrelated to insulin stimulation of glucose disposal [25]. This effect is partially independent of changes in heart rate, and therefore reflects direct desensitization of the autonomic neural reflex arch. In addition, the effect is more marked on the parasympathetic component of the autonomic arch (parasympathetic withdrawal), thereby giving rise to relative sympathetic dominance.

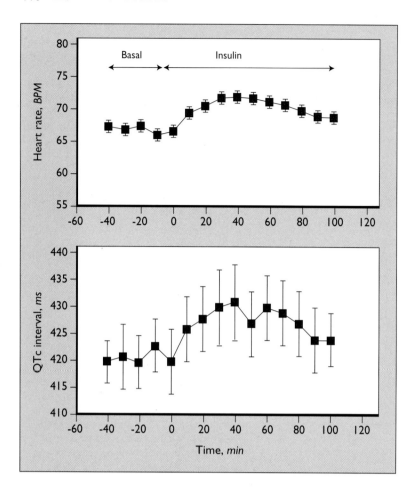

FIGURE 8-33. Electrophysiologic action of insulin. Insulin acutely hyperpolarizes plasma membranes, possibly through its stimulatory effect on ATP-dependent sodium-potassium exchange. The graph shows the changes in heart rate and corrected QT (QTc) interval on the electrocardiogram during a euglycemic insulin clamp in healthy volunteers. Despite a tachycardic effect (*top*), insulin causes a prolongation of the QTc interval (*bottom*), indicating a prolongation of the repolarization phase. In chronically hyperinsulinemic individuals, this action of insulin may sensitize the heart to arrhythmias, particularly in at-risk individuals. BPM—beats per minute. (*Adapted from* Gastaldelli *et al.* [26].)

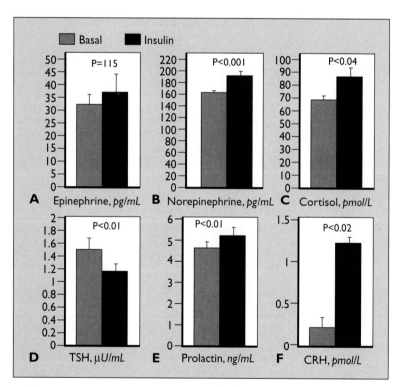

FIGURE 8-34. Insulin action and the central nervous system. Physiologic euglycemic hyperinsulinemia is associated with a rise in the circulating levels of norepinephrine (**A** and **B**), cortisol (**C**), prolactin (**E**), and corticotropin-releasing hormone (CRH) (**F**), and a decrease in thyroid-stimulating hormone (TSH) (**D**) [25]. This pattern of hormonal responses is compatible with a moderate stress reaction orchestrated by CRH. Thus, the hemodynamic, autonomic nervous, and hormonal responses to peripheral hyperinsulinemia coherently indicate that insulin acts in the central nervous system, most probably following transport from the plasma across the blood-brain barrier [27].

NATIVE AND EXPERIMENTAL INSULIN RESISTANCE

Physiologic	Nonendocrine
Puberty	Essential hypertension
Pregnancy	Chronic uremia
Bed rest	Liver cirrhosis
Contraceptives	Rheumatoid arthritis
High-fat diet	Acanthosis nigricans
Metabolic	Chronic heart failure
Type 2 diabetes	Myotonic dystrophia
Uncontrolled type 1 diabetes	Trauma, burns, sepsis
Diabetic ketoacidosis	Surgery
Obesity	Neoplastic cachexia
Severe malnutrition	Experimental
Hyperuricemia	Short-term hyperglycemia
Insulin-induced hypoglycemia	Short-term hypoglycemia
Excessive alcohol consumption	Short-term hyperinsulinemia
Endocrine	Short-term hypoinsulinemia
Thyrotoxicosis	Fat infusion
Hypothyroidism	Amino acid infusion
Cushing syndrome	Infusion of counterregulatory hormones
Pheochromocytoma	
Acromegaly	Acidosis

FIGURE 8-35. Native and experimental insulin resistance. This table lists conditions that have been found to be associated with insulin resistance or under which insulin resistance can be produced experimentally.

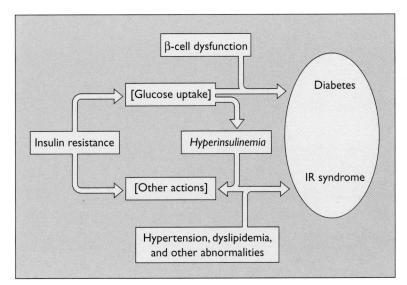

FIGURE 8-36. Insulin action and the insulin resistance syndrome: a working hypothesis. Insulin resistance (IR) in the glucose pathway combines with β-cell dysfunction to produce the hyperglycemia of diabetes. Insulin resistance also induces compensatory hyperinsulinemia. Insulin pathways other than glucose metabolism (lipids, blood pressure, endothelial function, autonomic nervous system) may themselves be resistant or, if normally sensitive, be overly stimulated by the hyperinsulinemia. The signs and symptoms of the IR syndrome develop from these pathways.

References

1. DeFronzo RA, Tobin J, Andres R: Glucose clamp technique: a method for quantifying insulin secretion and resistance. *Am J Physiol* 1979, 237:E214–E223.

2. Ferrannini E, Mari A: How to measure insulin sensitivity. *J Hypertens* 1998, 16:895–906.

3. Iozzo P, Beck-Nielsen H, Laakso M, *et al.*: Independent influence of age on basal insulin secretion in nondiabetic humans. *J Clin Endocrinol Metab* 1999, 84:863–868.

4. DeFronzo RA, Simonson D, Ferrannini E: Hepatic and peripheral insulin resistance: a common feature of insulin-independent and insulin-dependent diabetes. *Diabetologia* 1982, 23:313–320.

5. DeFronzo RA, Ferrannini E, Hendler R, *et al.*: Regulation of splanchnic and peripheral glucose uptake by insulin and hyperglycemia in man. *Diabetes* 1983, 32:35–45.

6. Landau BR, Wahren J, Chandramouli V, *et al.*: Use of 2H2O for estimating rates of gluconeogenesis. Application to the fasted state. *J Clin Invest* 1995, 95:172–178.

7. Gastaldelli A, Baldi S, Pettiti M, *et al.*: Influence of obesity and type 2 diabetes on gluconeogenesis and glucose output in hormones. *Diabetes* 2000, 49:1367–1373.

8. Paternostro G, Camici PG, Lammerstma AA, *et al.*: Cardiac and skeletal muscle insulin resistance in patients with coronary artery disease: a study with positron-emitting tomography. *J Clin Invest* 1996, 98:2094–2099.

9. Kelley DE, Mokan M, Simoneau JA, Mandarino LJ: Interaction between glucose and free fatty acid metabolism in human skeletal muscle. *J Clin Invest* 1993, 92:91–98.

10. Groop LC, Saloranta C, Schenk M, *et al.*: The role of free fatty acid metabolism in the pathogenesis of insulin resistance in obesity and non–insulin-dependent diabetes mellitus. *J Clin Endocrinol Metab* 1991, 72:96–102.

11. Ferrannini E, Camastra S, Coppack SW, *et al.*: Insulin action and non-esterified fatty acids. *Proc Nutr Soc* 1997, 56:753–761.

12. Randle PJ, Garland PB, Hales CN, Newsholme EA: The glucose fatty acid cycle: its role in insulin sensitivity and the metabolic disturbances of diabetes mellitus. *Lancet* 1963, i:785–789.

13. Golay A, Swilocky AL, Chen YD, Reaven GM: Relationship between plasma free fatty acid concentration, endogenous glucose production, and fasting hyperglycemia in normal and non–insulin-dependent diabetic individuals. *Metabolism* 1987, 36:692–696.

14. Bonadonna RC, Saccomani MP, Seely L, *et al.*: Glucose transport in human skeletal muscle: the in vivo response to insulin. *Diabetes* 1993, 42:191–198.

15. Bonadonna RC, Del Prato S, Cobelli C, *et al.*: Transmembrane glucose transport in skeletal muscle of patients with non–insulin-dependent diabetes. *J Clin Invest* 1993, 92:486–492.

16. Camastra S, Bonora E, Del Prato S, *et al.*: Effect of obesity and insulin resistance on resting and glucose-induced thermogenesis in man. EGIR (European Group for the Study of Insulin Resistance). *Int J Obes Relat Metab Disord* 1999, 23(12):1307–1313.

17. Ferrannini E, Vichi S, Beck-Nielsen H, *et al.*: Insulin action and age. *Diabetes* 1996, 45:947–953.

18. Ferrannini E, Natali A, Bell P, *et al.*: Insulin resistance and hypersecretion in obesity. *J Clin Invest* 1997, 100:1166–1173.

19. Greco AV, Mingrone G, Giancaterini A, *et al.*: Insulin resistance in morbid obesity: reversal with intramyocellular fat depletion. *Diabetes* 2002, 51(1):144–151.

20. Ferrannini E, Natali A, Capaldo B, *et al.*: Insulin resistance, hyperinsulinemia, and blood pressure. Role of age and obesity. *Hypertension* 1997, 30:1144–1149.

21. Yki-Järvinen H, Utriainen T: Insulin-induced vasodilatation: physiology or pharmacology? *Diabetologia* 1998, 41:369–379.

22. Taddei S, Virdis A, Mattei P, *et al.*: Effect of insulin on acetylcholine-induced vasodilation in normotensive subjects and patients with essential hypertension. *Circulation* 1995, 92:2911–2920.

23. Steinberg HO, Brechtel G, Johson A, *et al.*: Insulin-mediated skeletal muscle vasodilatation is nitric oxide dependent. A novel action of insulin to increase nitric oxide release. *J Clin Invest* 1994, 94:1172–1179.

24. Tack CJ, Lutterman JA, Vervoot G, *et al.*: Activation of the sodium-potassium pump contributes to insulin-induced vasodilatation in humans. *Hypertension* 1996, 28:426–432.

25. Muscelli E, Emdin M, Natali A, *et al.*: Autonomic and hemodynamic responses to insulin in lean and obese humans. *J Clin Endocrinol Metab* 1998, 83:2084–2090.

26. Gastaldelli A, Emdin M, Conforti F, *et al.*: Insulin prolongs the QTc interval in humans. *Am J Physiol Regul Integr Comp Physiol* 2000, 279(6):R2022–R2025.

27. Schwartz MW, Figlewicz DP, Baskin DB, *et al.*: Insulin in the brain: a hormonal regulator of energy balance. *Endocr Rev* 1992, 13:81–113.

HYPOGLYCEMIA

F. John Service

9

Hypoglycemia is a clinical syndrome, arising from diverse causes, in which low levels of plasma glucose eventually lead to neuroglycopenia. Symptoms of hypoglycemia begin at plasma glucose levels of approximately 60 mg/dL, and impairment of brain function begins at levels of approximately 50 mg/dL. The rate of decrease in plasma glucose levels does not influence the occurrence of symptoms. The symptoms of hypoglycemia have been classified into two major groups: autonomic and neuroglycopenic. The latter have been identified from experimental studies as the following: dizziness, confusion, difficulty in speaking, headache, inability to concentrate, warmth, weakness, confusion or difficulty in thinking, and fatigue or drowsiness. In a retrospective analysis of 60 patients with insulinoma, 85% of patients had various combinations of diplopia, blurred vision, sweating, palpitations, and weakness; 80% had confusion or abnormal behavior; 53% had amnesia or coma; and 12% had generalized seizures. Symptoms of hypoglycemia differ among patients but are consistent from episode to episode for each patient. Symptoms do not evolve in a consistent chronologic order; autonomic symptoms (sweating, trembling, anxiety, palpitation, hunger, tingling) do not always precede the neuroglycopenic symptoms. Many patients experience only neuroglycopenic symptoms. Persons with recurrent hypoglycemia may develop varying degrees of hypoglycemia unawareness analogous to that observed in persons with insulin-dependent diabetes. None of these symptoms is specific for hypoglycemia; the presence of one of several may be from other causes.

The long-established classification of hypoglycemia as either food-deprived (composed of organic diseases and manifested by neuroglycopenic symptoms) or food-stimulated (arising from functional disturbances and manifested by autonomic symptoms) is no longer useful.

Persons with insulinomas, the archetypical food-deprived hypoglycemic disorder, may have symptoms after eating (and in rare instances only at this time) as well as during fasting. Persons with factitious hypoglycemia have erratically occurring symptoms that are independent of food ingestion. Food-stimulated hypoglycemias, such as galactosemia, hereditary fructose intolerance, and ackee-fruit poisoning, result in neuroglycopenic symptoms. The disorders that supposedly arise from a functional disturbance of glucose homeostasis and produce only autonomic symptoms—functional hypoglycemia, early diabetes hypoglycemia, and alimentary hypoglycemia—were predicated on the now-discredited 5-hour oral glucose-tolerance test and have no scientific support.

A more useful approach is a classification based on clinical characteristics. Persons who appear healthy are likely to have hypoglycemic disorders different from those experienced by ill persons. Hospitalized patients are at additional risk for hypoglycemia, often from iatrogenic factors. Hypoglycemia may occur from accidental drug ingestion in healthy persons, the mistaken dispensing of a sulfonylurea, or the idiosyncratic actions of some of the drugs used to treat seriously ill patients. The occurrence of hypoglycemia in a patient with an illness known to be associated with this condition requires little, if any, investigation of its cause, only a recognition of the association of the disease with the risk for hypoglycemia. Healthy-appearing persons of all ages and both sexes are at risk for insulinomas. Factitious hypoglycemia due to self-administered insulin is often seen in female health care workers. These clinical patterns facilitate the differential diagnosis and help direct the diagnostic evaluation. Asymptomatic patients may have artifactual hypoglycemia because of leukemia or severe hemolysis or may have adapted to lifelong hypoglycemia caused by glycogen storage disease [1].

Symptoms, Classification, and Glucose Behavior in Hypoglycemic Disorders

CLINICAL CLASSIFICATION OF HYPOGLYCEMIC DISORDERS

Patient appears healthy*

No coexistent disease
  Drugs
    Ethanol
    Salicylates
    Quinine
    Haloperidol
  Insulinoma
  Insulin or sulfonylurea factitial hypoglycemia
  Severe exercise
  Ketotic hypoglycemia
    Insulin autoimmune hypoglycemia
    Islet hypertrophy/nesidioblastosis
      Persistent hyperinsulinemic hypoglycemia of infancy
      Noninsulinoma pancreatogenous hypoglycemia syndrome

Compensated coexistent disease
  Drugs
    Dispensing error
    Disopyramide
    β-adrenergic blocking agents

Patient appears ill

Drugs
  Pentamidine and *Pneumocystis carinii*
    pneumonia
  Trimethoprim–sulfamethoxazole and
    renal failure
  Propoxyphene and renal failure
  Quinine and cerebral malaria
  Quinine and malaria
  Topical salicylates and renal failure
    Unripe ackee fruit and undernutrition

Predisposing illness
  Children
    Small-for-gestational-age infant
    Beckwith-Wiedemann syndrome
    Erythroblastosis fetalis
    Infant of diabetic mother
    Glycogen storage disease
    Defects in amino acid and fatty acid
      metabolism
    Reye's syndrome
    Cyanotic congenital heart disease
    Hypopituitarism
    Isolated growth hormone deficiency
    Isolated adrenocorticotropic hormone
      deficiency
    Addison's disease
    Galactosemia
    Hereditary fructose intolerance
    Carnitine deficiency
    Defective type 1 glucose transporter
      in the brain
  Adults
    Acquired severe liver disease
    Large non–β-cell tumor
    Sepsis
    Renal failure
    Congestive heart failure
    Lactic acidosis
    Starvation
    Anorexia nervosa
    Following removal of pheochromocytoma
    Insulin receptor antibody hypoglycemia
    Mutations in the β-cell sulfonylurea
      receptor gene
    Glutamate dehydrogenase gene
    Glucokinase gene

Hospitalized patient
  Diseases predisposing to hypoglycemia
  Total parenteral nutrition and insulin therapy
  Questran interference with glucocorticoid
    absorption
  Shock

Mutations in the β-cell sulfonylurea receptor gene, glutamate dehydrogenase gene, and glucokinase gene are rare causes of hyperinsulinemic hypoglycemia usually manifested in infancy or childhood.

FIGURE 9-1. Clinical classification of hypoglycemic disorders.

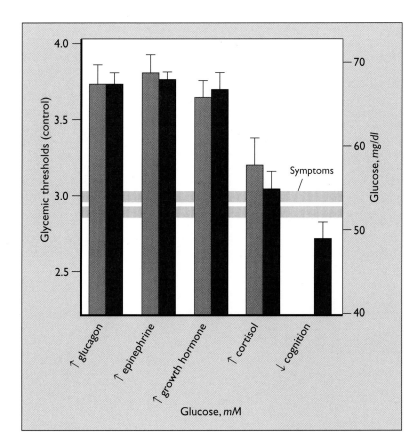

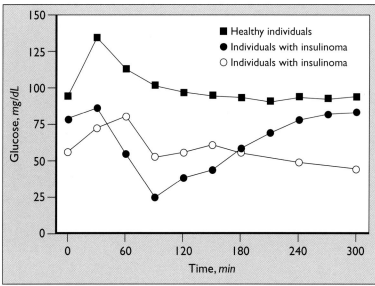

FIGURE 9-3. Plasma glucose responses to a mixed meal. *Squares* represent responses in healthy persons; *open* (fasting hypoglycemia profile) and *closed* (post-prandial hypoglycemia profile) *circles* represent responses in persons with insulinoma. Postprandial hypoglycemia with spontaneous resumption of normoglycemia infrequently can be seen in patients with this disorder. Therefore, categorization of patients by timing of hypoglycemic symptoms may not be useful for diagnosing the cause of the hypoglycemic disorder. (*Adapted from* Service [2].)

FIGURE 9-2. Mean arterialized venous glycemic thresholds of increments in plasma levels of glucagon, epinephrine, growth hormone, and cortisol for symptoms of hypoglycemia and for impairment of cognitive function during decrements in plasma glucose levels in control patients from two independent studies. *Light blue bars* represent data from a report by Series in 1995 [2]; *dark blue bars* represent data from a chapter by Series in 1989 [3]. Error bars are the upper boundary of the standard error. (*Adapted from* Cryer [4].)

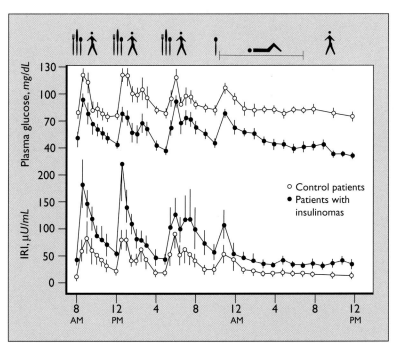

FIGURE 9-4. Serial measurements of plasma glucose and insulin were done in control patients and patients with insulinoma. Although plasma glucose levels increased after meal ingestion (represented by the knife, fork, and spoon symbol), they declined to hypoglycemic levels in the postabsorptive state and during fasting. Insulinomas were persistently hyperinsulinemic in the absorptive, postabsorptive, and fasting states (the striding symbol represents exercise, and the reclining symbol represents sleep) IRI—immunoreactive insulin. (*Adapted from* Service and Nelson [5].)

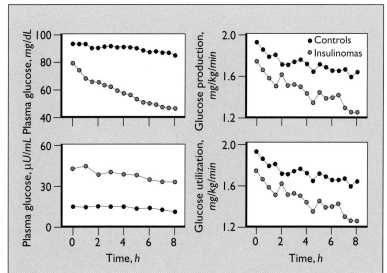

FIGURE 9-5. Glucose turnover was isotopically measured in control patients and patients with insulinoma during food deprivation. Patients with insulinomas became hypoglycemic primarily as a result of decreased glucose production rather than increased glucose utilization. Thus, the primary effect of persistent hyperinsulinemia in patients with insulinomas is to turn off hepatic glucose production. (*Adapted from* Rizza et al. [6].)

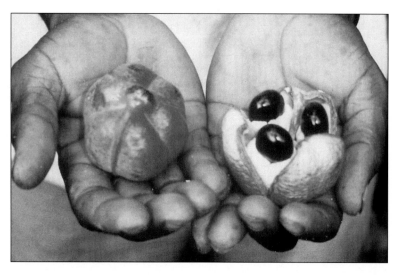

FIGURE 9-6. (*See Color Plate*) The ackee fruit in its unripe form (*left*) and ripe form (*right*). The ackee tree, indigenous to west Africa, was introduced to Jamaica in 1778 by Thomas Clarke. In Jamaica it is considered a dietary staple. It is well known in west Africa and Jamaica that the fruit may be poisonous during certain stages in its development.

Outbreaks of a disorder commonly called Jamaica vomiting sickness tend to occur during the colder months of the year, when other food is scarce and the fruit is still unripe. The major clinical features of this disorder, caused by ingestion of an unripe ackee fruit, include the sudden onset of vomiting and violent retching, which is preceded by generalized epigastric discomfort lasting 2 hours to 3 days. After a period of prostration averaging 10 hours, the second bout of vomiting may occur, followed by convulsions and sometimes death. The most striking finding is marked hypoglycemia. Well-nourished people may never develop manifestations of the disease, whereas those with chronic malnutrition, especially children between 2 and 5 years of age, are much more likely to become symptomatic. Hypoglycins A and B mediate the illness: they inhibit transport of long-chain fatty acids into the mitochondria, thereby suppressing their oxidation and resulting in depression of gluconeogenesis [3].

FIGURE 9-7. Protocol for prolonged 72-hour fast.

PROTOCOL FOR PROLONGED SUPERVISED FAST

1. Date the onset of the fast as of the last ingestion of calories. Discontinue use of all nonessential medications.

2. Allow the patient to drink calorie-free and caffeine-free beverages.

3. Ensure that the patient is active during waking hours.

4. Measure plasma levels of glucose, insulin, C-peptide, and, if an assay is available, proinsulin in the same specimen: repeat measurements every 6 hours until the plasma glucose level is <60 mg/dL. At this point, the interval should be reduced to every 1 to 2 hours.

5. End the fast when the plasma glucose level is <45 mg/dL and the patient has symptoms or signs of hypoglycemia.

6. At the end of the fast, measure plasma levels of glucose, insulin, C-peptide, proinsulin, β-hydroxy-butyrate, and sulfonylurea in the same specimen. Then inject 1 mg of glucagon intravenously and measure plasma glucose level after 10, 20, and 30 minutes. At this point the patient can be fed.

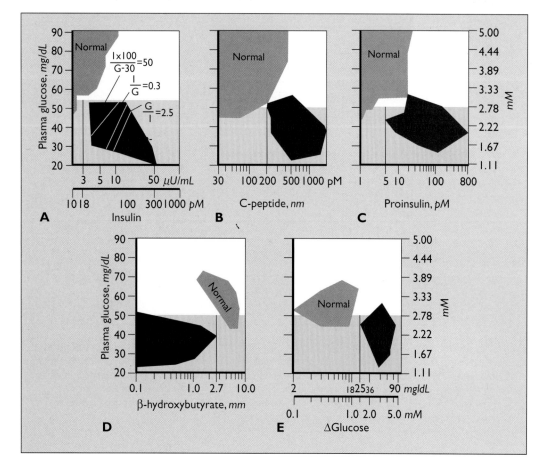

FIGURE 9-8. Limits of plasma levels of insulin (**A**), C-peptide (**B**), proinsulin (**C**), and β-hydroxy-butyrate (**D**), and changes in plasma glucose levels (**E**) in response to intravenous glucagon, according to 1) plasma glucose levels at the end of a 72-hour fast in 25 control patients and 2) the point at which the features of Whipple's triad were noted in 40 patients with histologically confirmed insulinomas. The shaded areas represent plasma glucose levels (50 mg/dL [2.8 mmol/L]). The vertical lines represent the diagnostic criteria for insulinoma: insulin level of at least 3 microunits per mL (18 pmol/L), C-peptide level of at least 200 pmol/L, proinsulin level of at least 5 pmol/L, β-hydroxybutyrate level of 2.7 mmol/L or less, and change in glucose level of at least 25 mg/dL (1.4 mmol/L). The ratios of glucose and insulin have no diagnostic utility.

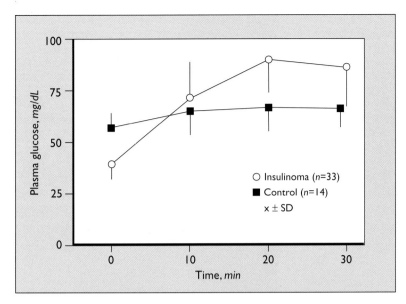

FIGURE 9-9. Plasma glucose responses to glucagon, 1 mg, administered intravenously at the end of the prolonged fast (0 minutes). These responses are greater in patients with insulinoma than in control patients. The rationale for this procedure is that insulin is glycogenic and antiglycogenolytic and therefore results in persistence of hepatic glycogen despite fasting. Patients with insulin-mediated hypoglycemia have a maximum increment of at least 25 mg/dL above the terminal fasting plasma glucose levels, whereas others (control patients or those with non–insulin-mediated hypoglycemia whose hepatic glycogen has been depleted by fasting) have lower increments [7]. Error bars represent the standard deviation. (*Adapted from* Service and Nelson [5].)

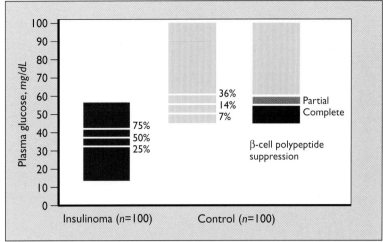

FIGURE 9-10. Plasma glucose levels at the end of a 72-hour fast. The *yellow panel* depicts the range (57 to 44 mg/dL) at the termination of the prolonged 72-hour fast (Whipple's triad) in 100 patients with insulinoma (the fast was terminated well before the 72-hour point because of the occurrence of symptomatic hypoglycemia confirmed biochemically). The 75th percentile (42 mg/dL), 50th percentile (38 mg/dL), and 25th percentile (33 mg/dL) are also shown. The *red panel* shows the plasma glucose levels at the 72-hour point in 100 control patients who underwent the 72-hour fast. Thirty-six percent of patients had a plasma glucose level of 60 mg/dL or less, 14% had a level of 55 mg/dL or less, and 7% had a level of 50 mg/dL or less. Two patients had terminal plasma glucose levels of 44 mg/dL. The *blue panel* depicts suppression of β-cell polypeptides in normal persons at the end of the 72-hour fast. One or two of the three β-cell polypeptides (insulin, C-peptide, and proinsulin) were suppressed below our diagnostic criteria for hyperinsulinemia in the range of 60 to 55 mg/dL, and all three were suppressed when the plasma glucose level was 55 mg/dL or lower.

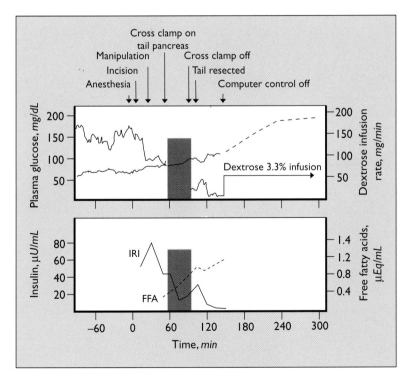

FIGURE 9-11. Artificial pancreas. The Biostator (Life Science Instruments, Elkhart, IN) has been used by some practitioners to maintain euglycemia in the preoperative and intraoperative period. A reduction in the glucose infusion rate after removal of the insulinoma indicates that all hyperfunctioning tissue has been removed. An alternate approach is to conduct frequent serial measurements of plasma glucose levels in the operating room. Patients are taken to the operating room without glucose running, and the plasma glucose level is permitted to decrease to a modestly hypoglycemic range. After tumor removal, an increase in the plasma glucose level can be expected within 30 minutes in most patients. In some patients, the plasma glucose level is increasing as a result of stress before tumor removal. Also after removal of the tumor, the slope of the elevation in the glucose level increases distinctly. FFA—free fatty acids; IRI—insulin resistance index. (*Adapted from* Kudlow *et al.* [8].)

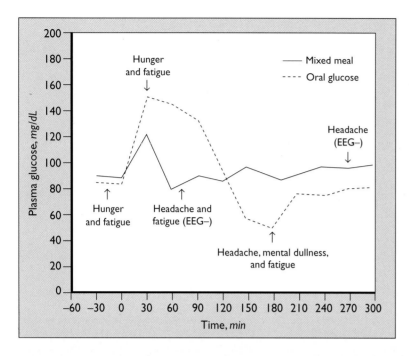

FIGURE 9-12. The oral glucose tolerance test. This test has been used to evaluate patients with suspected reactive hypoglycemia. Unfortunately, this test is of no use because a high percentage of normal persons have a post–oral glucose testing nadir of 50 mg/dL or less. The preferred assessment is a mixed-meal test. As shown in this figure, individual symptoms occurred throughout the oral glucose tolerance test, both at the nadir and at the apogee. In addition, symptoms were present during the mixed-meal test when no evidence of hypoglycemia was noted. These observations provide strong evidence that symptoms could not be ascribed to hypoglycemia. EEG—electroencephalogram. (*Adapted from* Service [3].)

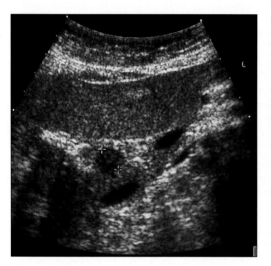

FIGURE 9-13. Hypoechogenicity of insulinomas. The ultrasonographic characteristic of insulinoma is hypoechogenicity. The insulinoma is marked with white crosses and is distinctly hypoechogenic in contrast to surrounding tissue.

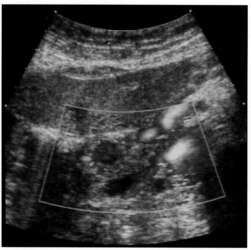

FIGURE 9-14. (See Color Plate) Hypoechogenicity of insulinomas. Color Doppler analysis shows the hypervascularity of the insulinoma noted in Figure 9-13.

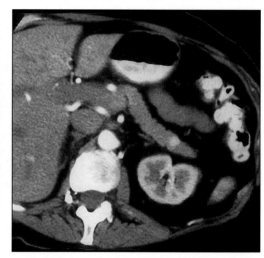

FIGURE 9-15. Insulinoma. A 0.8-cm insulinoma is seen in the arterial phase of the spiral CT scan, which was obtained by using triple-phase agent.

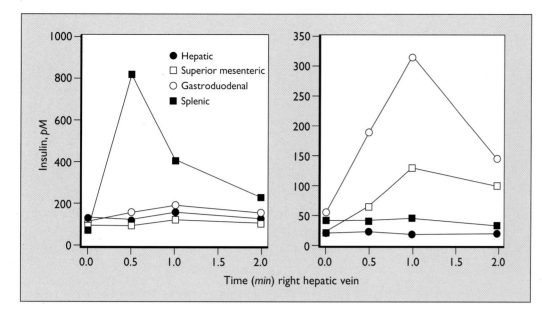

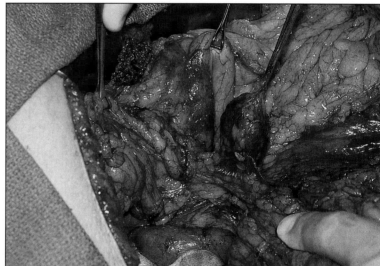

FIGURE 9-16. The selective arterial calcium stimulation test. This is both a localization (actually a regionalization) procedure and a dynamic test. The principle of this procedure is that hyperfunctioning β cells release insulin in response to the injection of a small dose of calcium intra-arterially, whereas normal β cells do not. During this procedure, the insulin level is measured before and at fixed time sequences after the injection of 0.025 mEq of calcium per kg of body weight sequentially into the splenic, gastroduodenal, and superior mesenteric arteries. A two- to threefold increment in the level of insulin in the right hepatic vein indicates hyperfunctioning β cells—either insulinoma or hypertrophic islets—in the arterial distribution of the injected artery. In the left panel, the positive response after injection into the splenic artery indicates that hyperfunctioning β cells (presumably an insulinoma) are present in the tail of the pancreas. In the right panel, the positive responses to injections into the superior mesenteric and gastroduodenal arteries suggest that the insulinoma is likely to be in the head of the pancreas. (*Adapted from* Doppman *et al.* [9].)

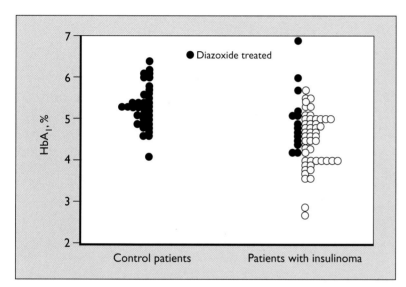

FIGURE 9-17. Glycated hemoglobin values (measured by affinity chromatography) for control patients evaluated for potential hypoglycemic disorder and insulinomas, some of whom had been treated with diazoxide. Although glycated hemoglobin values are lower in patients with insulinoma than in control patients, the values overlap too much to allow a diagnostic level to be established. Twenty-five percent of the patients with insulinoma had glycated hemoglobin values of 4.1% or less; this was at the lower limit of values observed in control patients. (*Adapted from* Hassoun *et al.* [10].)

FIGURE 9-18. (See Color Plate) Insulinomas. Insulinomas vary in size, from a few millimeters to several centimeters. The median is 1.5 cm. This figure shows a 4-cm tumor. In a large series of patients (*n* = 224) observed at the Mayo Clinic from 1927 to 1986 [11], 86.6% of patients had a single benign tumor, 5.9% had malignant tumors, 8.9% had multiple tumors, and 7.6% had multiple endocrine neoplasia type syndrome. The estimated incidence in the northern European population is 4 cases per 1 million patient-years. The median age in the Mayo Clinic series was 47 years (range, 8 to 82 years), and 59% of patients were women. During the study period, one patient had islet hyperplasia.

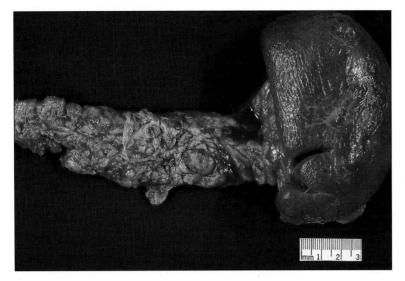

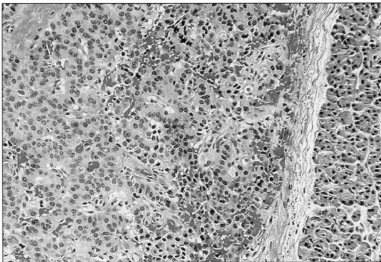

FIGURE 9-19. (See Color Plate) Removal of the distal pancreas and spleen in a patient with multiple islet cell tumors as part of the multiple endocrine neoplasia (MEN) I syndrome. Insulinoma constitutes the second most common pancreatic tumor in the MEN I syndrome. In a study from the Mayo Clinic [11], more than 50% of patients with insulinoma as part of MEN I syndrome had multiple tumors. The associated endocrinopathies have primarily been hyperparathyroidism, prolactinoma, gastrinoma, and Cushing disease. The standard operative approach is to enucleate tumors in the head of the pancreas and, if tumors are present in the rest of the pancreas, to conduct a partial pancreatectomy.

FIGURE 9-20. (See Color Plate) Pancreatic tissue showing normal exocrine pancreas on the right side of the figure. The left side of the figure shows an islet cell tumor composed of uniform cells with round nuclei and eosinophilic cytoplasm. The tumor is highly vascular, and small clusters of red blood cells are present throughout the neoplasm. Mitotic figures are not identified, and there is no invasive growth of the neoplasm. These findings suggest that this tumor is probably benign. (Hematoxylin and eosin; original magnification, ×6.)

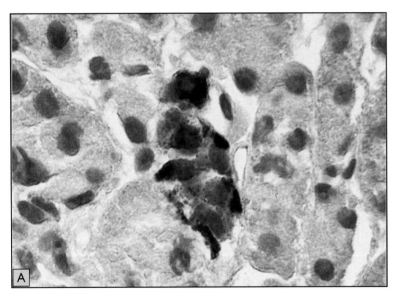

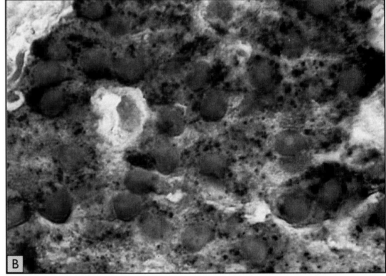

FIGURE 9-21. (See Color Plate) Higher magnification of an insulin-producing islet cell tumor after immunostaining. **A,** Normal exocrine and endocrine pancreatic tissues. An islet cell staining positively for insulin is present in the middle of the pancreatic exocrine tissue. **B,** An

insulinoma with strong diffuse positive immunoreactivity after staining with an insulin antibody. The tumor cells reveal diffuse granular cytoplasmic staining. The blue staining of the nuclei is from the hematoxylin counterstain. (×40)

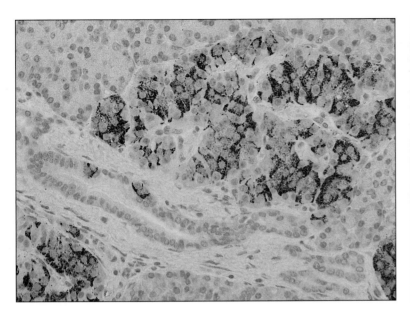

FIGURE 9-22. (See Color Plate) Islet hyperplasia/nesidioblastosis, a rare cause of hyperinsulinemic hypoglycemia in adults. This slide shows large islets immunostained with insulin, as well as two β cells budding from the acinar duct. The latter is the characteristic of nesidioblastosis [12]. (×150)

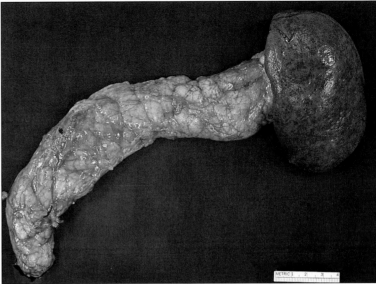

FIGURE 9-23. (See Color Plate) Islet hyperplasia/nesidioblastosis. When hyperinsulinemic hypoglycemia in an adult is suspected to be due to islet hyperplasia/nesidioblastosis and an insulinoma cannot be identified by intraoperative ultrasonography or complete mobilization and palpation of the pancreas, gradient-guided partial pancreatectomy is indicated. In this patient, a selective arterial calcium stimulation test indicated hyperfunctioning β cells in the region of the splenic and gastroduodenal arteries. As a result, resection was performed to the right of the superior mesenteric vein [12].

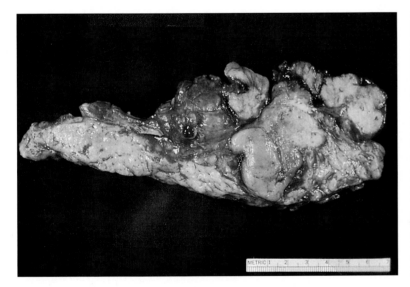

FIGURE 9-24. (See Color Plate) Islet-cell carcinoma in the body of the pancreas. The tail of the pancreas is to the right. The tumor has a paler appearance than the surrounding pancreas. In addition, the tumor involves adjacent nodes shown on the inferior portion of the resected tissue. In general, islet-cell carcinomas are larger than benign tumors and metastasize regionally to nodes. The life expectancy of patients with islet-cell carcinoma is considerably longer than that of patients with acinar-cell pancreatic carcinoma [11].

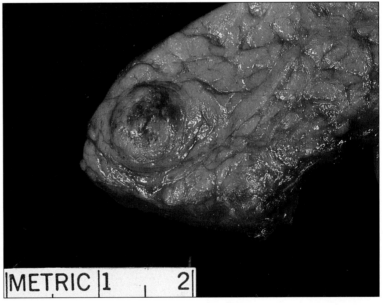

FIGURE 9-25. (See Color Plate) Solitary insulinoma slightly less than 2 cm in diameter embedded in the tail of the pancreas. The pancreatic duct is adjacent to the tumor, and the proximity of the tumor to the duct mandated distal pancreatectomy. Insulinomas are reddish-brown or gray, which distinguishes them from normal pancreatic tissue. In this case, the tumor is reddish-brown. These tumors also have a firmer consistency than normal pancreatic tissue.

Survival Rates and Recurrence

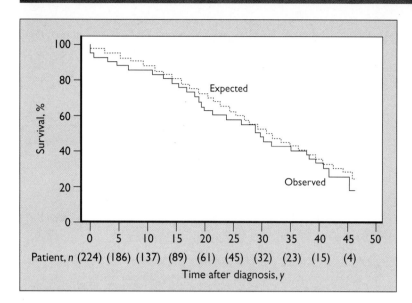

FIGURE 9-26. Survival after diagnosis of insulinoma (Mayo Clinic patients: 1927–1986). Among 224 patients whose initial surgery resulted in removal of an insulinoma at the Mayo Clinic, the overall survival rate (including the small number of patients with malignant insulinoma) was no different from the rate expected for the general population. (*Adapted from* Service *et al.* [11].)

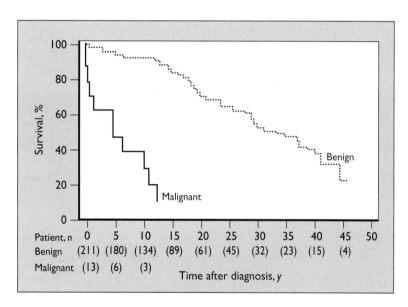

FIGURE 9-27. Survival rates for malignant insulinoma diagnosed on the basis of the presence of metastases at the time of pancreatic exploration (Mayo Clinic patients: 1927–1986). The 10-year rate was approximately 40%. Although this is far less than the survival rate seen in patients with benign insulinoma, it does exceed the rate associated with acinar-cell pancreatic carcinoma. (*Adapted from* Service *et al.* [11].)

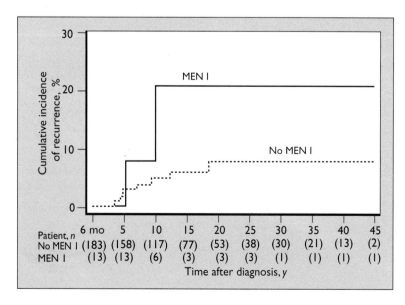

FIGURE 9-28. Recurrence rates in 224 patients whose initial surgery resulted in the removal of an insulinoma at the Mayo Clinic observed over a 60-year period (1927 to 1986) and followed for 45 years. Insulinomas did not recur within the first 4 years of follow-up, indicating that subsequent hyperinsulinemic hypoglycemia was not caused by persistent insulinoma. The recurrence rates were 7% for patients without multiple endocrine neoplasia (MEN) I syndrome and 21% for those with MEN I syndrome. No patient had a documented recurrence 20 years after the initial surgery. (*Adapted from* Service *et al.* [11].)

References

1. Service FJ: Hypoglycemic disorders. *N Engl J Med* 1995, 332:1144–1152.

2. Service FJ: Hypoglycemias. In *Cecil's Textbook of Medicine, Update 4*. Edited by Smith LH Jr. Philadelphia: WB Saunders; 1989.

3. Service FJ: Clinical presentations and laboratory evaluation of hypoglycemic disorders in adults. In *Hypoglycemic Disorder: Pathogenesis, Diagnosis and Treatment*. Edited by Service FJ. Boston: GK Hall; 1983:73–95.

4. Cryer PE: Glucose counter-regulation: the physiological mechanisms that prevent or correct hypoglycemia. In *Hypoglycaemia and Diabetes: Clinical and Physiological Aspects*. Edited by Frier BM, Fisher BM. London: Edward Arnold; 1993:34–55.

5. Service FJ, Nelson RL: Insulinoma. *Compr Ther* 1980, 6:70–74.

6. Rizza RA, Haymond MW, Verdonk CA, *et al.*: Pathogenesis of hypoglycemia in insulinoma patients: suppression of hepatic glucose production by insulin. *Diabetes* 1981, 30:377–381.

7. O'Brien T, O'Brien PC, Service FJ: Insulin surrogates in insulinoma. *J Clin Endocrinol Metab* 1993, 77:448–451.

8. Kudlow JE, Albisser AM, Angel A, *et al.*: Insulinoma resection facilitated by the artificial endocrine pancreas. *Diabetes* 1978, 27:774–777.

9. Doppman JL, Chang R, Fraker DL, *et al.*: Localization of insulinomas to regions of the pancreas by intra-arterial stimulation with calcium. *Ann Intern Med* 1995, 123:269–273.

10. Hassoun AAK, Service FJ, O'Brien PC: Glycated hemoglobin in insulinoma. *Endocr Pract* 1998, 4:181–183.

11. Service FJ, O'Brien PC, Kao PC, *et al.*: C-peptide suppression test: effects of gender, age and body mass index. Implications for the diagnosis of insulinoma. *J Clin Endocrinol Metab* 1992, 74:204–210.

12. Service FJ, Natt N, Thompson GB, *et al.*: Non-insulinoma pancreatogenous hypoglycemia: a novel syndrome of hyperinsulinemic hypoglycemia in adults independent of mutations in Kir6.2 and SUR1 genes. *J Clin Endocrin Metab* 1999, 84(5):1582–1589.

MECHANISMS OF HYPERGLYCEMIC DAMAGE IN DIABETES

Michael Brownlee

10

In the 21st century, the central therapeutic problem in diabetes mellitus is not management of its acute metabolic derangements but prevention and treatment of its chronic complications. In the United States, diabetes is the leading cause of new blindness in people ages 20 to 74 years, and the leading cause of end-stage renal disease. Diabetic patients are the fastest growing group of renal dialysis and transplant recipients. The life expectancy for patients with diabetic end-stage renal failure is only 3 or 4 years. Over 60% of diabetic patients are affected by neuropathy, which includes distal symmetrical polyneuropathy, mononeuropathies, and a variety of autonomic neuropathies causing erectile dysfunction, urinary incontinence, gastroparesis, and nocturnal diarrhea. Approximately 60% of type 2 diabetic patients have hypertension. Accelerated lower extremity arterial disease in conjunction with neuropathy makes diabetes account for 50% of all nontraumatic amputations in the United States. Diabetic patients have

a death rate from coronary heart disease that is two to four times that of nondiabetic patients. A similar increased risk occurs with stroke. Heart disease in diabetic patients appears earlier in life and more often is fatal. Life expectancy is about 7 to 10 years shorter for diabetic patients than for people without diabetes [1].

Epidemiologic studies show a strong relationship between glycemia and diabetic complications in both type 1 and type 2 diabetes. There is a continuous relationship between the level of glycemia and the risk of development and progression of complications. In this chapter, we review the mechanisms of hyperglycemic damage in diabetes. The discussion includes the specificity of target organ damage, the major mechanisms of hyperglycemic tissue damage, the relationship of various mechanisms to each other, the potential role of insulin resistance, the genetics of complication susceptibility, and the development of complications during post-hyperglycemic euglycemia.

Target-Organ Specificity of Hyperglycemic Damage

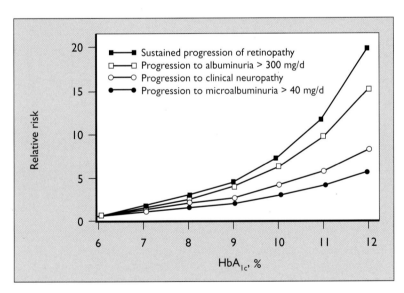

FIGURE 10-1. Relative risks for the development of diabetic complications at different levels of mean hemoglobin A_{1c} (HbA$_{1c}$, glycated hemoglobin), obtained from the Diabetes Control and Complications Trial. Patients with insulin-dependent diabetes whose intensive insulin therapy resulted in HbA$_{1c}$ values 2% lower than those receiving conventional insulin therapy had a **76%** lower incidence of retinopathy, a **54%** lower incidence of nephropathy, and a **60%** reduction in neuropathy. A relationship between level of chronic hyperglycemia and diabetic macrovascular disease has also been found in several recent studies. Thus, hyperglycemia is the primary initiating factor in the pathogenesis of diabetic complications. (*Adapted from* Skyler [1].)

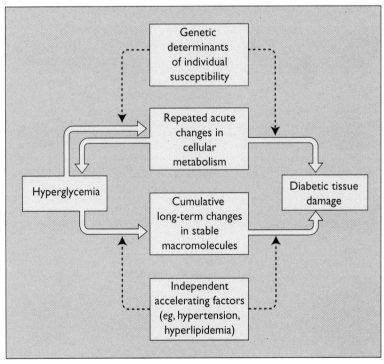

FIGURE 10-2. The mechanisms by which hyperglycemia and independent risk factors interact to cause chronic diabetic complications. One group of mechanisms involves repeated acute changes in cellular metabolism that are reversible when euglycemia is restored. Another group of mechanisms involves cumulative changes in long-lived macromolecules that persist despite restoration of euglycemia. These mechanisms are influenced by genetic determinants of susceptibility or resistance to hyperglycemic damage and by independent risk factors such as hypertension. (*Adapted from* Giardino and Brownlee [2].)

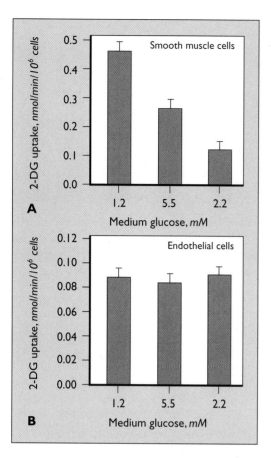

A

B

FIGURE 10-3. Lack of downregulation of glucose transport in cells affected by diabetic complications. Vascular smooth muscle cells, which are not damaged by hyperglycemia, show an inverse relationship between glucose concentration and glucose transport measured as 2-deoxyglucose (2-DG) uptake (**A**). In contrast, vascular endothelial cells, a major target of hyperglycemic damage, show no significant change in glucose transport when the glucose level is elevated (**B**). Thus, intracellular hyperglycemia appears to be the major determinant of diabetic tissue damage. (*Adapted from* Kaiser *et al.* [3].)

Major Mechanisms of Hyperglycemic Damage

MECHANISMS OF HYPERGLYCEMIA-INDUCED TISSUE DAMAGE

Formation of reactive oxygen species
Aldose reductase activity/redox changes
Diacylglycerol–protein kinase C activation
Formation of advanced glycation end products

FIGURE 10-4. Mechanisms of hyperglycemia-induced tissue damage. Four major hypotheses about how hyperglycemia causes diabetic complications have generated extensive data, as well as several clinical trials based on specific inhibitors of these mechanisms.

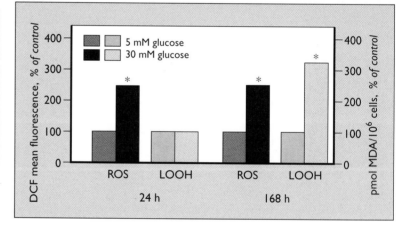

FIGURE 10-5. Hyperglycemia increases intracellular reactive oxygen species (ROS) and lipid peroxidation (LOOH). In aortic endothelial cells, 30 mmol of glucose/L increased ROS formation (measured as dichlorofluorescein [DCF]) by 250% within 24 hours, and resultant lipid peroxidation (measured as malondialdehyde [MDA]) by 330% within 168 hours. Thus, hyperglycemia rapidly increases intracellular ROS production in cells affected by diabetic complications. (*Adapted from* Giardino *et al.* [4].)

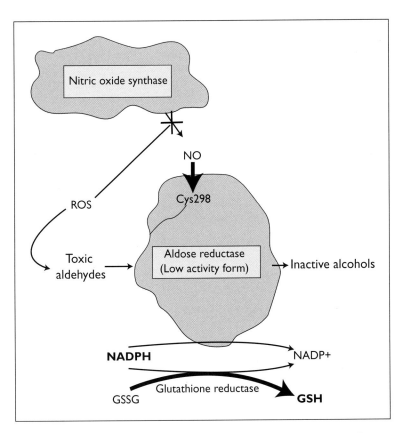

FIGURE 10-6. Potential function of aldose reductase in nondiabetic cells. The enzyme aldose reductase converts a variety of toxic aldehydes (such as 2-oxo-aldehydes and those derived from lipid peroxidation) to inactive alcohols. The reduced form of nicotinamide adenine dinucleotide phosphate (NADPH) is the cofactor in both this reaction and in the regeneration of glutathione by glutathione reductase. Reactive oxygen species (ROS) appear to reduce nitric oxide (NO) levels. The activity of aldose reductase is reversibly downregulated by nitric oxide modification of a cysteine residue in the enzyme's active site. GSH—reduced glutathione; GSSG—oxidized glutathione; NADP—nicotinamide adenine dinucleotide phosphate, oxidized form. (*Adapted from* Chandra et al. [5], Pieper et al. [6], and King and Brownlee [7].)

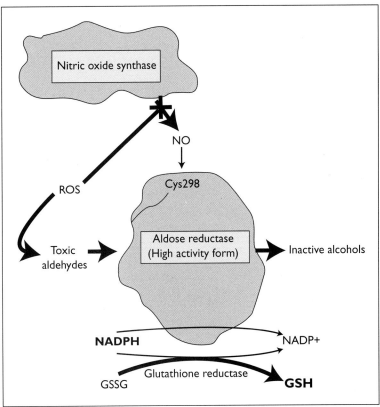

FIGURE 10-7. Potential function of aldose reductase in nondiabetic cells under oxidative stress. In a euglycemic environment, reactive oxygen species (ROS) increase the concentration of toxic aldehydes. At the same time, nitric oxide (NO) levels are reduced, thereby converting aldose reductase to a high activity form. Glutathione levels are unaffected. GSH—reduced glutathione; GSSG—oxidized glutathione; NADP—nicotinamide adenine dinucleotide phosphate, oxidized form; NADPH—nicotinamide adenine dinucleotide phosphate, reduced form. (*Adapted from* Chandra et al. [5], Pieper et al. [6], and King and Brownlee [7].)

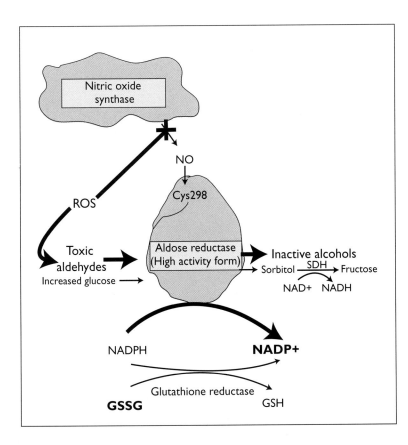

FIGURE 10-8. Potential function of aldose reductase in diabetic cells. In a hyperglycemic environment, reactive oxygen species (ROS) are increased, with the same consequences described in Figure 10-7. In addition, increased intracellular glucose levels result in increased enzymatic conversion to polyalcohol sorbitol and in concomitant decreases in levels of the reduced form of nicotinamide adenine dinucleotide phosphate (NADPH) and glutathione. In cells in which aldose reductase activity is sufficient to deplete glutathione, hyperglycemia-induced oxidative stress would be augmented. Sorbitol is oxidized to fructose by the enzyme sorbitol dehydrogenase (SDH). GSH—reduced glutathione; GSSG—oxidized glutathione; NAD—nicotinamide adenine dinucleotide; NADH—nicotinamide adenine dinucleotide, reduced form; NADP—nicotinamide adenine dinucleotide phosphate. (*Adapted from* Chandra et al. [5], Pieper et al. [6], and King and Brownlee [7].)

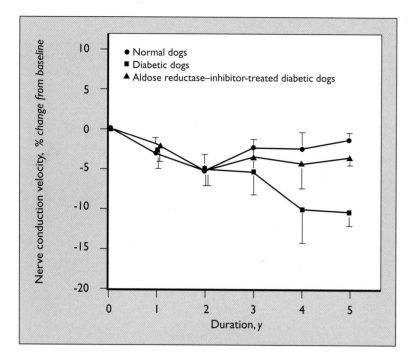

FIGURE 10-9. Effect of aldose reductase inhibition on diabetes-induced decreases in nerve conduction velocity. In diabetic dogs, conduction became significantly less than normal within 42 months. Conduction velocity in dogs treated with aldose reductase inhibitors remained statistically equal to normal throughout the 5-year study. In contrast, aldose reductase inhibition had no effect on the development of diabetic retinopathy. (*Adapted from* Engerman *et al.* [8].)

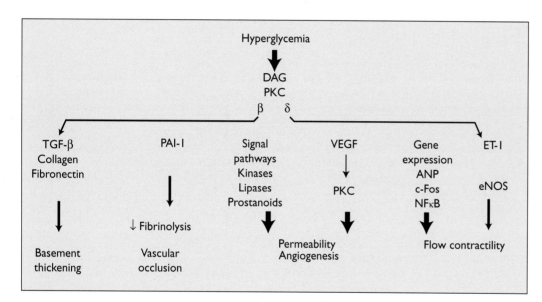

FIGURE 10-10. Potential consequences of hyperglycemia-induced diacylglycerol-protein kinase C activation. Hyperglycemia increases diacylglycerol (DAG) content, in part by de novo synthesis, and possibly also by phosphatidylcholine hydrolysis. Increased DAG activates protein kinase C (PKC), primarily the beta and delta isoforms. Activated PKC increases the production of cytokines and extracellular matrix, the fibrinolytic inhibitor PAI-1, and the vasoconstrictor endothelin-1 (ET-1). Protein kinase C is also a mediator of vascular endothelial growth factor (VEGF) activity. These changes would contribute to basement membrane thickening, vascular occlusion, increased permeability, and activation of angiogenesis. ANP—atrial natriuretic peptide; eNOS—endothelial nitric oxide synthase; TGF—transforming growth factor. (*Adapted from* Koya and King [9].)

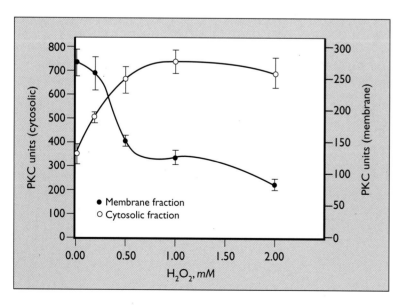

FIGURE 10-11. Reactive oxygen species (ROS) activate protein kinase C (PKC) in vascular endothelial cells. As ROS-producing H_2O_2 increases, it activates PKC. The mechanism appears to involve direct or indirect activation of phospholipase D, which hydrolyzes phosphatidylcholine to produce diacylglycerol (DAG). Reactive oxygen species could also increase DAG through increased de novo synthesis resulting from ROS inhibition of the enzyme glyceraldehyde-3-phosphate dehydrogenase. (*Adapted from* Taher *et al.* [10] and Schuppe-Koistinen *et al.* [11].)

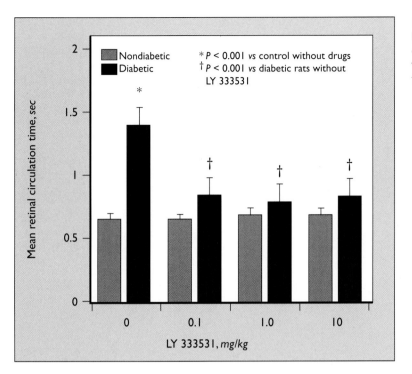

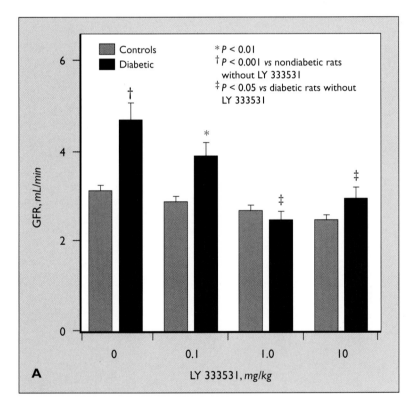

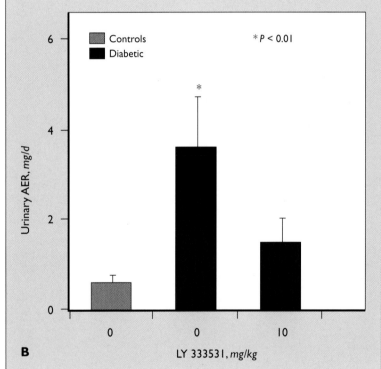

FIGURE 10-12. Amelioration of diabetes-induced retinal vascular dysfunction by an inhibitor of protein kinase C beta. In rats, diabetes increased mean retinal circulation time from 0.67 seconds to 1.40 seconds. In diabetic patients, treatment with the highest dose of the protein kinase C beta inhibitor LY 333531 reduced the time to 0.87 seconds. (*Adapted from* Ishii *et al.* [12].)

FIGURE 10-13. Amelioration of diabetes-induced renal dysfunction by an inhibitor of protein kinase C (PKC) beta. In rats, diabetes increased the glomerular filtration rate (GFR) from a mean of 3.0 to 4.6 mL/min. In diabetic patients, treatment with the highest dose of the PKC beta inhibitor LY 333531 normalized the mean GFR (**A**). Similarly, diabetes increased the albumin excretion rate in rats from a mean of 1.6 to 11.7 mg/d. Treatment of diabetic patients with the highest dose of LY 333531 reduced the mean albumin excretion rate to 4.9 mg/d (**B**). (*Adapted from* Ishii *et al.* [12].)

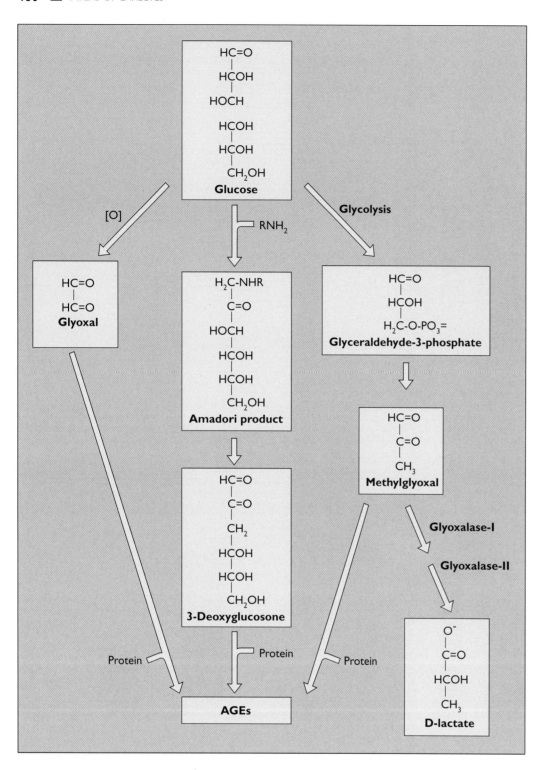

FIGURE 10-14. Potential pathways leading to the formation of advanced glycation end products (AGEs). The latter can arise from autoxidation of glucose to glyoxal, decomposition of the Amadori product to 3-deoxyglucosone, and fragmentation of glyceraldehyde-3-phosphate to methylglyoxal. These reactive dicarbonyls react with amino groups of proteins to form AGEs. Methylglyoxal and glyoxal are detoxified by the glyoxalase system. All three AGE precursors are also substrates for other reductases. (*Adapted from* Shinohara *et al.* [13] and Vander Jagt *et al.* [14])

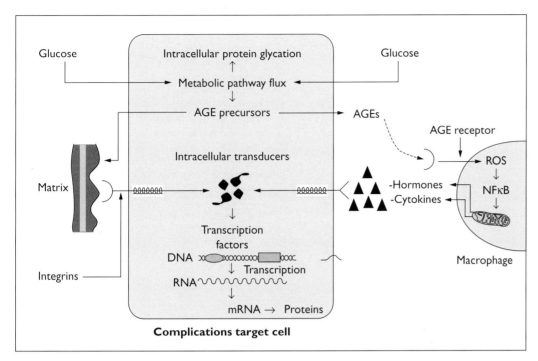

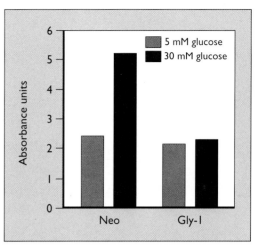

FIGURE 10-15. Intracellular production of advanced glycation end product (AGE) precursors damages target cells by three general mechanisms. First, intracellular protein glycation alters protein function. Second, extracellular matrix modified by AGE precursors has abnormal functional properties. Third, plasma proteins modified by AGE precursors bind to AGE receptors on adjacent cells, such as macrophages, thereby inducing receptor-mediated production of reactive oxygen species (ROS). The latter, in turn, activates NFκB and expression of pathogenic gene products, including cytokines and hormones. mRNA—messenger RNA. (*Adapted from* Brownlee [15].)

FIGURE 10-16. Intracellular protein glycation by the advanced glycation end product precursor methylglyoxal increases macromolecular endocytosis in endothelial cells. After exposure to 30 mmol of glucose/L, macromolecular endocytosis by GM7373 endothelial cells that were stably transfected with neomycin resistance gene (Neo) were increased 2.2-fold. In contrast, when increased methylglyoxal accumulation was prevented by overexpressing the enzyme glyoxalase I (Gly-1) in these cells, 30 mmol of glucose/L did not increase macromolecular endocytosis. (*Adapted from* Shinohara *et al.* [13].)

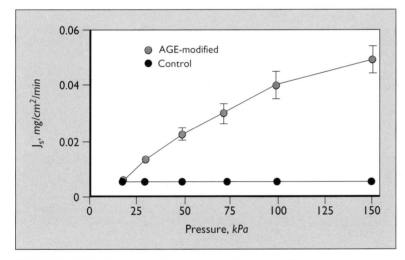

FIGURE 10-17. Glomerular basement membrane modified by advanced glycation end products (AGEs) has increased permeability to albumin. Ultrafiltration of albumin (J_s) by AGE-modified glomerular basement membrane is significantly increased compared with ultrafiltration of albumin by unmodified glomerular basement membrane over a range of different filtration pressures. (*Adapted from* Cochrane and Robinson [16].)

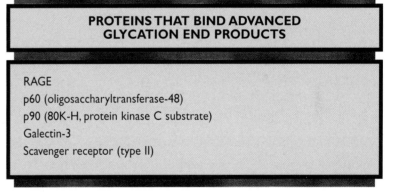

PROTEINS THAT BIND ADVANCED GLYCATION END PRODUCTS

RAGE

p60 (oligosaccharyltransferase-48)

p90 (80K-H, protein kinase C substrate)

Galectin-3

Scavenger receptor (type II)

FIGURE 10-18. Advanced glycation end product (AGE)–binding proteins and putative receptors. Five AGE-binding proteins have been identified. 1) RAGE (receptor for AGE) is a novel member of the immunoglobulin superfamily; its ligation generates reactive oxygen species and activates the pleiotropic transcription factor NFκB; 2) p60 exhibits 95% identity to OST-48, a component of the oligosaccharyltransferase complex in microsomal membranes; 3) p90 has significant sequence homology with human 80K-H, a substrate of protein kinase C; 4) galectin-3, a carbohydrate-binding protein, also binds AGEs; 5) the type II macrophage scavenger receptor binds AGEs and mediates their uptake by endocytosis. RAGE—receptor for AGE. (*Adapted from* Yan *et al.* [17], Li *et al.* [18], Vlassara *et al.* [19], and Araki *et al.* [20].)

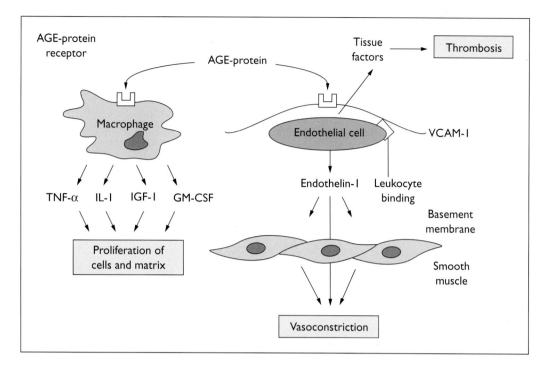

FIGURE 10-19. The mechanisms by which advanced glycation end product (AGE)–modified protein binding to specific receptors on macrophages and endothelial cells may cause pathologic changes in diabetic blood vessels. On macrophages and mesangial cells, binding stimulates production of tumor necrosis factor (TNF)-α, interleukin-1 (IL-1), insulin-like growth factor-1 (IGF-1), and granulocyte-macrophage colony-stimulating factor (GM-CSF) at levels that increase proliferation of smooth muscle cells and increase matrix production. On endothelial cells, binding induces procoagulatory changes in gene expression and increased expression of leukocyte-binding vascular adhesion molecule-1 (VCAM-1). (*Adapted from* Brownlee [21].)

EFFECT OF AMINOGUANIDINE TREATMENT ON DIABETIC TARGET TISSUES

Variable	Nondiabetic Animals	Diabetic Animals	Diabetic Animals Receiving Aminoguanidine Treatment
Retinal acellular capillaries, mm^2	9±2	167±27	33±11
Retinal microaneurysms, % *positive*	0	37.5	0
Urinary albumin excretion, *mg/24 h*	2.4±1.3	38.9±1.4	5.1±1.5
Mesangial volume fraction, %	12.5±2.5	18.8±2.5	13.7±0.6
Motor nerve conduction velocity, *m/sec*	65.5±2	52.4±3	64±2
Nerve action potential amplitude, %	100	63	97
Arterial elasticity, *nL/mm Hg/mm*	–	7.5±1.5	10.8±3
Arterial fluid filtration, *nL/mm*	–	0.9	0.45

FIGURE 10-20. Amelioration of abnormalities in diabetic target tissues by an advanced glycation end product inhibitor. The effects of this inhibitor (aminoguanidine) on diabetic abnormalities have been investigated in the retina, kidney, nerve, and artery. In experimental animals, the development of all pathognomonic abnormalities examined was inhibited by 85% to 90%. In a large randomized, double-blind, placebo-controlled, multicenter study of type 1 diabetic patients with overt nephropathy, aminoguanidine treatment lowered total urinary protein and slowed progression of nephropathy. In addition, aminoguanidine reduced the progression of diabetic retinopathy (Bolton *et al.*, unpublished data). (*Adapted from* Brownlee [15].)

Interrelationship of Mechanisms of Hyperglycemic Damage

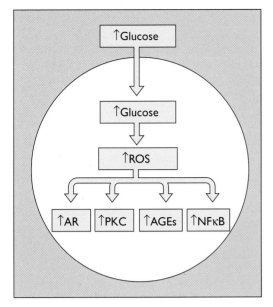

FIGURE 10-21. Overproduction of superoxide by the mitochondrial electron transport chain. Until recently, there has been no apparent common element linking the different biochemical mechanisms underlying diabetic complications. This issue has now been resolved by the recent discovery that each of the different pathogenic mechanisms reflects a single hyperglycemia-induced process: overproduction of superoxide by the mitochondrial electron transport chain. In cells in which intracellular glycemia reflects blood glucose (like endothelial cells), increased generation of nicotinamide adenine dinucleotide in the tricarboxylic acid cycle results in excess mitochondrial superoxide generation. This superoxide increases flux through aldose reductase (AR), activates protein kinase C (PKC), increases intracellular formation of advanced glycation end product (AGE) precursors, and activates the pleiotrophic transcription factor NFκB. Superoxide also increases flux through the hexosamine pathway (not shown) [22]. ROS—reactive oxygen species.

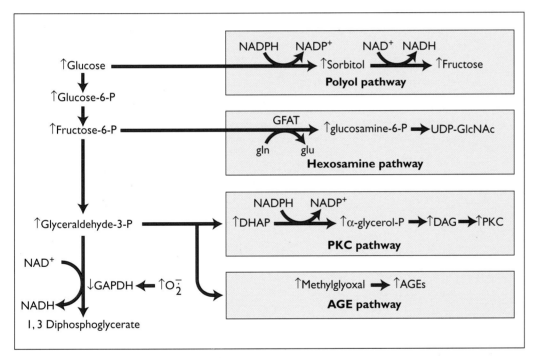

FIGURE 10-22. Potential mechanism by which hyperglycemia-induced mitochondrial superoxide overproduction activates four pathways of hyperglycemic damage. Excess superoxide partially inhibits the glycolytic enzyme-reduced glyceraldehyde-phosphate dehydrogenase (GAPDH), thereby diverting upstream metabolites from glycolysis into pathways of glucose overutilization. This results in increased flux of dihydroxyacetone phosphate (DHAP) to diacylglycerol (DAG), an activator of protein kinase C (PKC), and of triose phosphates to methylglyoxal, the main intracellular advanced glycation end product (AGE) precursor. Increased flux of fructose-6-phosphate to UDP-N-acetylglucosamine increases modification of proteins by N-acetylglucosamine (GlcNAc), and increased glucose flux through the polyol pathway consumes nicotinamide adenine dinucleotide phosphate (NADPH) and depletes the intracellular antioxidant-reduced glutathione. GFAT—glutamine: fructose-6-phosphate amidotransferase; gln—glucosamine; glu—glutamine; NAD—nicotinamide adenine dinucleotide; NADH—nicotinamide adenine dinucleotide, reduced form; NADP—nicotinamide adenine dinucleotide phosphate; UDP—uridine diphosphate.

Potential Role of Insulin Resistance

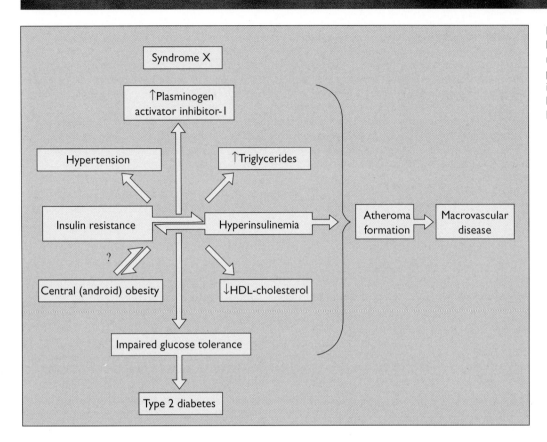

FIGURE 10-23. Insulin resistance may exacerbate known risk factors for vascular damage. Insulin resistance is associated with atherogenic changes in plasma lipoproteins, increased plasminogen activator inhibitor-1 levels, and hypertension. This association has been termed "syndrome X." HDL—high-density lipoprotein. (*Adapted from* Gray and Yudkin [23].)

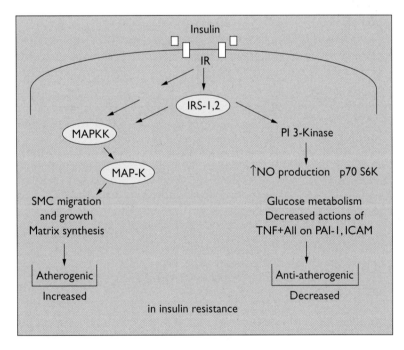

FIGURE 10-24. Insulin resistance (IR) in vascular cells may promote damage by inhibiting antiatherogenic gene expression. Selective resistance to insulin action in the phosphatidylinositol (PI) 3-kinase signaling pathway may reduce antiproliferative nitric oxide (NO) production and interfere with insulin's inhibitory effect on tumor necrosis factor (TNF) and the stimulation of PAI-1 and intracellular adhesion molecule (ICAM) expression by angiotensin II. IRS—insulin receptor substrate; MAP-K—mitogen-activated protein kinase; MAPKK—mitogen-activated protein kinase kinase; SMC—smooth muscle cell. (*Adapted from* King and Brownlee [7].)

Genetics of Susceptibility to Complications

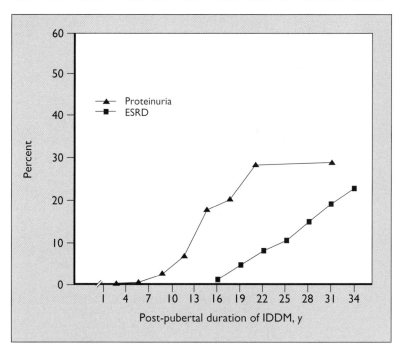

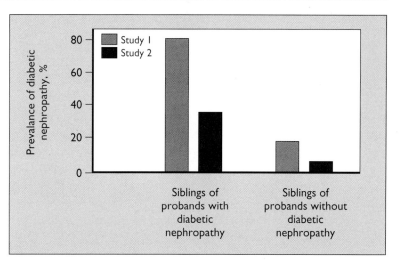

FIGURE 10-25. Prevalence of clinically significant diabetic nephropathy in patients with insulin-dependent diabetes (IDDM) according to diabetes duration. The cumulative incidence of overt proteinuria levels off at 27%. After 34 years of diabetes, the cumulative incidence of end-stage renal disease (ESRD) is 21.4%. These data suggest that only a subset of patients are susceptible to the development of clinical nephropathy. (*Adapted from* Krolewski *et al.* [24].)

FIGURE 10-26. Familial clustering of diabetic nephropathy suggests a major genetic effect. In one study, the risk for nephropathy was 83% in diabetic siblings of an affected patient compared with 16% in diabetic siblings of an unaffected patient. In another study, the risks were 33% and 10%, respectively. Familiar clustering has also been reported for diabetic retinopathy and for coronary artery calcification. (*Adapted from* Trevisan *et al.* [25].)

Development of Complications During Posthyperglycemic Euglycemia

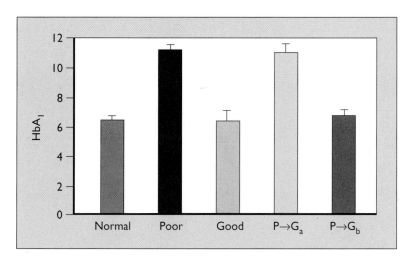

FIGURE 10-27. Development of retinopathy during posthyperglycemic normoglycemia ("hyperglycemic memory"). Shown are mean hemoglobin A(HbA_1) values for dogs in one study [26]. Normal dogs were compared to diabetic dogs that had had poor control for 5 years, good control for 5 years, or poor control for 2.5 years ($P{\rightarrow}G_a$) followed by good control for the next 2.5 years ($P{\rightarrow}G_b$). Values for both the good control group and the $P{\rightarrow}G_b$ group were identical to those in the normal group. (*Adapted from* Engerman and Kern [26].)

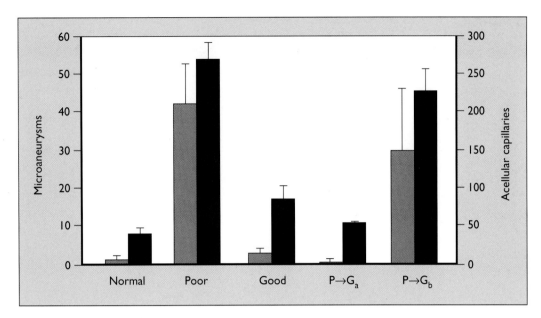

FIGURE 10-28. Development of retinopathy during posthyperglycemic normoglycemia ("hyperglycemic memory"). Shown is quantitation of retinal microaneurysms and acellular capillaries in one study [26]. Lesions of diabetic retinopathy developed during 5 years of poor control. Good control almost always prevented this abnormality. After 2.5 years of poor control (P→G_a), retinopathy was absent. However, despite the institution of good control in this group after 2.5 years (P→G_b), retinopathy developed over the next 2.5 years to an extent almost equal to that seen in the 5-year poor control group. (*Adapted from* Engerman and Kern [26].)

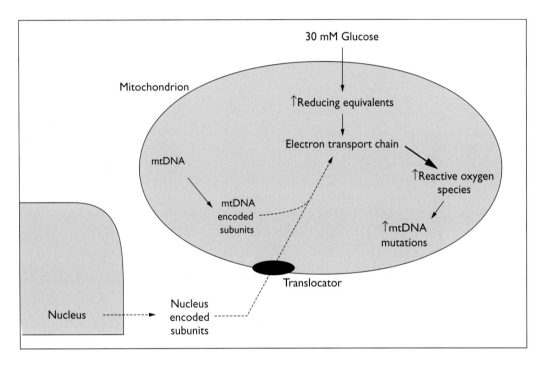

FIGURE 10-29. Potential mechanism for hyperglycemic memory. Hyperglycemia-induced increases in reactive oxygen species are a consequence of increased reducing equivalents generated from increased glucose metabolism flowing through the mitochondrial electron transport chain. The increased production of reactive oxygen species would not only increase aldose reductase activity, protein kinase C activity, and formation of advanced glycation end products, but would also induce mutations in mitochondrial DNA (mtDNA). (*Adapted from* Wei [27] and Nishikawa *et al.* [28].)

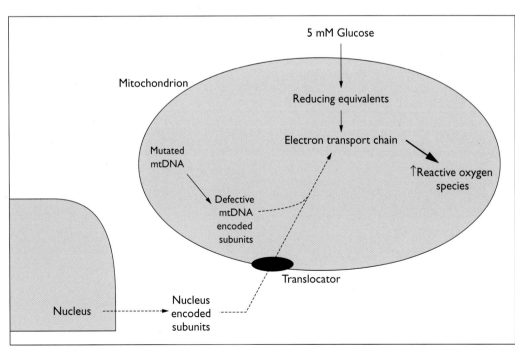

FIGURE 10-30. Potential mechanism for hyperglycemic memory. Mitochondrial DNA (mtDNA) mutated by hyperglycemia-induced reactive oxygen species would encode defective electron transport chain subunits. These defective subunits would cause increased production of reactive oxygen species by the electron transport chain at physiologic concentrations of glucose and glucose-derived reducing equivalents. (*Adapted from* Wei [27] and Nishikawa *et al.* [28].)

References

1. Skyler J: Diabetic complications: the importance of glucose control. *Endocrinol Metab Clin North Am* 1996, 25(2):243–245.

2. Giardino J, Brownlee M: Mechanisms of chronic diabetic complications. In *Textbook of Diabetes,* vol 1. Edited by Pickup JC, Williams G. London: Blackwell Scientific; 1997.

3. Kaiser N, Sasson S, Feener EP: Differential regulation of glucose transport and transporters by glucose in vascular endothelial and smooth muscle cells. *Diabetes* 1993, 42:80–89.

4. Giardino I, Edelstein D, Brownlee M: BCL-2 expression or antioxidants prevent hyperglycemia-induced formation of intracellular advanced glycation endproducts in bovine endothelial cells. *J Clin Invest* 1996, 97:1422–1428.

5. Chandra A, Srivastava S, Petrash JM: Active site modification of aldose reductase by nitric oxide donors. *Biochim Biophys Acta* 1997, 131:217–222.

6. Pieper GM, Langenstroer P, Siebeneich W: Diabetic-induced endothelial dysfunction in rat aorta: role of hydroxyl radicals. *Cardiovasc Res* 1997, 34:145–156.

7. King GL, Brownlee MB: The cellular and molecular mechanisms of diabetic complications. *Endocrinol Metab Clin North Am* 1996, 25(2):255–270.

8. Engerman RL, Kern TS, Larson ME: Nerve conduction and aldose reductase inhibition during 5 years of diabetes or galactosaemia in dogs. *Diabetologia* 1994, 37:141–144.

9. Koya D, King GL: Protein kinase C activation and the development of diabetic complications. *Diabetes* 1998, 47:859–867.

10. Taher MM, Garcia JG, Natarajian V: Hydroperoxide-induced diacylglycerol formation and protein kinase C activation in vascular endothelial cells. *Arch Biochem Biophys* 1993, 303:260–266.

11. Schuppe-Koistinen I, Modéus P, Bergman T, Cotgreave IA: S-thiolation of human endothelial cell glyceraldehyde-3-phosphate dehydrogenase after hydrogen peroxide treatment. *Eur J Biochem* 1994, 221:1033–1037.

12. Ishii H, Jirousek MR, Koya D, et al.: Amelioration of vascular dysfunctions in diabetic rats by an oral PKC beta inhibitor. *Science* 1996, 272:728–731.

13. Shinohara M, Thornalley PJ, Giardino I, et al.: Overexpression of glyoxalase-1 in bovine endothelial cells inhibits intracellular advanced glycation endproduct formation and prevents hyperglycemia-induced increases in macromolecular endocytosis. *J Clin Invest* 1998, 101(5):1142–1147.

14. Vander Jagt DL, Torres JE, Hunsaker LA, et al.: Physiological substrates of human aldose and aldehyde reductases. *Adv Exp Med Biol* 1997, 414:491–497.

15. Brownlee M: Glycation and diabetic complications. *Diabetes* 1994, 43:836–841.

16. Cochrane SM, Robinson GB: In vitro glycation of glomerular basement membrane alters its permeability: a possible mechanism in diabetic complications. *FEBS Lett* 1995, 375:41–44.

17. Yan SD, Schmidt AM, Anderson GM, et al.: Enhanced cellular oxidant stress by the interaction of advanced glycation end products with their receptors/binding proteins. *J Biol Chem* 1994, 269:9889–9897.

18. Li YM, Mitsuhashi T, Wojciechowicz D, et al.: Molecular identity and cellular distribution of advanced glycation endproduct receptors: relationship of p60 to OST-48 and p90 to 80K-H membrane proteins. *Proc Natl Acad Sci U S A* 1996, 93:11047–11052.

19. Vlassara H, Li YM, Imani F, et al.: Identification of galectin-3 as a high-affinity binding protein for advanced glycation end products (AGE): a new member of the AGE-receptor complex. *Mol Med* 1995, 1:634–646.

20. Araki N, Higashi T, Mori T, et al.: Macrophage scavenger receptor mediates the endocytic uptake and degradation of advanced glycation end products of the Maillard reaction. *Eur J Biochem* 1995, 230:408–415.

21. Brownlee M: Advanced glycation end products in diabetic complications. *Curr Opin Endocrinol Diabetes* 1998, 3:291–297.

22. Brownlee M: Biochemistry and molecular cell biology of diabetic complications. *Nature* 2001, 414:813–820.

23. Gray RP, Yudkin JS: Cardiovascular disease in diabetic mellitus. In *Textbook of Diabetes*, vol. 1. Edited by Pickup JC, Williams G. London: Blackwell Scientific; 1997.

24. Krolewski SA, Warram JH, Freire MB, et al.: Epidemiology of late diabetic complications: a basis for the development and evaluation of prevention programs. *Endocrinol Metab Clin North Am* 1996, 25(2):217–242.

25. Trevisan R, Barnes DJ, et al.: Pathogenesis of diabetic nephropathy. In *Textbook of Diabetes*, vol. 2. Edited by Pickup JC, Williams G. London: Blackwell Scientific; 1997.

26. Engerman RL, Kern TS: Progression of incipient diabetic retinopathy during good glycemic control. *Diabetes* 1987, 36:808–812.

27. Wei Y: Oxidative stress and mitochondrial DNA mutations in human aging. *Soc Exp Biol Med* 1998, 217:53–63.

28. Nishikawa T, Edelstein D, Brownlee MB, et al.: Reversal of hyperglycemia-induced PKC activation, intracellular AGE formation, and sorbitol accumulation by inhibition of electron transport complex II. *Diabetes* 1999, 48(Suppl):A73.

EYE COMPLICATIONS OF DIABETES

Lloyd Paul Aiello

11

Diabetic retinopathy is a well-characterized, sight-threatening, chronic, ocular disorder that eventually develops to some degree in nearly all patients with diabetes mellitus. With experienced ophthalmic evaluation, diabetic retinopathy can be detected in its early stages. Existing therapies are remarkably effective when administered at the appropriate time in the disease process. In addition, improvement of systemic glycemic control is associated with a delay in onset and slowing of progression of diabetic retinopathy. Nevertheless, diabetic retinopathy is the leading cause of new cases of legal blindness among Americans between the ages of 20 and 74 years. The pathologic changes associated with diabetic retinopathy are similar in types 1 and 2 diabetes mellitus, although there is a higher risk of more frequent and severe ocular complications in type 1 diabetes [1]. However, because more patients have type 2 than type 1 disease, patients with type 2 disease account for a higher proportion of those with visual loss.

Most visual loss associated with diabetes results from either new vessel growth on the retina (proliferative diabetic retinopathy [PDR]) or increased retinal vascular permeability (diabetic macular edema). The clinical stage associated with the greatest risk of severe visual loss is termed *high-risk PDR*, while the stage with the greatest risk of moderate visual loss is termed *clinically significant macular edema* (CSME). In the United States, an estimated 700,000 persons have PDR, 130,000 have high-risk PDR, 500,000 have macular edema, and 325,000 have CSME [2–5]. An estimated 63,000 cases of PDR, 29,000 of high-risk PDR, 80,000 of macular edema, 56,000 of CSME, and 5000 new cases of legal blindness occur yearly as a result of diabetic retinopathy [1,6]. Blindness has been estimated to be 25 times more common in persons with diabetes than in those without the disease [7,8].

Estimates of the medical and economic impact of retinopathy-associated morbidity have been performed using computer simulations. The models predict that if patients with type 1 disease receive treatment as recommended in the clinical trials in the absence of good glycemic control, a savings of $624 million and 173,540 person-years of sight would be realized [3,4]. The Diabetes Control and Complication Trial (DCCT) showed that the rate of development of any retinopathy and, once present, the rate of retinopathy progression were significantly reduced after 3 years of intensive insulin therapy [9,10]. Subsequent studies have confirmed a continuing benefit of intensive insulin therapy [11]. Applying DCCT intensive insulin therapy to all persons with insulin-dependent diabetes mellitus in the United States would result in a gain of 920,000 person-years of sight, although the costs of intensive therapy are three times that of conventional therapy [12,13].

An understanding of the pathogenesis, natural history, and available treatment options for patients with diabetic retinopathy is critical for all health care providers, because current therapeutic options can be remarkably effective at preventing severe visual loss when administered in an appropriate and timely manner. Indeed, with appropriate medical and ophthalmologic care, over 90% of visual loss resulting from diabetic retinopathy can be prevented [14,15].

Anatomy, Symptoms, and Pathology

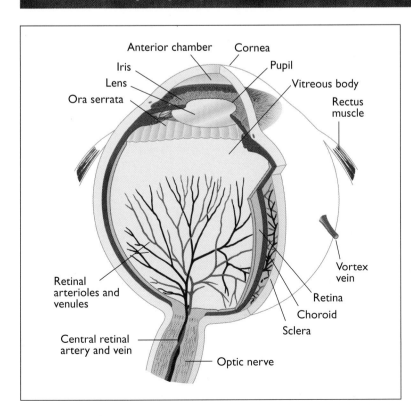

FIGURE 11-1. Normal ocular anatomy. This schematic cross-section shows the normal anatomy of the human eye. Diabetes can affect almost all ocular structures (*see* Fig. 11-2). However, the characteristic and most common changes occur in the retina and are termed *diabetic retinopathy*. Most of the severe sight-threatening complications involve either pathologic growth of vessels (neovascularization) in the retina or increased retinal vessel permeability [15]. These conditions are termed *proliferative diabetic retinopathy* and *diabetic macular edema*, respectively. Neovascularization also can arise at the iris, potentially leading to neovascular glaucoma.

Labels in figure: Anterior chamber, Cornea, Iris, Pupil, Lens, Vitreous body, Ora serrata, Rectus muscle, Vortex vein, Retinal arterioles and venules, Retina, Choroid, Sclera, Central retinal artery and vein, Optic nerve

OCULAR STRUCTURES AFFECTED BY DIABETES

Ocular Structure	Diabetes-associated Pathology
Lids, nerves, and muscles	Palsy of cranial nerves III, IV, or VI
Cornea	Reduced sensitivity
	Increased susceptibility to corneal erosions
	Increased susceptibility to infection (corneal ulcers)
Anterior chamber	Hyphema (blood)
	Shallowing with longer disease duration
Iris	Neovascularization
	Depigmentation
Lens	Increased susceptibility to cataract
Vitreous	Vitreous hemorrhage
	Early posterior vitreous detachment
	Asteroid hyalosis
Retina	Retinal hemorrhages
	Microaneurysms
	Venous beading
	Intraretinal microvascular abnormalities
	Capillary vessel loss
	Neovascularization
	Edema
	Lipid deposits
Optic disc	Neovascularization
	Diabetic papillopathy (swelling)
Sclera and other tissues	Delayed wound healing

FIGURE 11-2. Diabetes can affect most structures of the human eye [16]. Diabetes-induced ischemia of cranial nerves III, IV, and VI can result in drooping of the lids, ocular motility abnormalities, or both as a result of impaired innervation of the ocular muscles. Corneal erosions, corneal ulcers, cataracts, and delayed wound healing also reflect the general diabetic state. However, most visual loss associated with diabetes arises from complications involving neovascularization of the retina (or iris) or increased vasopermeability of the retinal vasculature.

CLINICAL PRESENTATIONS OF DIABETIC EYE COMPLICATIONS

Diabetes-associated Pathology	Clinical Symptoms
Palsy of cranial nerves III, IV, VI	Diplopia: binocular
	Ptosis
	Anisocoria
	"Blurred vision"
Reduced corneal sensitivity or corneal erosions or corneal infections	Ocular pain
	Ocular discharage
	Corneal opacification
	Decreased vision
Hyphema	Decreased vision
	Blood layering in anterior chamber
Angle closure glaucoma	Ocular pain
	"Halos" around lights
	Decreased vision
Iris neovascularization	Ocular pain
	Decreased vision
	Blood layering in anterior chamber
Cataract	Decreased vision
	Glare with bright lights
Vitreous hemorrhage	"Spots," "cobwebs," "lines" in vision (floaters)
	Decreased vision
Macular edema	Moderately decreased vision
	Image distortion
Proliferative diabetic retinopathy	Symptoms associated with vitreous hemorrhage and macular edema
Retina detachment	Photopsia
	Floaters
	Scotoma
	Decreased vision
	Image distortion
Diabetic papillopathy	Visual field change

FIGURE 11-3. Clinical presentations associated with diabetic eye complications. Each of the numerous diabetes-associated ocular pathologies can present with a diverse array of symptoms. Only a partial list is presented here. It is important to realize that serious diabetic eye disease may exist *without any discernible symptoms.* This fact underscores the essential need for regular, routine, lifelong follow-up regardless of the presence or absence of visual symptoms.

OCULAR PATHOLOGY ASSOCIATED WITH RETINOPATHY PROGRESSION

Disease Stage	Common Pathologic Changes
Preclinical stages	Alterations in cellular biochemistry
	Alterations in retinal blood flow
	Loss of retinal pericytes
	Thickening of basement membranes
Early stages	Retinal vascular microaneurysms
Mild NPDR	and blot hemorrhages
	Increased retinal vascular permeability
	Cotton wool spots
Middle stages	Venous caliber changes or beading
Moderate NPDR	IRMAs
Severe NPDR	Retinal capillary loss
Very severe NPDR	Retinal ischemia
	Extensive intraretinal hemorrhages and microaneurysms
Advanced stages	Neovascularization of the disc
PDR	Neovascularization elsewhere
	Neovascularization of the iris
	Neovascular glaucoma
	Pre-retinal and vitreous hemorrhage
	Fibrovascular proliferation
	Retinal traction, retinal tears, retinal detachment

FIGURE 11-4. Ocular pathology associated with progression of diabetic retinopathy. Diabetic retinopathy generally progresses through well-characterized stages. Each stage is associated with typical pathologic changes. Some degree of clinically apparent retinopathy occurs in nearly all patients with diabetes of 20 or more years' duration, although preclinical alterations in blood flow, pericyte number, and basement membrane thickness can occur much earlier [17]. The clinical stages before the development of neovascularization are termed *nonproliferative diabetic retinopathy* (NPDR). NPDR is subdivided into mild, moderate, severe, or very severe categories, depending on the type and extent of clinical pathology present. Increased vascular permeability can occur at this or any later stage. As the disease progresses, gradual loss of the retinal microvasculature results in retinal ischemia. Venous caliber abnormalities, intraretinal microvascular abnormalities (IRMAs), and more severe vascular leakage are common reflections of this increasing retinal nonperfusion (*see* Fig. 11-7). Once ischemia-induced neovascularization occurs, the disease is referred to as proliferative diabetic retinopathy (PDR) (*see* Fig. 11-9). Neovascularization can arise at the optic disc (neovascularization of the disc) or elsewhere in the retina (neovascularization elsewhere). The new vessels are fragile and prone to bleeding, resulting in vitreous hemorrhage. With time, the neovascularization tends to undergo fibrosis and contraction, resulting in retinal traction, retinal tears, vitreous hemorrhage, and retinal detachment (*see* Fig. 11-13). New vessels also can arise on the iris, resulting in neovascular glaucoma (*see* Fig. 11-14). (*Adapted from* Aiello *et al.* [15].)

Nonproliferative Diabetic Retinopathy

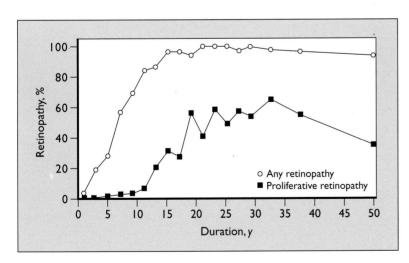

FIGURE 11-5. Incidence of diabetic retinopathy by duration of diabetes. The percentage of patients developing either any diabetic retinopathy or proliferative diabetic retinopathy is presented as a function of duration of type 1 diabetes in years. Note that almost all patients have some evidence of diabetic retinopathy once the duration of diabetes exceeds 15 years. In addition, the incidence of proliferative diabetic retinopathy (PDR) is negligible within 5 years of the onset of diabetes, although nearly 60% of patients eventually will develop PDR. These observations serve as the foundation for clinical care recommendations concerning the appropriate timing of initial ophthalmologic evaluation, as detailed in Figure 11-6. (*Adapted from* Krolewski *et al.* [18].)

INITIAL OPHTHALMOLOGIC EXAMINATION SCHEDULE

Age at Onset of Diabetes Mellitus	Recommended First Examination	Minimum Routine Follow-up*
29 years or younger	Within 3–5 years after diagnosis of diabetes Once patient is age 10 years or older	Yearly
30 years or older	At time of diagnosis of diabetes	Yearly
Patient becomes pregnant	Before conception and during first trimester	Physician discretion pending results of first trimester examination

*Abnormal findings necessitate more frequent follow-up.

FIGURE 11-6. Only about 25% of patients with type 1 diabetes will have any retinopathy after 5 years, although most eventually will develop the disease (see Fig. 11-5) [19]. The prevalence of PDR is less than 2% at 5 years. For patients with type 2 disease, however, the onset date of diabetes frequently is not known precisely, and thus, more severe disease can be observed soon after diagnosis. Up to 3% of patients first diagnosed after age 30 may have clinically significant macular edema or high-risk PDR at the time of initial diagnosis of diabetes [20]. Thus, in patients over age 10, the initial ophthalmic examination is recommended beginning 5 years after the diagnosis of type 1 diabetes mellitus and on diagnosis of type 2 diabetes mellitus [15]. The onset of vision-threatening retinopathy is rare in children before puberty, regardless of the duration of diabetes; however, if diabetes is diagnosed between the ages of 10 and 30 years, significant retinopathy may arise within 6 years [2]. Puberty can accelerate the progression of retinopathy. Thus, the initial ophthalmic evaluation is recommended within 3 to 5 years of diagnosis, once the patient is aged 10 years or older [15,21]. The onset of puberty is occurring progressively earlier, and consequently the timing of initial evaluation of children is under periodic review. Diabetic retinopathy also can become particularly aggressive during pregnancy in women with diabetes [22]. Ideally, patients with diabetes who are planning pregnancy should have an eye examination within 1 year of conception. Pregnant women should have a comprehensive eye examination in the first trimester of pregnancy. Close follow-up throughout pregnancy is indicated, with subsequent examinations determined by the findings present at the first trimester examination. This guideline does not apply to women who develop gestational diabetes because they are not at increased risk of developing diabetic retinopathy. (*Adapted from* Aiello *et al.* [15].)

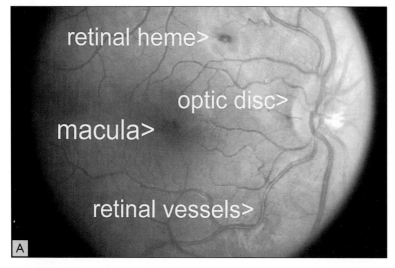

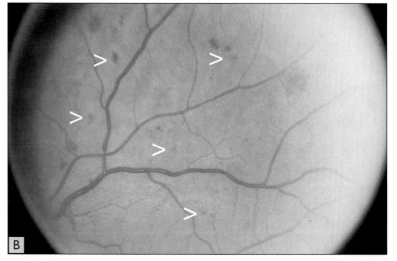

FIGURE 11-7. (See Color Plate) Characteristic findings in nonproliferative diabetic retinopathy (NPDR). The classic findings associated with NPDR are demonstrated. **A,** The central region of the human retina is called the macula and is responsible for detailed vision. This patient's right eye has minimal diabetic retinopathy, and the retina is normal except for a single retinal hemorrhage (retinal heme). The optic disc is located nasal to the macula, and the retinal vessels emanate from the optic disc and surround the macula. **B,** Retinal blot hemorrhages (*arrows*) and microaneurysms, which are saccular dilations of the vessel wall. These lesions often are two of the earliest clinically observed abnormalities. The patient has severe NPDR when hemorrhages and microaneurysms of this extent or greater in all four quadrants of the retina are observed.

(Continued on next page)

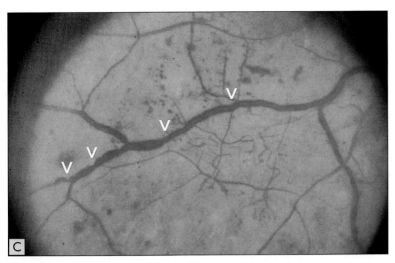

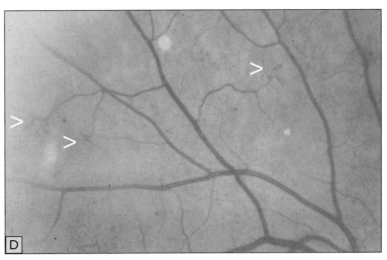

FIGURE 11-7. (*Continued*) **C,** Venous caliber changes referred to as *venous beading*. This finding often represents more advanced retinopathy, as is evident in this photograph (*arrows*). Two or more retinal quadrants of any venous beading (not necessarily as pronounced as shown) signify severe NPDR. **D,** *Arrows* show intraretinal microvascular abnormalities (IRMAs). IRMAs are abnormalities within the retina and may be a harbinger of early retinal neovascularization. IRMAs

often are associated with more advanced NPDR, and only one or more retinal quadrants of IRMAs of this or greater extent represent severe NPDR. Note that the clinical findings associated with severe NPDR therefore may be quite subtle. Any two or more of the findings associated with severe NPDR place the patient in the very severe category of NPDR. (*Panels B, C,* and *D from* The Early Treatment Diabetic Retinopathy Study Research Group [23]; with permission.)

Proliferative Diabetic Retinopathy and Macular Edema

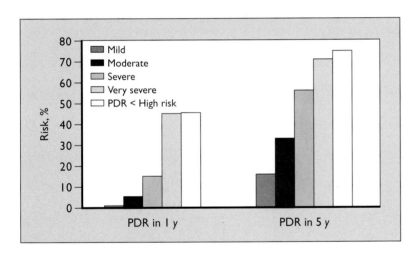

FIGURE 11-8. Progression to high-risk proliferative diabetic retinopathy (PDR) becomes more likely as the severity of nonproliferative diabetic retinopathy (NPDR) increases. Demonstrated is the likelihood of developing high-risk PDR (see Fig. 11-9) within 1 or 5 years for patients with mild, moderate, severe, and very severe levels of NPDR or PDR with less than high-risk characteristics. High-risk PDR is associated with the greatest incidence of severe and irreversible visual loss. Each increase in NPDR severity level is associated with an increase in progression to the sight-threatening proliferative stage of the disease. The known progression rates permit determination of appropriate intervals between follow-up ocular evaluations for patients with differing levels of diabetic retinopathy. Typically, follow-up ocular evaluations are performed as follows: annually for no retinopathy, every 6 to 12 months for mild to moderate NPDR, every 3 to 4 months for severe to very severe NPDR, and every 2 to 3 months for PDR that is less than high risk [15]. (*Adapted from* The Early Treatment Diabetic Retinopathy Study Research Group [24].)

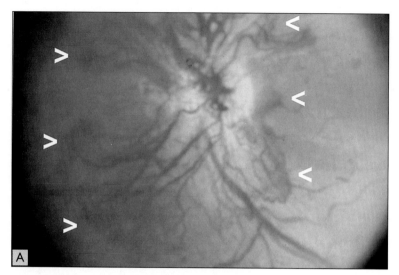

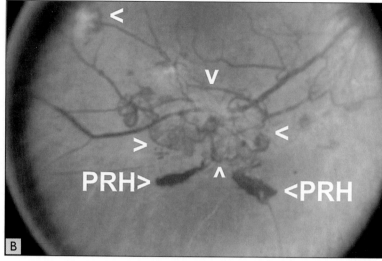

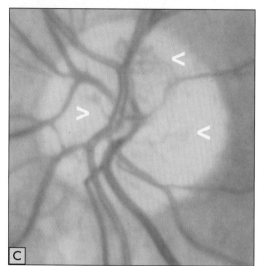

FIGURE 11-9. (See Color Plate) Characteristic clinical manifestations of proliferative diabetic retinopathy (PDR). When any neovascularization is present, diabetic retinopathy is termed *proliferative diabetic retinopathy*. The extent and location of neovascularization determine whether the PDR is considered to be high risk or less than high risk. Neovascularization at the optic disc (NVD), larger areas of vessels, and the presence of concurrent vitreous hemorrhages are the critical findings. Without laser photocoagulation, patients with high-risk PDR have a 28% risk of severe visual loss (<5/200, which is worse than legally blind) within 2 years. This risk compares with a 7% risk of severe visual loss after 2 years for patients with PDR without the high-risk characteristics [25,26]. **A,** Extensive NVD. **B,** Extensive neovascularization at an area remote (>1500 m) from the optic disc, referred to as neovascularization elsewhere (NVE). Pre-retinal hemorrhage (PRH) also is present. **C,** NVD approximately equal to one third to one fourth of the disc area. The following are the risk factors: presence of any neovascularization within the eye, NVD, pre-retinal (or vitreous) hemorrhage, and large areas of neovascularization. NVD equal to or greater than that shown in *panel C* is considered large. NVE greater than or equal to half of the disc area is considered large. When three or more of the risk factors listed previously are present, the patient has PDR with high-risk characteristics (PDR-HRC). Thus, the patient in *panel A* has PDR-HRC because neovascularization is present, located at the disc, and large in extent. The patient in *panel B* also has PDR-HRC because neovascularization is present, the extent of NVE is large, and pre-retinal hemorrhage is present. *Panel C* represents the minimal amount of NVD required for PDR-HRC. (*Panels B and C from* The Early Treatment Diabetic Retinopathy Study Research Group [23]; with permission.)

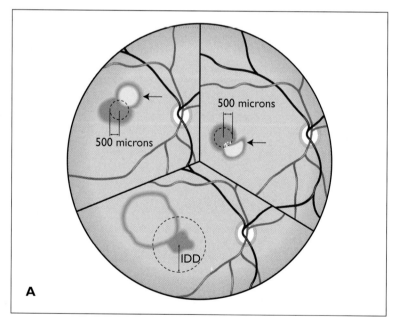

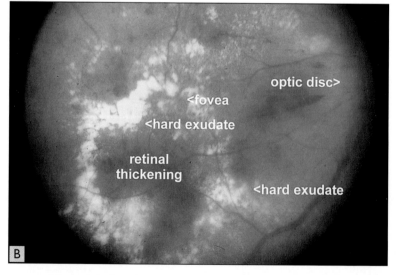

FIGURE 11-10. (See Color Plate) Clinical manifestations of diabetic macular edema. Increased permeability of the retinal microvasculature can result in transudation of serum and other blood components into the substance of the retina, often with deposition of lipid in the form of hard exudates. Retinal edema and thickening result. Macular edema may be present at any level of diabetic retinopathy and is defined as retinal thickening within 3000 μm of the

center of the macula (fovea). Macular edema that threatens the center of vision is termed *clinically significant macular edema* (CSME) [24,27]. **A,** Situations in which macular edema (*white*) is of sufficient extent and correct location to be termed *CSME*. Specifically, edema qualifies as CSME when it is at or within 500 μm of the fovea; associated with hard exudates (*arrows*) at or within 500 μm of the fovea; or one disc area in size, with any part of the edema at or within 1500 μm of the fovea. **B,** CSME owing to extensive hard exudate and thickening involving the fovea and surrounding retina. 1DD—one disk diameter. (*Panel A adapted from* Cavallerano [28].)

Complications and Causes of Visual Loss

CAUSES OF VISUAL LOSS IN DIABETIC RETINOPATHY

Complication Threatening Vision	Common Therapeutic Approach
Clinically significant macular edema (CSME)	Focal and/or grid laser photocoagulation surgery
Macular capillary nonperfusion	No currently effective therapy
High-risk proliferative diabetic retinopathy	Scatter (panretinal) laser photocoagulation surgery (PRP)
Vitreous hemorrhage	Careful observation or vitrectomy
Traction, rhegmatogenous retinal detachment, or both	Vitrectomy
Traction distorting the macula	Careful observation or vitrectomy
Fibrovascular tissues obscuring the retina	Careful observation or vitrectomy
Neovascular glaucoma	PRP, cryotherapy plus intraocular pressure management, or both

FIGURE 11-11. Diabetic retinopathy can result in permanent visual loss by several mechanisms. Long-standing CSME induces moderate visual loss from edema in the foveal region (see Fig. 11-10). If extensive capillary closure occurs in the macular region, vision can be permanently affected from the loss of blood supply to the fovea (see Fig. 11-12). Untreated high-risk proliferative diabetic retinopathy (PDR) primarily causes severe visual loss either by vitreous hemorrhage or retinal traction. Vitreous hemorrhage can reduce vision markedly owing to obscuration of the visual axis by blood (see Fig. 11-12). However, because the blood itself is relatively benign, vision will be recovered (in the absence of other ocular damage) once the hemorrhage clears either spontaneously or, when not resolving, after vitrectomy surgery (see Fig. 11-19). In contrast, neovascularization eventually tends to undergo a scarring process with fibrosis and contraction, resulting in retinal traction (see Fig. 11-13). Such traction can cause visual loss by distorting the macula; tearing the retina; or precipitating retinal detachment, further vitreous hemorrhage, or both. Rarely, fibrovascular tissue itself may obscure the visual axis (see Fig. 11-12). If neovascularization of the iris occurs, neovascular glaucoma may result and lead to permanent visual loss (see Fig. 11-14). (*Adapted from* Aiello *et al.* [15].)

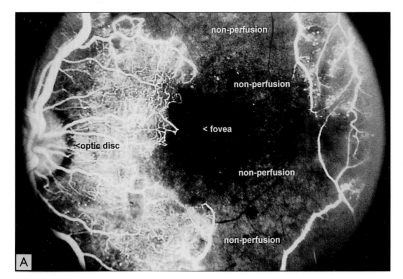

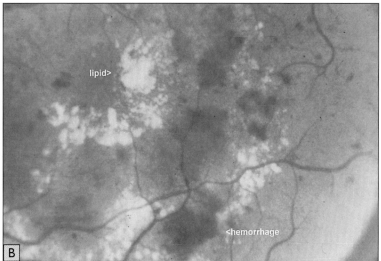

FIGURE 11-12. (See Color Plate) Ophthalmic complications associated with visual loss in diabetic retinopathy. Visual loss associated with diabetic retinopathy can arise from multiple complications of the disease. If the characteristic progressive capillary loss eventually involves a large portion of the central macula, then visual acuity is compromised. **A,** Fluorescein angiogram showing extensive macular capillary nonperfusion. Fluorescent dye (fluorescein) was injected into the patient's antecubital vein, and photographs were taken of the retina as the dye was passing through the retinal vessels. This technique, called *fluorescein angiography*, allows excellent visualization of the retinal vasculature. In this instance, the dye in the retinal vessels appears white, and the photograph shows nearly complete loss of the retinal vasculature perfusion in the macular region. These anatomic changes and their visual sequelae are irreversible. **B,** Extensive retinal vascular leakage into the macular region with retinal thickening, lipid deposits, and retinal hemorrhage. This patient has severe macular edema, with associated visual loss.

(Continued on next page)

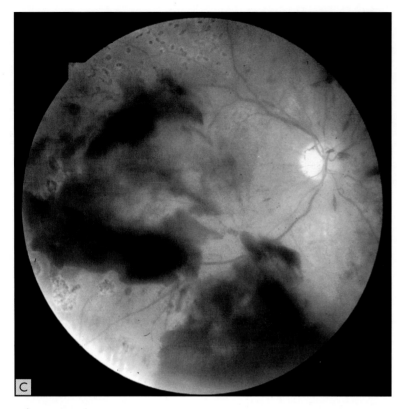

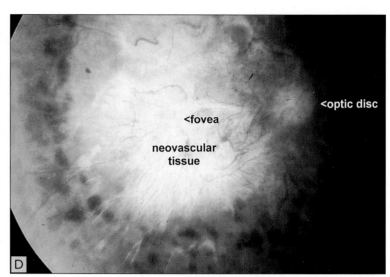

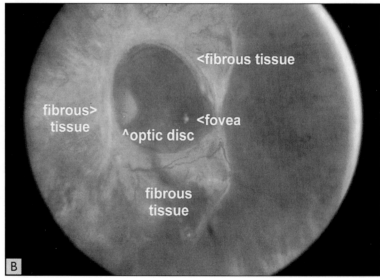

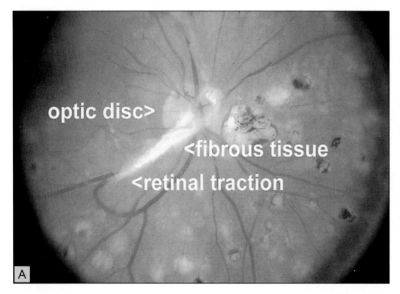

FIGURE 11-12. (*Continued*) **C**, Blood in the vitreous, a condition termed *vitreous hemorrhage* or *preretinal hemorrhage*. Preretinal hemorrhage refers specifically to blood immediately in front of the retina, whereas vitreous hemorrhage may be anywhere in the vitreous cavity. Vitreous hemorrhages are common in diabetic retinopathy owing to the fragility of new vessels and traction often exerted on these vessels by progressive retinal fibrosis. Although the hemorrhages usually clear spontaneously, surgical intervention may be required if they persist (*see* Fig. 11-19). Not only can vitreous hemorrhage obscure the patient's vision, but also the ophthalmologist's view of the retina, which may necessitate evaluation of the retinal anatomy using ultrasonography if the hemorrhage is severe (*see* Fig. 11-13). **D**, A rare form of visual loss in diabetes in which a sheet of neovascular tissue obscures the visual axis. Removal of the tissue by vitrectomy surgery often can restore useful vision (*see* Fig. 11-19). (*Panels A, B, and D courtesy of* The Wilmer Ophthalmological Institute.)

FIGURE 11-13. (See Color Plate) Ophthalmic complications associated with retinal traction in diabetic retinopathy. Some of the most severe visual losses associated with diabetic retinopathy result from the complications of traction exerted on the retina by fibrosing neovascular tissue. Initially, the traction can result in localized retinal detachment that, when distant from the critical areas of the retina, has little visual significance. **A**, A localized traction retinal detachment from the optic disc to an inferior retinal vessel. Note the elevation and distortion of the retinal vessel at the area of traction. As seen here, the detachment does not threaten the macula but should be examined carefully at regular intervals for progression toward the fovea. **B**, More extensive fibrovascular tissue and traction along the vascular arcades of the retina surrounding the macula. This configuration is typical of retinal traction in diabetic retinopathy because of the predilection for fibrovascular tissues to form along the vascular arcades. This configuration has been termed *wolf-jaw* owing to its apparent imminent "bite" on the macula.

(*Continued on next page*)

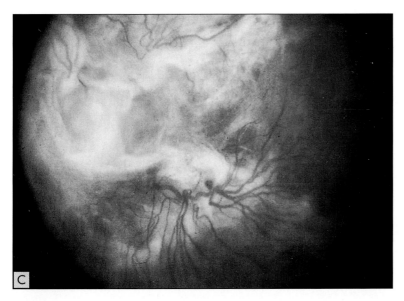

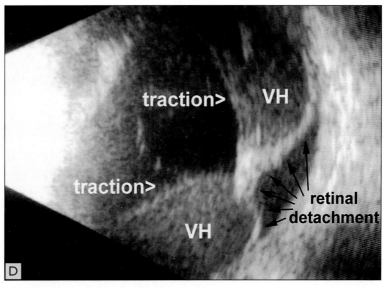

FIGURE 11-13. (*Continued*) **C,** A nearly total retinal detachment with extensive fibrovascular proliferation. Large retinal detachments also may occur when the tractional forces are sufficient to tear a hole in the retina, allowing vitreous fluid to pass into the subretinal space (rhegmatogenous detachment). If vitreous hemorrhage obscures the view of the retina, ultrasonography is indicated to monitor ocular status. **D,** Ultrasonography of vitreous hemorrhage (VH), retinal traction, and traction retinal detachment. When traction retinal detachment threatens the macula, vitrectomy surgery usually is indicated (*see* Fig. 11-19). (*Panel D courtesy of* R. Calderon, OD.)

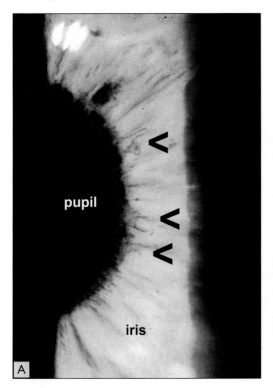

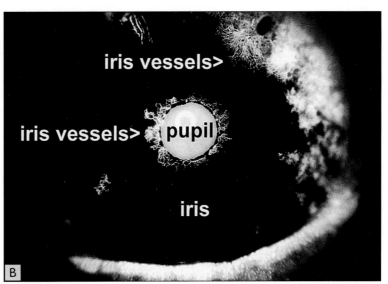

FIGURE 11-14. (See Color Plate) Neovascularization of the iris. In proliferative diabetic retinopathy, neovascularization can occur not only on the retina but also on the iris. Neovascularization of the iris sometimes is referred to as rubeosis iridis. If the neovascularization progresses to the base of the iris, the normal outflow channels for the aqueous fluid from the anterior chamber can become occluded and the intraocular pressure can increase dramatically. This condition, called *neovascular glaucoma*, can result in severe and permanent visual loss. Treatment involves prompt scatter laser photocoagulation as done for proliferative diabetic retinopathy (*see* Fig. 11-15). **A,** Neovascularization of the iris (NVI), with the iris vessels marked by arrows. **B,** Iris neovascularization using fluorescein angiography (*see* Fig. 11-12A). Fluorescein dye in the iris vessels (*white*) demonstrates the extent of the neovascularization on the iris.

Treatment

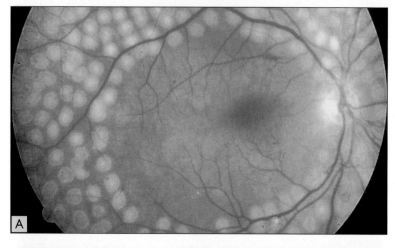

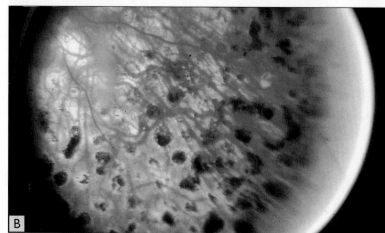

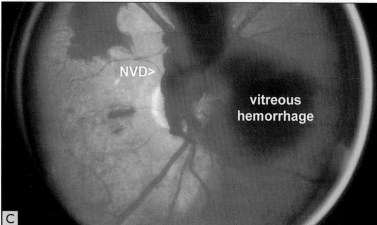

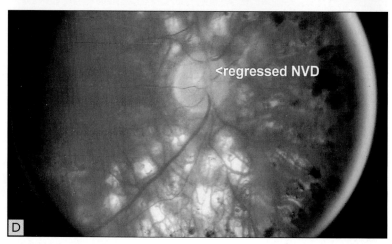

FIGURE 11-15. (See Color Plate) Panretinal laser photocoagulation for proliferative diabetic retinopathy (PDR). The primary therapy for PDR is scatter (panretinal) laser photocoagulation. However, cryotherapy or vitrectomy with endophotocoagulation may be effective when photocoagulation is not feasible. Treatment entails using a laser to place multiple burns throughout the midperiphery of the retina in an attempt to reduce the risk of visual loss. In general, prompt treatment is advised for patients with high-risk PDR. Some patients with PDR that is less than high-risk or with severe or very severe NPDR also may benefit from panretinal photocoagulation, depending on factors such as type of diabetes, medical status, access to care, compliance with follow-up, status and progression of the fellow eye, and family history [24,29]. **A,** Clinical appearance of the retina shortly after panretinal photocoagulation in PDR. The 500-μm-diameter retinal burns appear moderately white in intensity and one-half burn width apart. Laser burns are not placed over the retinal vessels, optic disc, or within the macular region. A total of 1200 to 1800 retinal burns generally are applied over two to three sessions occurring a few days to weeks apart. The procedure is done on an outpatient basis and generally requires only topical anesthesia. **B,** Panretinal photocoagulation scars as they appear months to years after their application. Note the areas of increased retinal pigmentation, atrophy, and spreading of the area of each retinal scar. **C,** PDR, neovascularization of the disk, and vitreous hemorrhage before laser panretinal photocoagulation. **D,** The same patient 2 years after panretinal photocoagulation. Note the resolution of the vitreous hemorrhage and regression of the neovascularization with only a small, fibrotic, nonperfused remnant of the original neovascular frond at the optic disc. Such remnants often do not regress completely and usually do not threaten vision. NVD—neovascularization at the disk. (Panels B, C, and D from The American Academy of Ophthalmology Diabetes 2000 Diabetic Retinopathy Course; with permission.)

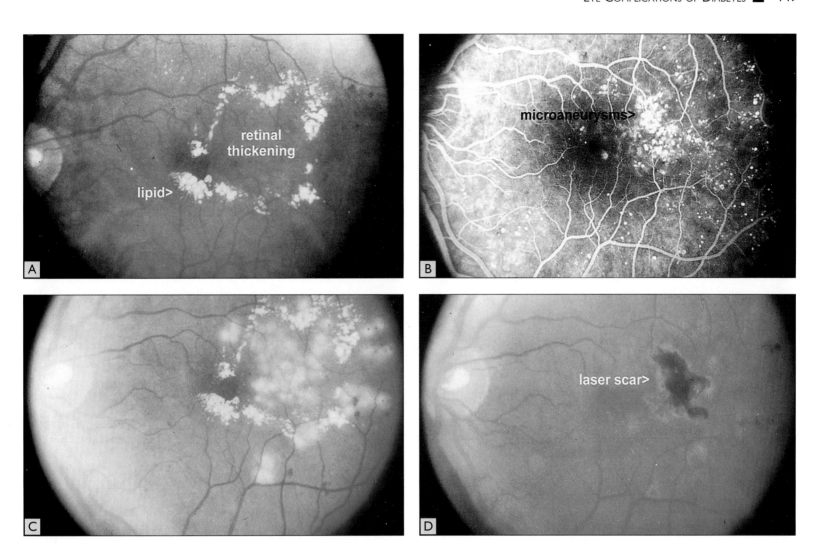

FIGURE 11-16. (See Color Plate) Focal laser photocoagulation for clinically significant diabetic macular edema. The primary therapy for clinically significant diabetic macular edema is focal laser photocoagulation. Treatment entails placing light 50- to 100-μm-diameter burns focally over leaking microaneurysms or in a grid pattern if retinal leakage is diffuse. Once the need for treatment is determined clinically, fluorescein angiography often is used to identify the type of leakage and specific microaneurysms for treatment. If treatment is successful, resolution of the macular edema may be expected 3 or more months after therapy. Treatment may be reapplied if the edema persists or recurs. **A**, Circinate lipid deposits, clinically significant macular edema, and reduced visual acuity. **B**, Fluorescein angiogram demonstrating multiple microaneurysms in the area of thickening within the circinate ring. **C**, Clinical appearance of the retina immediately after focal laser photocoagulation to the leaking microaneurysms. The retinal burns applied in this case are more intense than is optimal. **D**, Clinical appearance of the eye several months after laser therapy. The lipid and edema have resolved, and no thickening of the retina is present. Likewise, visual acuity has improved. The residual scarring of the retina is heavier than desired owing to the intensity of the initial laser burns. (*From* the American Academy of Ophthalmology Diabetes 2000 Program; with permission.)

THERAPEUTIC EFFICACY IN THE TREATMENT OF DIABETIC RETINOPATHY

Indication	Treatment	Efficacy
Clinically significant macular edema	Focal laser photocoagulation	50% reduction in moderate visual loss* after 3 y
High-risk proliferative diabetic retinopathy (PDR)	Scatter photocoagulation	60% reduction in severe visual loss† after 3 y
Development of high-risk PDR	Scatter photocoagulation	87% reduction in severe visual loss† after 3 y
		97% reduction in bilateral severe visual loss† after 3 y
		90% reduction in legal blindness after 5 y
Severe PDR and severe vitreous hemorrhage‡	Vitrectomy	60% increased chance of 20/40 or better after 2 y
Severe PDR and vision 10/200 or better‡	Vitrectomy	34% increased chance of 20/40 or better after 2 y
No diabetic retinopathy	Intensive glycemic control	76% reduction in onset of retinopathy
Nonproliferative diabetic retinopathy	Intensive glycemic control	63% reduction in retinopathy progression
		47% reduction in severe nonproliferative diabetic retinopathy and PDR
		26% reduction in development of macular edema
		51% reduction in need for laser treatment

*Moderate visual loss is defined as at least doubling of the visual angle (eg, 20/40 to 20/80).
†Severe visual loss is defined as best corrected acuity of 5/200 or worse on two consecutive visits 4 months apart.
‡For patients with type 1 diabetes only; no benefit was observed in the group having type 2 diabetes.

FIGURE 11-17. The only patient-initiated efforts proven to reduce the risk of visual loss include maintenance of optimal glycemic control and insistence on routine ophthalmologic evaluation [10,30]. Once visually significant complications of diabetes have arisen, the mainstay of therapy is laser photocoagulation. Scatter (panretinal) photocoagulation for the treatment of proliferative diabetic retinopathy is remarkably effective in preventing severe visual loss when patients at risk receive therapy in an appropriate and timely manner. Indeed, with appropriate medical and ophthalmologic care, over 95% of visual loss resulting from diabetic retinopathy can be prevented [14]. Focal photocoagulation for the treatment of clinically significant macular edema is somewhat less effective, although half of moderate visual loss can be prevented in this manner. If the application of laser photocoagulation is not possible or is ineffective, pars plana vitrectomy surgery also is useful in preventing visual impairment (see Fig. 11-19). (*Adapted from* Aiello *et al.* [15].)

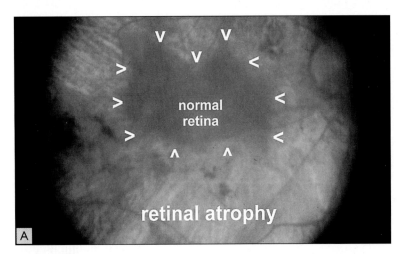

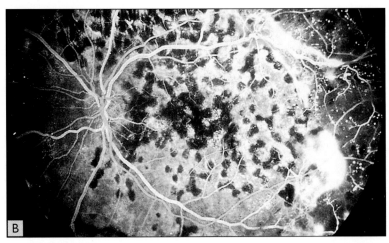

FIGURE 11-18. (See Color Plate) Side effects and complications of laser photocoagulation. Although laser photocoagulation is remarkably effective at preventing the visual loss associated with diabetic retinopathy, the therapy itself is inherently destructive. Each retinal laser burn destroys a portion of previously viable retina in an attempt to maintain better visual function than would be achieved without treatment. Thus, the therapy itself is associated with unavoidable side effects, most notably constriction of peripheral visual field and reduced night vision. These symptoms result from the selective destruction of the retinal midperiphery that subserves these functions. Unexpected complications also can arise from laser photocoagulation. **A,** Appearance of the retina several years after excessive laser panretinal photocoagulation. Note that the atrophy resulting from individual laser scars has spread to the point at which confluent loss of the peripheral retina occurs. Only the central aspect of the macula (*arrows*) remains intact. As expected, this patient has severe constriction of the visual field and significant difficulty with night vision. **B,** Fluorescein angiogram of panretinal photocoagulation mistakenly applied directly through the macula. The dark laser scars in this macular area, which is critical for detailed vision, cause permanent blind spots in the center of vision and reduced visual acuity.

(Continued on next page)

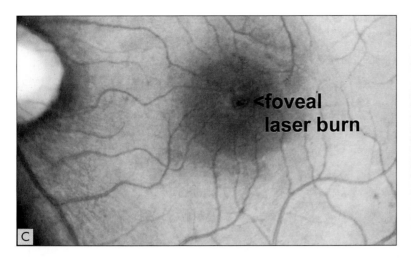

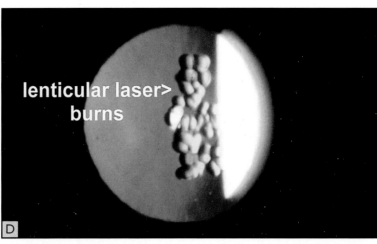

FIGURE 11-18. (*Continued*) **C**, A single laser burn mistakenly applied to the fovea. This area of retina subserves central vision, accounting for the large central blind spot and poor detailed vision experienced by this patient, who now is legally blind. **D**, Laser photocoagulation focused too far anteriorly may result in vaporization of the crystalline lens, as observed in this retroilluminated photograph of the human lens. Visual loss associated with this rare complication can be corrected by cataract surgery. (*Panels B–D courtesy of* the Wilmer Ophthalmological Institute.)

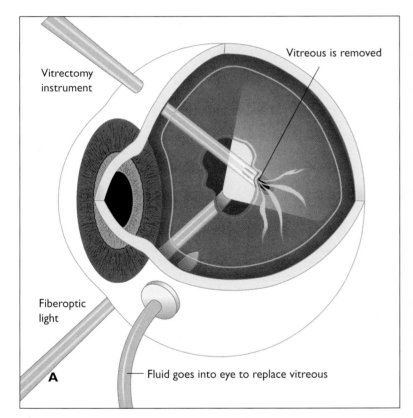

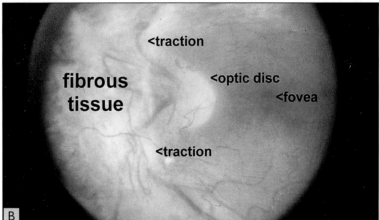

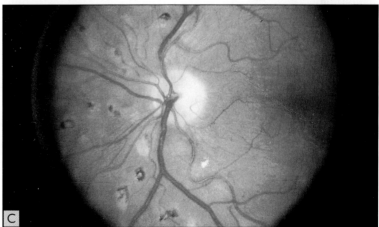

FIGURE 11-19. (See Color Plate) Pars plana vitrectomy surgery. Instances occur when high-risk proliferative diabetic retinopathy (PDR) is not amenable to laser photocoagulation and may arise as a result of the following: advanced disease, poor retinal visualization (*ie*, severe vitreous hemorrhage or cataract), active neovascularization despite complete laser treatment, traction-macular detachment, or combined traction-rhegmatogenous retinal detachment. In such cases, pars plana vitrectomy surgery may offer a therapeutic option. Vitrectomy surgery has the potential for serious complications, including profound visual loss and permanent pain and blindness. Thus, surgery should be undertaken only after careful consideration of the potential risks and benefits [31]. Vitrectomy performed by an experienced vitreoretinal surgeon, however, often can maintain vision in patients who otherwise almost certainly would have severe visual loss. **A**, Schematic representation of the pars plana vitrectomy procedure. Three openings are made from the outside of the eye into the vitreous cavity. An infusion line is placed in one opening to maintain pressure within the eye during surgery. The other two openings are used for the variety of instruments that can manipulate the vitreous and retina. Fiberoptic instruments allow for illumination, and the surgery is monitored by visualization through the pupil using an operating microscope. **B**, Proliferative diabetic retinopathy and extensive fibrovascular neovascularization before vitrectomy surgery. Note the fibrous tissue surrounding the optic disc that is exerting traction on the major superior and inferior retinal vessels, dragging them nasally. **C**, The same retina after vitrectomy surgery. Note the removal of the fibrous tissue that had surrounded the optic disc with return of the major retinal vessels to a more normal anatomic position after removal of the traction. (*Panel A from* "For my patient: retinal detachment and vitreous surgery," The Retina Research Fund; *panels B and C from* the American Academy of Ophthalmology Diabetic Retinopathy Vitrectomy Study course; with permission.)

SYSTEMIC FACTORS POTENTIALLY AFFECTING DIABETIC RETINOPATHY

Glycemic control	Pregnancy
Hypertension	Smoking
Renal disease	Anemia
Dyslipidemia	

FIGURE 11-20. Systemic factors affecting retinopathy. Although great emphasis is placed on the clinical evaluation of the retina and the adherence to rigorous treatment algorithms, concomitant systemic disorders can exert significant influence on the development, progression, and ultimate outcome of diabetic eye disease. Optimized control of systemic disorders can improve the visual prognosis of the patient with diabetes [11]. Such care often involves an intensive, multifaceted, health care team approach to the treatment of patients with diabetes [32]. A list of systemic disorders potentially affecting diabetic retinopathy is presented; these disorders should be managed carefully.

Growth Factors and Potential Novel Therapies

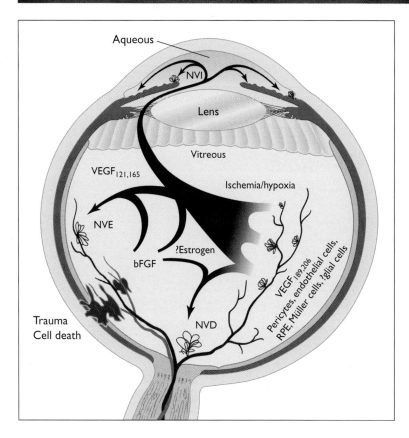

FIGURE 11-21. Model of growth factor action in diabetic retinopathy. For the past half century, investigators have recognized that numerous ischemic retinopathies result in retinal neovascularization and vascular leakage similar to that observed in diabetic retinopathy. These findings have suggested that common inciting events and mediating factors may be responsible for these complications. The potential role of growth factors in mediating retinal neovascularization was first suggested by Michaelson in 1948 and later refined by numerous investigators [33]. A schematic representation of the growth factor model of intraocular neovascularization is shown. Damage to the retinal tissues, probably caused by capillary loss and subsequent hypoxia in the case of diabetes, results in the release of growth factors from the retina. These growth factors are secreted by a variety of retinal cell types and may act locally to produce neovascularization and vascular permeability or may diffuse through the vitreous cavity to induce these complications at distant sites. The presence of two or more growth factors may actually augment the induction of neovascular activity, as is the case with basic fibroblast growth factor (bFGF) and vascular endothelial growth factor (VEGF). In addition, the growth factors may diffuse down a concentration gradient from the vitreous cavity into the aqueous cavity where they are eventually cleared through the trabecular meshwork at the base of the iris. This diffusion path would account for neovascularization observed at the iris. Numerous growth factors have been implicated in this process. Molecules that probably contribute to the neovascularization in diabetic retinopathy include VEGF, growth hormone, insulin-like growth factor-1, and bFGF. Of these, VEGF is the only molecule that possesses all the expected characteristics of a major mediator of intraocular neovascularization and vasopermeability, although many factors are likely to contribute to such complex processes. The relative growth factor concentrations and angiogenic potency are represented by arrow width. NVD—neovascularization at the disc; NVE—neovascularization elsewhere; NVI—neovascularization at the iris; RPE–retinal pigment epithelium. (*Adapted from* Aiello et al. [34].)

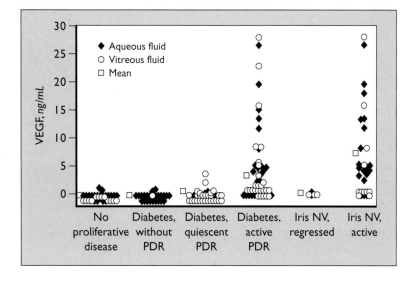

FIGURE 11-22. Angiogenic growth factors increase when neovascularization is present. For a growth factor to mediate intraocular neovascularization in diabetic retinopathy, it should be present at elevated concentrations during or shortly before the onset of active neovascularization. Demonstrated are the results of a study in which intraocular fluids were obtained from 136 patients with diabetes who were undergoing intraocular surgery. The concentration of vascular endothelial growth factor (VEGF) in the intraocular fluids was evaluated and the results plotted by extent of retinopathy. Concentrations of VEGF were low in patients who did not have diabetes or who had diabetes but no proliferative diabetic retinopathy (PDR). However, when patients had active neovascularization either of the retina or iris, concentrations of VEGF were greatly elevated. Once neovascularization had become quiescent, concentrations of vascular endothelial factor returned to baseline. The study also demonstrated the predicted concentration gradient between the vitreous and aqueous cavities and a 75% decrease in VEGF levels after successful laser panretinal photocoagulation. NV–neovascularization. (*Adapted from* Aiello et al. [35].)

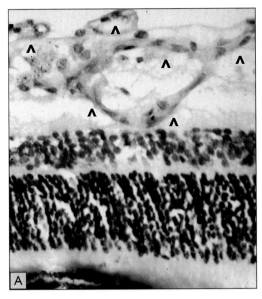 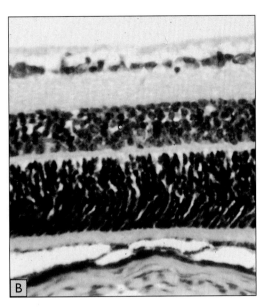

FIGURE 11-23. (See Color Plate) Inhibition of vascular endothelial growth factor (VEGF) suppresses retinal neovascularization in animals. If vascular endothelial growth factor is responsible for a significant portion of the neovascular response in ischemic retinopathies, then inhibition of this molecule should result in suppression of retinal neovascularization. Several investigators have now evaluated this causal relationship. Inhibition of VEGF using three different techniques has resulted in suppression of retinal and

iris neovascularization in murine and primate models [36–38]. Demonstrated are the results from one of these studies using the chimeric receptor antagonists in a murine model of ischemia-induced retinopathy [36,39]. When these inhibitors of VEGF are injected into the neonatal eye at the time when the retinas become hypoxic, suppression of subsequent retinal neovascularization occurs in 95% to 100% of animals. The magnitude of inhibition is approximately 50%. **A,** Histologic cross-section of a neonatal mouse retina that received an intraocular injection of an inactive control compound. The *arrows* show the extensive inner retinal neovascularization. **B,** Corresponding area of retina in the contralateral eye of the same animal that received an active inhibitor of VEGF. Note the suppression of inner retinal neovascularization and normal appearance of the retina by light microscopic examination without evidence of retinal toxicity. These data suggest that growth factor inhibitors eventually may prove useful as novel therapies for diabetic retinopathy and macular edema. Such therapeutic approaches theoretically would eliminate the side effects inherent in the retinal-destructive treatments in use today (*see* Figs. 11-15 and 11-18). (*From* Aiello [40]; with permission.)

NOVEL THERAPEUTIC APPROACHES UNDER INVESTIGATION FOR DIABETIC RETINOPATHY

Prevention	Intervention	Restoration
Antihyperglycemics	Anti-permeability	Medical approaches
ARI*	PKC inhibitors,* antihistamines,* anti-AGE*	Stem cell utilization
Anti-AGE*		Gene therapy
PKC inhibitors*	Anti-angiogenesis	Surgical approaches
Preservation of function	GH/IGF-1 inhibitors,* PKC inhibitors,* angiostatin/endo-	Retinal transplantation
Antioxidants*	statin, ribozymes, aptamers,*	Ocular transplantation
Hemostabilization	antibodies,* chimeric recep-	Artificial visual
Neuroprotection	tors, PEDF	prosthetics*
	Anti-proliferation	
	Anti-integrins,* metalloproteinases*	
	Vitreal lysis*	

*Compounds in or pending clinical trials.

FIGURE 11-24. Novel therapeutic approaches for diabetic retinopathy. The possibility of preventing the visual loss from diabetes in a nondestructive manner utilizing a pharmacologic approach has become the focus of intensive investigations. Multiple approaches have been proposed, and many preclinical results have appeared promising. Several clinical trials are underway to evaluate the efficacy of these new therapeutic modalities. A partial list of approaches under investigation is presented. AGE—advanced glycation end products; ARI—aldose reductase inhibitors; IGF-1—insulin-like growth factor-1; GH—growth hormone; PEDF—pigment-epithelium derived factor; PKC—protein kinase C.

Acknowledgments

The excellent technical and editorial assistance of Jerry D. Cavallerano, OD, PhD, is gratefully acknowledged.

Portions of this chapter are adapted from Aiello *et al.* [15] and the American Academy of Ophthalmology Diabetes 2000 Diabetic Retinopathy course.

References

1. Klein R, BE Klein, Moss SE: Visual impairment in diabetes. *Ophthalmology* 1984, 91:1–9.

2. Klein R, Klein BE, Moss SE, Cruickshanks KJ: The Wisconsin Epidemiologic Study of Diabetic Retinopathy. XV. The long-term incidence of macular edema. *Ophthalmology* 1995, 102:7–16.

3. Javitt JC, Aiello LP, Bassi LJ, *et al.*: Detecting and treating retinopathy in patients with type I diabetes mellitus. Savings associated with improved implementation of current guidelines. American Academy of Ophthalmology. *Ophthalmology* 1991, 98:1565–1573.

4. Javitt JC, Aiello LP, Chiang Y, *et al.*: Preventive eye care in people with diabetes is cost-saving to the federal government. Implications for health-care reform. *Diabetes Care* 1994, 17:909–917.

5. Javitt JC, Aiello LP: Cost-effectiveness of detecting and treating diabetic retinopathy [see comments]. *Ann Intern Med* 1996, 124:164–169.

6. Javitt, JC, Canner JK, Sommer A: Cost effectiveness of current approaches to the control of retinopathy in type I diabetics. *Ophthalmology* 1989, 96:255–264.

7. Kahn HA, Hiller R: Blindness caused by diabetic retinopathy. *Am J Ophthalmol* 1974, 78:58–67.

8. Palmberg PF: Diabetic retinopathy. *Diabetes* 1977, 26:703–709.

9. The Diabetes Control and Complications Trial Research Group: The effect of intensive treatment of diabetes on the development and progression of long-term complications in insulin-dependent diabetes mellitus [see comments]. *N Engl J Med* 1993, 329:977–986.

10. The relationship of glycemic exposure (HbA1c) to the risk of development and progression of retinopathy in the Diabetes Control and Complications Trial. *Diabetes* 1995, 44:968–983.

11. Retinopathy and nephropathy in patients with type I diabetes four years after a trial of intensive therapy. *Am J Ophthalmol* 2000, 129(5):704–705.

12. Lifetime benefits and costs of intensive therapy as practiced in the Diabetes control and complications trial. The Diabetes Control and Complications Trial Research Group [see comments]. *JAMA* 1996 276:1409–1415; published erratum, *JAMA* 1997, 278:25.

13. Resource utilization and costs of care in the Diabetes Control and Complications Trial. *Diabetes Care* 1995, 18:1468–1478.

14. Ferris FL: How effective are treatments for diabetic retinopathy? *JAMA* 1993, 269:1290–1291.

15. Aiello LP, Gardner TW, King GL, *et al.*: Diabetic retinopathy: technical review. *Diabetes Care* 1998, 21:143–156.

16. National Diabetes Data Group: Diabetes in America. Washington, DC: US Government Printing Office; 1995.

17. Bursell SE, Clermont AC, Kinsley BT, *et al.*: Retinal blood flow changes in patients with insulin-dependent diabetes mellitus and no diabetic retinopathy. *Am J Physiol* 1996, 270:R61–R70.

18. Krolewski AS, Warram JH, Rand LI, *et al.*: Risk of proliferative diabetic retinopathy in juvenile-onset type I diabetes: a 40-yr follow-up study. *Diabetes Care* 1984, 9:443–452.

19. Klein R, Klein BE, Moss SE, *et al.*: The Wisconsin epidemiologic study of diabetic retinopathy. II. Prevalence and risk of diabetic retinopathy when age at diagnosis is less than 30 years. *Arch Ophthalmol* 1984, 102:520–536.

20. Klein R, Moss SE, Klein BE, *et al.*: New management concepts for timely diagnosis of diabetic retinopathy treatable by photocoagulation. *Diabetes Care* 1987, 10:633–638.

21. American Academy of Pediatrics: Screening for retinopathy in the pediatric patient with type I diabetes mellitus. *Pediatrics* 1998, 101:313–314.

22. Klein BE, Moss SE, Klein R: Effect of pregnancy on progression of diabetic retinopathy. *Diabetes Care* 1990, 13:34–40.

23. The Early Treatment Diabetic Retinopathy Study Research Group: Grading diabetic retinopathy from stereoscopic color fundus photographs: an extension of the modified Airlie House classification. ETDRS report number 10. *Ophthalmology* 1991, 98:786–806.

24. The Early Treatment Diabetic Retinopathy Study Research Group: Early photocoagulation for diabetic retinopathy. ETDRS report number 9. *Ophthalmology* 1991, 98:766–785.

25. The Diabetic Retinopathy Study Research Group: Photocoagulation treatment of proliferative diabetic retinopathy. Clinical application of Diabetic Retinopathy Study (DRS) findings, DRS Report Number 8. *Ophthalmology* 1981, 88:583–600.

26. The Diabetic Retinopathy Study Research Group: Indications for photocoagulation treatment of diabetic retinopathy: Diabetic Retinopathy Study Report no. 14. *Int Ophthalmol Clin* 1987, 27:239–253.

27. The Early Treatment Diabetic Retinopathy Study Research Group: Photocoagulation for diabetic macular edema. Early Treatment Diabetic Retinopathy Study report number 1. *Arch Ophthalmol* 1985, 103:1796–1806.

28. Cavallerano J: Diabetic retinopathy. *Clinical Eye and Vision Care* 1990, 2:4–14.

29. Ferris F: Early photocoagulation in patients with either type 1 or type 2 diabetes. *Trans Am Ophthalmol Soc* 1996, 94:505–537.

30. The Diabetes Control and Complications Trial Research Group: The effect of intensive diabetes treatment on the progression of diabetic retinopathy in insulin-dependent diabetes mellitus: the Diabetes Control and Complications Trial. *Arch Ophthalmol* 1995, 113:36–51.

31. The Diabetic Retinopathy Vitrectomy Study Research Group: Early vitrectomy for severe proliferative diabetic retinopathy in eyes with useful vision. Clinical application of results of a randomized trial: Diabetic Retinopathy Vitrectomy Study Report 4. *Ophthalmology* 1988, 95:1321–1334.

32. Aiello LP, Cahill MT, Wong JS: Systemic considerations in the management of diabetic retinopathy. *Am J Ophthalmol* 2001, 132(5):760–776.

33. Michaelson IC: The mode of development of the vascular system of the retina, with some observations on its significance for certain retinal diseases. *Trans Ophthalmol Soc UK* 1948, 68:137–180.

34. Aiello LP, Northrup JM, Keyt BA: Hypoxic regulation of vascular endothelial growth factor in retinal cells. *Arch Ophthalmol* 1995, 113:1538–1544.

35. Aiello LP, Avery RL, Arrigg PG, et al.: Vascular endothelial growth factor in ocular fluid of patients with diabetic retinopathy and other retinal disorders [see comments]. N Engl J Med 1994, 331:1480–1487.

36. Aiello LP, Pierce EA, Foley ED, et al.: Suppression of retinal neovascularization in vivo by inhibition of vascular endothelial growth factor (VEGF) using soluble VEGF-receptor chimeric proteins. Proc Natl Acad Sci USA 1995, 92:10457–10461.

37. Adamis AP, Shima DT, Tolentino MJ, et al.: Inhibition of vascular endothelial growth factor prevents retinal ischemia-associated iris neovascularization in a nonhuman primate. Arch Ophthalmol 1996, 114:66–71.

38. Robinson GS, Pierce EA, Rook SL, et al.: Oligodeoxynucleotides inhibit retinal neovascularization in a murine model of proliferative retinopathy. Proc Natl Acad Sci USA 1996, 93:4851–4856.

39. Smith LE, Wesolowski E, McLellan A, et al.: Oxygen-induced retinopathy in the mouse. Invest Ophthalmol Vis Sci 1994, 35:101–111.

40. Aiello LP: Vascular endothelial growth factor. 20th-century mechanisms, 21st-century therapies. Invest Ophthalmol Vis Sci 1997, 38:1647–1652.

41. Gaede P, Vedel P, Parving HH, Pedersen O: Intensified multifactorial intervention in patients with type 2 diabetes mellitus and microalbuminuria: the Steno type 2 randomised study. Lancet 1999, 353:617–622.

DIABETES AND THE KIDNEY

Robert C. Stanton

12

Diabetic nephropathy is a serious public health concern because it has become the major cause of end-stage renal disease in the United States (see Fig. 12-1). It is characterized primarily by the clinical presentation of microalbuminuria, which slowly progresses to frank proteinuria, followed by a gradual decline in glomerular filtration rate, eventually leading to renal failure. Nodular sclerosis of the mesangium in the glomerular tuft is the characteristic pathologic change seen in diabetic nephropathy. A minority of patients with diabetes mellitus develop renal failure, but the number of cases of diabetic nephropathy is increasing every year, mostly because of the aging of patients with type 2 diabetes mellitus. Success in prolonging the lives of patients with both type 1 and type 2 diabetes mellitus has led to an increase in the numbers of patients with complications of the disease. In the past 15 years, much has been learned about the possible causes of diabetic nephropathy. This understanding has led to the development and use of specific therapies that have been effective in slowing the progression to renal failure. Although effective, these therapies are not cures. Thus, there is an ongoing effort to further identify 1) the factors predisposing to renal failure; 2) the causes of diabetic nephropathy; and 3) the factors that lead to progression to renal failure. This chapter presents an overview of the demographics, diagnosis, and natural history as well as current ideas about the pathogenesis underlying the development and progression of diabetic nephropathy. An understanding of these mechanisms has provided specific directions for the development of new, effective treatments that hold promise for the development of new clinically applicable therapies in the next 10 years. This chapter does not differentiate between the nephropathy of type 1 diabetes mellitus and the nephropathy of type 2 diabetes mellitus because recent evidence suggests that both pathogenesis and therapy for diabetic nephropathy in type 1 and type 2 diabetes mellitus are similar. Although there are clear differences in susceptibility to diabetic nephropathy, and there are some differences in the approach to screening and therapy, it is believed that there are more similarities than differences. Reviews by Ruggenenti and Remuzzi [1] and Ritz and Orth [2] provide more information on diabetic nephropathy in patients with type 2 diabetes mellitus.

Demographics and Prevalence

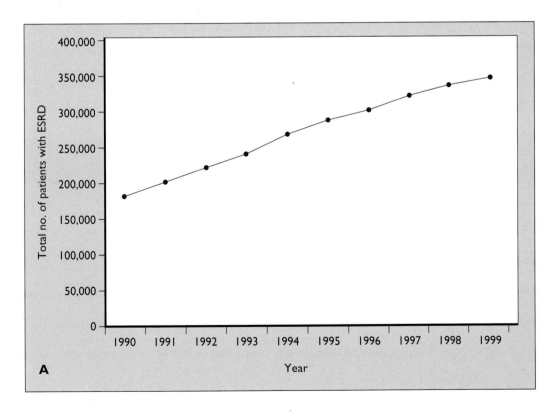

A

FIGURE 12-1. Demographics of end-stage renal disease (ESRD). **A,** Diabetic nephropathy occurs in about 20% to 40% of patients with type 1 diabetes mellitus and 10% to 15% of patients with type 2 diabetes mellitus. It is a significant cause of morbidity in these patients; the appearance of nephropathy leads to both a significant decrease in life expectancy and a significant increase in hospitalizations and medical care costs.

(Continued on next page)

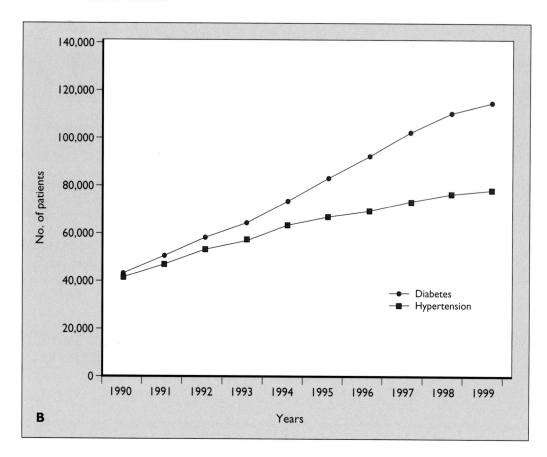

B

FIGURE 12-1. (Continued) **B**, The major causes of ESRD in the United States are diabetes, hypertension, and glomerulonephritis, and since the late 1980s, diabetes has become the leading cause [3]. The 1998 report of the U.S. Renal Data System shows that over the past 10 years, the percentage of patients with ESRD has increased from 24% to 37%. This figure also shows that the rate of increase in ESRD due to diabetes is greater than the increase for hypertension.

PREVALENCE AND INCIDENCE OF ESRD BY CAUSE

Cause	Prevalence	Incidence
Diabetes mellitus	114,478	38,160
Hypertension	77,978	23,133
Glomerulonephritis	53,994	8038

FIGURE 12-2. Prevalence and incidence of end-stage renal disease (ESRD) by top three causes in 1999 [3]. Prevalence—number of patients with ESRD on December 31, 1999; incidence—number of patients starting in ESRD in all of 1999.

Diagnosis of Diabetic Nephropathy

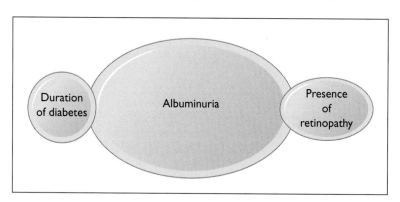

FIGURE 12-3. Diagnosis of diabetic nephropathy. The hallmark of the diagnosis of diabetic nephropathy is albuminuria. Microalbuminuria is the earliest detectable clinical sign of diabetic nephropathy. Typically, microalbuminuria progresses to frank proteinuria over a period of years. The rate of progression is based on a number of factors, which are discussed later in this chapter. In addition to microalbuminuria, patients with early diabetic nephropathy have increased glomerular filtration rates, and their kidneys undergo hypertrophy. Thus, increased creatinine clearance and increased kidney size are additional signs of early diabetic nephropathy. There are clear associations between diabetic nephropathy and two other diagnostically important factors: 1) the duration of diabetes and 2) pre-existing retinopathy. It is unusual for diabetic nephropathy to appear in patients who have had type 1 diabetes for less than 5 years. Most patients (as many as 90%) with diabetic nephropathy also have retinopathy [4]. Thus, either short duration of diabetes or no evidence of retinopathy in a patient with evidence of renal dysfunction should lead the clinician to consider other renal diseases.

REASONS TO CONSIDER OTHER RENAL DISEASES IN PATIENTS WITH DIABETES MELLITUS

Absence of albuminuria

Diabetes mellitus present for less than 5 years

Rapidly increasing serum creatinine

Presence of active urinary sediment

FIGURE 12-4. Reasons to consider other renal diseases in patients with diabetes mellitus. If there is no albuminuria/proteinuria, then the patient does not have diabetic nephropathy. Less definite but still important considerations in the diagnosis of diabetic nephropathy are listed. Worsening renal function in a patient with diabetes mellitus for less than 5 years should prompt the physician to consider other causes of renal failure. Typically, the decrease in glomerular filtration rate occurs over years. If a patient has a decreasing creatinine clearance or increasing serum creatinine that occurs over weeks to months, other renal diseases should be considered. The presence of an active urinary sediment (ie, the presence of such elements as red blood cells, white blood cells, and red blood cell casts) should lead the physician to consider other renal diseases. Although most patients with diabetic nephropathy have a relatively inactive urinary sediment, as many as 25% to 30% of patients with diabetic nephropathy may have hematuria and even red blood cell casts [5]. The finding of an active sediment, therefore, should alert the physician to consider other causes, but by itself it may not be a reason to strongly pursue evidence for other renal diseases.

MICROALBUMINURIA AND MACROALBUMINURIA

Definition of microalbuminuria
  < 30 mg/24 h or > 20 μg/min
  Albumin/creatinine ratio of > 30 mg/g
Definition of frank albuminuria or macroalbuminuria
  > 300 mg/24 h or > 200 μg/min
Common causes of transient increases in albuminuria
  Exercise
  Pregnancy
  Poor glycemic control
  Congestive heart failure
  Hypertension
  Urinary tract infection

FIGURE 12-5. Detection of albuminuria. Microalbuminuria is the hallmark of early diabetic nephropathy, so all diabetic patients should be routinely screened for the presence of microalbuminuria. Although a timed urine collection is a very effective way to determine albumin excretion accurately, it is neither convenient nor cost-effective. Recent studies have shown that the albumin/creatinine ratio, obtained by measuring a spot urine sample for albumin and creatinine, is a highly accurate method for screening and following patients with diabetes mellitus [6]. The dipsticks used for the determination of protein in the urine are not sensitive enough to measure protein excretion less than 300 mg per 24 hours, however, so direct laboratory measurement of albumin is required to detect microalbuminuria. A spot measurement of albumin alone is affected by the urine volume, but normalizing to the amount of creatinine in the urine eliminates this concern. As shown, a value of 30 mg/g is suggestive of the presence of microalbuminuria. A number of studies have shown that the albumin/creatinine ratio is a highly accurate and effective test for the detection and following of patients with diabetes mellitus.

In determining the presence of microalbuminuria, causes of transient increases in albuminuria must be considered. Macroalbuminuria reflects progressive diabetic nephropathy. Increased attention to treatment (see Fig. 12-21) should be given. Thus, repeat measurements of albumin excretion are recommended before labeling a patient with a diagnosis of early diabetic nephropathy.

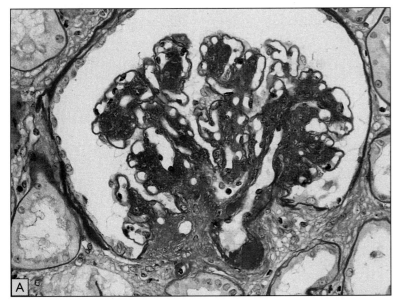

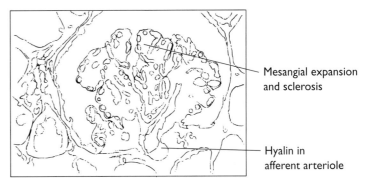

Mesangial expansion and sclerosis

Hyalin in afferent arteriole

FIGURE 12-6. (See Color Plate) Pathology of diabetic nephropathy. Typical changes of diabetic nephropathy are seen in the light micrograph (**A**) and in the electron micrograph (**B**) [7]. *Panel A* shows nodular sclerosis, mesangial expansion, and hyalin deposition in the afferent arteriole.

(Continued on next page)

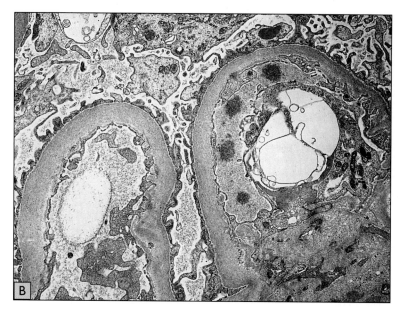

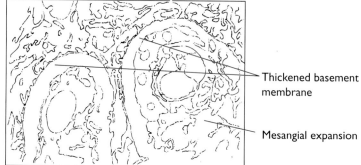

Thickened basement membrane

Mesangial expansion

FIGURE 12-6. (Continued) *Panel B* shows two capillary loops. The capillary loop on the right shows basement membrane thickening and mesangial expansion. Although these changes are typical of diabetic nephropathy, they are not pathognomonic. Two other diseases also must be considered in a patient with these renal biopsy findings: light chain deposition disease and amyloid. It is possible to differentiate among these diseases by specific stains and history. (*Courtesy of* Dr. Helmut Rennke, Boston, MA.)

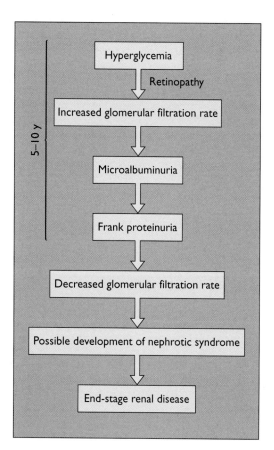

FIGURE 12-7. Natural history of diabetic nephropathy. If a patient with diabetes mellitus develops microalbuminuria, the progression to renal failure tends to be inexorable unless specific interventions are done. This schematic shows the likely progression in an idealized patient. As previously noted, the presence of microalbuminuria is the first easy and reliably detectable evidence of renal failure. A patient who is going to develop renal failure usually has detectable retinopathy and will show evidence of renal failure 5 to 10 years after the diagnosis of diabetes mellitus. Interestingly, if the patient has not developed proteinuria after 15 to 20 years of diabetes, the likelihood of the development of renal disease with progression to renal failure is greatly reduced [8]. The reasons for progression are multifactorial. The ensuing figures discuss both the possible causes of the development of diabetic nephropathy and the reasons for the progression of diabetic nephropathy.

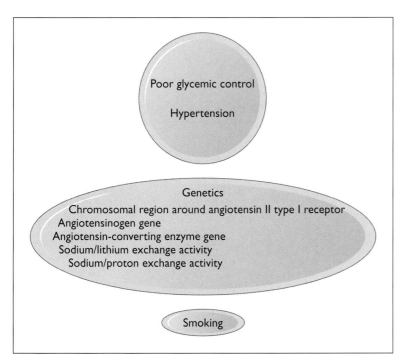

FIGURE 12-8. Risk factors for development of diabetic nephropathy. Poor glycemic control and hypertension have been shown to increase the likelihood of developing diabetic nephropathy [9]. Both of these factors are independently correlated with the development of diabetic nephropathy. Patients with poor glycemic control also are more likely to have hypertension than are patients with good glycemic control [9]. In addition, there has been a concerted effort to detect specific genes that predispose patients to the development of diabetic nephropathy. The existence of such genes is supported by a number of findings. A family history of diabetic nephropathy increases the likelihood of developing nephropathy [10]. In addition, certain genetically similar groups are more susceptible to nephropathy than are other groups. For example, members of the Pima Indian tribe in Arizona have a high rate of development of type 2 diabetes, and above age 45 more than 60% have developed nephropathy, a percentage that is much higher than the average [11]. Specific genes listed in this figure have been suggested to be associated with the development of nephropathy. Smoking, probably because of its deleterious effects on vascular endothelial cells, also has been shown to increase the likelihood of developing diabetic nephropathy in patients with both type 1 and type 2 diabetes mellitus [12].

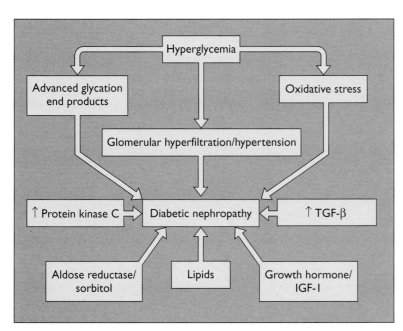

FIGURE 12-9. Suggested mechanisms underlying the development and progression of diabetic nephropathy. A number of mechanisms have been proposed to be responsible for the development of diabetic nephropathy. None of these are mutually exclusive, and it is likely that interactions of among many of these factors contribute to diabetic nephropathy. An understanding of these mechanisms is essential so that appropriate therapies may be produced to prevent both the development and progression of diabetic nephropathy. A number of existing therapies, as well as treatments currently in development or in clinical trials, are based on altering one or more of the mechanisms shown in this figure. The ensuing figures provide a brief review of each of these mechanisms. IGF-1—insulin-like growth factor-1; TGF-β—transforming growth factor-beta.

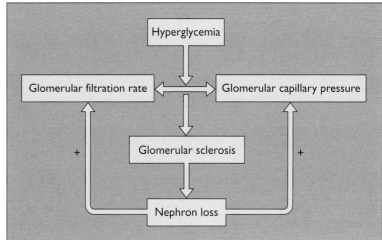

FIGURE 12-10. Glomerular hyperfiltration. Glomerular hyperfiltration is a hallmark of diabetic nephropathy. Glomerular filtration rates (GFR) of 150 mL/min and greater are seen in early diabetic nephropathy. Zatz *et al.* [13] were the first to show that intervention directed at decreasing hyperfiltration significantly slowed the progression of diabetic nephropathy in rats. The hypothesis is that the increased GFR is associated with increased pressure in the glomerular capillary tuft. This glomerular hypertension then leads to glomerular sclerosis and loss of functioning nephrons. Although the total glomerular filtration rate eventually decreases when enough nephrons undergo sclerosis, the hypothesis suggests that the filtration and, thus, the pressure in the remaining functioning glomeruli will be high because the filtered load delivered to the kidney is the same as it was when there were more functioning glomeruli. Much research supports this general hypothesis. More importantly, efforts to use interventions that lead specifically to a reduction in glomerular capillary pressure are now mainstays of treatment for diabetic nephropathy (eg, angiotensin-converting enzyme inhibitors, angiotensin-receptor blockers, and low-protein diets). An extension of this hypothesis was recently suggested by Brenner and Mackenzie [14], who proposed that one predisposing factor for the progression of renal disease and possibly for the development of diabetic nephropathy is the number of glomeruli one is born with. That is, the presence of fewer glomeruli would lead to relative glomerular hyperfiltration/hypertension, which would slowly lead to renal failure. This hypothesis is still controversial.

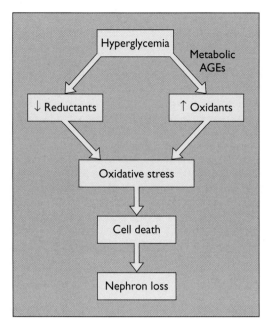

FIGURE 12-11. Oxidative stress. Many studies in both humans and animals have determined that patients with diabetes have evidence of increased oxidant stress [15]. Intracellular oxidants can increase as a result of intracellular production of oxidants or by exposure to extracellular oxidants. The cell carefully regulates the level of intracellular oxidants by a series of enzymes that reduce the oxidants. Defects in the actions of these enzymes also would contribute to an excessive level of intracellular oxidants. Hyperglycemia alone can increase the level of intracellular oxidants. Increased oxidants can cause defects in a number of intracellular events and cause cell death. In addition, increased oxidants lead to increased activity of protein kinase C, thus linking two pathophysiologic mechanisms. A number of studies currently underway are aimed at determining whether antioxidants such as vitamin E have a therapeutic role in the treatment of diabetic nephropathy. AGE—advanced glycation end products.

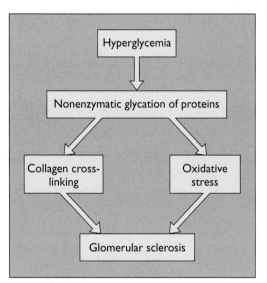

FIGURE 12-12. Advanced glycation end products. Advanced glycation end products (AGEs) are proteins that have reacted nonenzymatically with glucose. Although they exist normally, the number of AGEs increases significantly in patients with diabetic nephropathy. AGEs have been implicated in the development of complications of diabetes [16]. In particular, AGE production leads to increased oxidant stress. AGEs also can cause collagen cross-linking and, by binding to specific receptors, can lead to intracellular increases in oxidants. Administration of AGEs to animals can cause a number of changes that are seen in animals with diabetes, including glomerular sclerosis [17]. Accumulation of AGEs parallels the severity of diabetic nephropathy [18]. A number of trials currently are underway using an inhibitor of the formation of AGEs, aminoguanidine, to determine whether this drug can help patients with established nephropathy and also help prevent diabetic nephropathy.

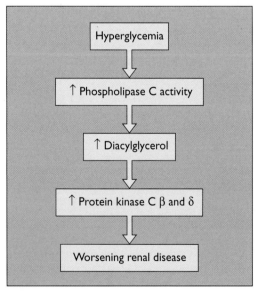

FIGURE 12-13. Protein kinase C. Protein kinase C (PKC) is a serine/threonine kinase that has been shown to play important roles in normal cell growth, in cancerous cell growth, and in a number of other intracellular processes. Work by Koya and King [19] has shown that hyperglycemia leads to activation of PKC. More detailed work has demonstrated that specific isoforms of PKC are specifically activated by hyperglycemia. The prevention of PKC activation may reduce mesangial expansion and prevent the progression of renal disease. The deleterious effects of PKC on the kidney may be the result of stimulation of the production of the cytokine transforming growth factor (TGF)-β (see Fig. 12-14). In particular, PKC β has been suggested to play an important pathophysiologic role in the development of vascular, retinal, and other complications of diabetes mellitus. Ishii et al. [20] showed in diabetic rats that an inhibitor that specifically blocks PKC greatly reduced the increase in renal TGF-β and also reduced the increase in other proteins associated with sclerosis. This suggests that PKC inhibitors may play an important role in future treatments for diabetic nephropathy.

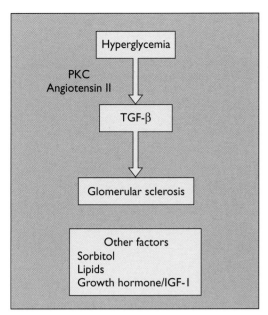

FIGURE 12-14. Transforming growth factor-β. Transforming growth factor-β (TGF-β) is a cytokine that can stimulate some cells to grow and inhibit the growth of other cells. Ziyadeh *et al.* [21] have provided a strong body of work that supports the hypothesis that TGF-β is an important mediator of the lesions seen in diabetic nephropathy. The suggestion that TGF-β plays a role in the pathogenesis of diabetic nephropathy is supported by the following evidence: 1) patients with diabetic nephropathy have increased levels of TGF-β; 2) TGF-β can cause glomerular sclerosis in animal models of diabetic nephropathy; and 3) neutralizing antibodies to TGF-β have prevented the development of diabetic nephropathy in an animal model. An interesting speculation is that increased activity of protein kinase C (PKC) leads to increased expression of TGF-β. Thus, hyperglycemia could be the initiating point that leads to increased oxidative stress, which leads to increased activity of PKC, which leads to increased expression of TGF-β. In addition, hyperglycemia leads to the production of advanced glycation end products. Thus, all of these mechanisms, separately and together, contribute to the development and progression of diabetic nephropathy.

Other factors have been implicated as well. Aldose reductase activity and the production of sorbitol have been implicated in diabetic nephropathy. Sorbitol is produced by the reduction of glucose by aldose reductase. Sorbitol is osmotically active, and, thus, increased sorbitol may lead to cell swelling and cell death. In addition, the action of aldose reductase leads to the loss of intracellular antioxidants, thereby increasing oxidative stress. Although increased aldose reductase activity appears to play a significant role in the pathogenesis of diabetic neuropathy, it remains to be shown whether it plays an important role in diabetic nephropathy. Epidemiologic studies have implicated increased lipids as possible mediators. Although it seems clear that increased lipids are associated with progression of diabetic nephropathy, the mechanism underlying this association has not been well defined. The important association of worsening vascular disease with increased lipids may be the mechanism by which lipids contribute to the progression of diabetic nephropathy. Lastly, a growing body of research suggests that growth hormone/insulin-like growth factor-1 (IGF-1) may play an important role in the pathogenesis of diabetic nephropathy. A study showed a strong positive correlation between urinary levels of growth hormone and IGF-1 with the development of microalbuminuria and increased kidney size in patients with type 1 diabetes mellitus [21].

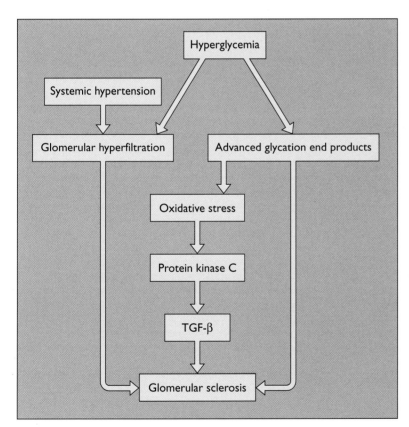

FIGURE 12-15. Possible connections between various mechanisms that may contribute to diabetic nephropathy. This model suggests that controlling the blood sugar is of paramount importance. Research from the Diabetes Control and Complications Trial (DCCT) strongly supports this idea [22]. Nevertheless, after there is evidence of diabetic nephropathy, many of these mechanisms may occur independent (to some extent) of the current blood glucose control. For example, if nephron loss has occurred, then glomerular hyperfiltration/hypertension will continue even in the presence of tight control of blood sugar. Other mechanisms shown in the figure also may become somewhat autonomous after initial damage to the glomerulus is accomplished. Thus, tight control of the blood sugar as well as other interventions that block mechanisms shown in this figure probably are needed to prevent the progression of diabetic nephropathy. TGF-β—transforming growth factor-beta.

TREATMENT FOR DIABETIC NEPHROPATHY

Mechanism	Treatment	Efficacy in Humans
Hyperglycemia	Tight control of blood sugar	Proven
Systemic hypertension	Antihypertensive agents	Proven
Glomerular hypertension	ACE inhibitors	Proven
	ARB	Proven
	Calcium channel blockers	
	Low-protein diet	
Lipids/cholesterol	Lipid-lowering agents	Important adjunctive therapy
Advanced glycation end products	Aminoguanidine	In trials
Oxidative stress	Antioxidants (eg, Vitamin E)	In trials
Increased protein kinase C	PKC inhibitors	Unknown
TGF-β	?Antibodies to TGF-β	Unknown
	PKC inhibitors	
Increased aldose reductase/sorbitol	Aldose reductase inhibitors	Questionable
Growth hormone/IGF-1	No obvious therapy	Unknown

FIGURE 12-16. The efficacy in humans of various treatments for diabetic nephropathy, listed according to mechanism. As previously noted, a combined therapeutic approach probably is the most beneficial. ACE—angiotensin-converting enzyme; ARB—angiotensin-receptor blockers; IGF—insulin-like growth factor; PKC—protein kinase C; TGF—transforming growth factor.

Treatment and Prevention

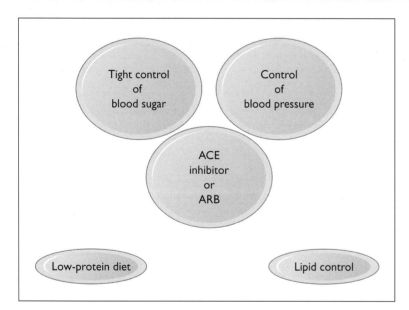

FIGURE 12-17. Treatment and prevention of diabetic nephropathy. The mainstay of prevention is tight control of the blood sugar and control of hypertension. The Diabetes Control and Complications Trial Research Group clearly showed that control of the blood sugar is very beneficial in preventing both the onset and the progression of diabetic nephropathy [22]. This is entirely consistent with the information presented in Figures 12-10 through 12-15 suggesting that hyperglycemia can be the predominant mechanism that leads to the activation of the other proposed mechanisms. In addition, many studies clearly have indicated that hypertension both predisposes to and worsens

diabetic nephropathy [23]. Thus, before microalbuminuria has developed, all patients should be urged to monitor blood sugar closely and to control blood pressure. The current recommendation is to aim for a blood pressure lower than 135/85 [23].

When microalbuminuria develops, the principal therapies are those shown here. In addition to tight control of the blood glucose and control of hypertension, all patients should be taking an angiotensin-converting enzyme inhibitor (ACE I). The ACE I drugs, although not a cure, clearly have been shown to slow the progression of diabetic nephropathy. These drugs reduce the levels of angiotensin II. A reduction in angiotensin II leads to a decrease in glomerular filtration and a decrease in glomerular pressure. In addition to its vasoactive properties, angiotensin II is also a growth factor. Thus, it has been proposed that ACE I drugs also work by inhibiting the growth-promoting effects of angiotensin II [24]. Angiotensin II receptor blockers (eg, Valsartan and Losartan), are now available. Studies have shown that angiotensin-receptor blockers (ARB) are effective in type 2 diabetic nephropathy [30–32]. The angiotensin II receptor-blocker drugs are especially useful in patients who develop a cough while taking ACE I. In addition, for unclear reasons, the hyperkalemia that can occur in patients taking ACE I is much less common in patients taking angiotensin II receptor blockers.

Other recommended treatments are adherence to a low-protein diet and control of lipids. A low-protein diet probably acts similarly to ACE I by decreasing intraglomerular pressure. In practical terms, it is somewhat difficult to achieve a low enough intake of protein, because the diet is rather bland. Nevertheless, it is recommended that diet counseling be done for both blood sugar control and low protein intake so that the patients do not ingest a high-protein diet that could potentially accelerate progression of renal disease. When patients are nearing end-stage renal disease, it is important for protein intake to be liberalized, because at this point there is little benefit to a low-protein diet and the risk of malnutrition is significant.

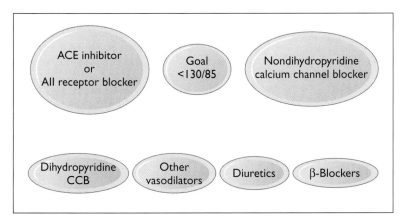

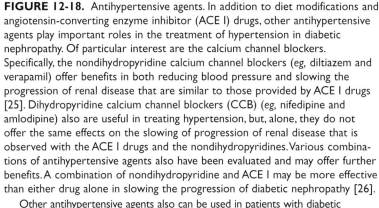

FIGURE 12-18. Antihypertensive agents. In addition to diet modifications and angiotensin-converting enzyme inhibitor (ACE I) drugs, other antihypertensive agents play important roles in the treatment of hypertension in diabetic nephropathy. Of particular interest are the calcium channel blockers. Specifically, the nondihydropyridine calcium channel blockers (eg, diltiazem and verapamil) offer benefits in both reducing blood pressure and slowing the progression of renal disease that are similar to those provided by ACE I drugs [25]. Dihydropyridine calcium channel blockers (CCB) (eg, nifedipine and amlodipine) also are useful in treating hypertension, but, alone, they do not offer the same effects on the slowing of progression of renal disease that is observed with the ACE I drugs and the nondihydropyridines. Various combinations of antihypertensive agents also have been evaluated and may offer further benefits. A combination of nondihydropyridine and ACE I may be more effective than either drug alone in slowing the progression of diabetic nephropathy [26].

Other antihypertensive agents also can be used in patients with diabetic nephropathy, such as diuretics, β-blockers, and vasodilators, but used alone they do not have the same effects on diabetic nephropathy as do ACE I and nondihydropyridines. AII—angiotensin II.

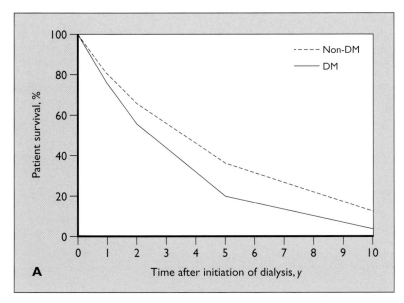

FIGURE 12-19. Survival estimates for patients on dialysis. As noted in Figure 12-1, diabetic nephropathy is the leading cause of end-stage renal disease (ESRD) in the United States. In addition, the rate of increase in ESRD resulting from diabetes is significantly greater than that for the other leading causes of renal failure. Most of this increase reflects an aging population in which type 2 diabetes mellitus (DM) is prevalent. A review covers the general issues of ESRD in the diabetic population [27]. Probably because of the many comorbid conditions that are present in diabetic patients, diabetic patients on dialysis (**A**) or post-transplantation (**B**) have a lower rate of survival than do nondiabetic ESRD patients [27]. It is not clear whether the mode of dialysis has any effects, positive or negative, on morbidity or mortality, although most ESRD diabetic patients are treated by hemodialysis [27]. The decision to use hemodialysis versus peritoneal dialysis should be made on consideration of such factors as lifestyle, overall health of the patient, and comorbid conditions (eg, vision impairment). The use of peritoneal dialysis may simplify or complicate glucose management. Because peritoneal dialysate contains varying concentrations of glucose (1.5%. 2.5%, and 4.25%), glucose control can be significantly affected when dialysate exchanges occur. This problem is minimized by injecting insulin directly into the dialysate solution. This insulin delivery method can be used not only to counteract the effects of the acute exposure to the high glucose concentrations but also as a way to provide a constant level of insulin that may help in maintaining a reasonably stable blood glucose throughout the day. This method of insulin delivery is effective for overall blood glucose maintenance only for patients who do fluid exchanges during the day. Many patients prefer to do peritoneal dialysis by repeated nighttime exchanges using a machine that cycles the fluid in and out of the abdomen. During the day these patients have no fluid exchanges. The insulin injected in each bag at night is dosed to maintain a steady glucose concentration through the night, and the patient follows a standard schedule of subcutaneous injections throughout the day. (*Data from* U. S. Renal Data System [28].)

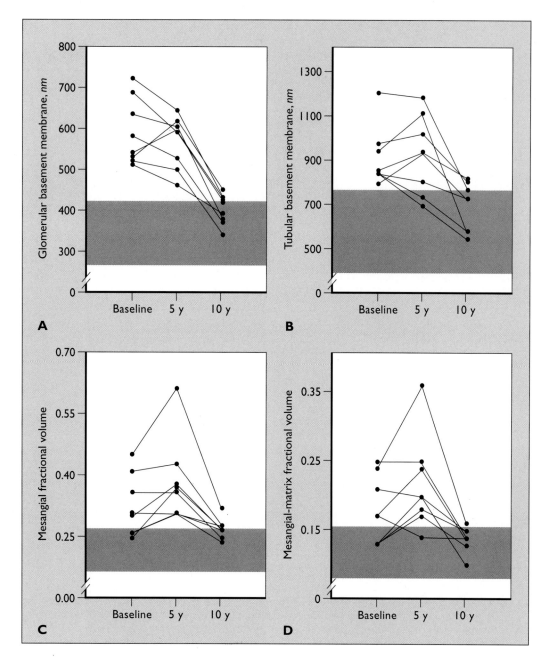

FIGURE 12-20. Kidney and pancreas transplantation. Kidney or kidney/pancreas transplantation generally is believed to be the preferred therapy for patients with end-stage renal disease. Survival rates after transplantation are higher than those for patients who remain on dialysis (see Fig. 12-19). Diabetic nephropathy recurs in most kidney transplant recipients, although it usually is many years before diabetic nephropathy is severe enough to cause loss of the transplant (**A** through **D**). Loss of the transplant because of the recurrence of diabetic nephropathy is rare, therefore.

Pancreas transplantation usually is done only in conjunction with a kidney transplant. It has been believed that because blood glucose levels can be controlled with insulin, pancreas transplantation offers too many risks compared to its benefits. The biggest risks relate to immunosuppression and the increased risk of life-threatening infections. In addition, there has been little evidence showing that early pancreas transplant would affect the progression of diabetic nephropathy. An intriguing study by Fioretto *et al.* [29] shows, however, that pancreas transplantation alone can cause actual reversal in the lesions of diabetic nephropathy that become evident only after 5 years of normoglycemia. This finding may increase interest in pancreas transplantation as a way to prevent the development of diabetic nephropathy. (*Adapted from* Fioretto *et al.* [29].)

JOSLIN DIABETES CENTER SCREENING AND TREATMENT RECOMMENDATIONS FOR MICROPROTEINURIA AND MACROPROTEINURIA

Screening

Screen for microalbuminuria by checking for albumin/creatinine (A/C) ratio:

Annually in patients 10–65 years of age

As clinically indicated in patients >65 years of age

Continue use of routine urinalysis as clinically indicated

Treatment

If A/C ratio <20 μg/mg (30 mg/24 h)

Recheck in 1 year

If A/C ratio 20–300 μg/mg (30–300 mg/24 h)

Confirm presence of microalbuminuria with at least 2 positive collections done within 3–6 mo. In the process rule out confounding factors that cause false positive results, eg, urinary tract infection, pregnancy, excessive exercise

Once confirmed

Initiate/modify use of ACE inhibitor. Consider use for type 2 diabetes. If side effects to ACE inhibitor occur, consider angiotensin II receptor antagonist treatment.

Initiate/modify hypertension treatment with a goal blood pressure under 130/80 mm Hg or MAP <90

Encourage home blood pressure monitoring

Refer to diabetes education

Refer to registered dietitian for dietary management

Strive to improve glycemic control with an optimal goal of HbA_{1c} <8% or as otherwise clinically indicated

Monitor serum creatinine and potassium, and treat appropriately

Repeat A/C ratio testing at least every 12 mo. Consider testing more often when changes in medication are made

If A/C ratio >300 μg/mg (>300 mg/24 h) or overt proteinuria

Follow all guidelines as stated for A/C ratio 20–300 μg/mg

Consider a consultation with nephrology team when:

A/C ratio is >300 μg/mg

Rapid rise in creatinine (eg, 0.8 to 1.4 in 12 mo); presence of hematuria, or sudden increase in proteinuria

Questioning etiology of nephropathy

For refinement of treatment program to prevent further decline in renal function

Refer to renal team for collaborative care when:

Creatinine is elevated (>1.8 women, >2.0 in men)

Problems with ACE inhibitors, difficulties in management of hypertension or hyperkalemia

FIGURE 12-21. Screening and treatment recommendations for proteinuria. The current recommendations for treatment for proteinuria at the Joslin Diabetes Center in Boston, Massachusetts are based on the level of proteinuria. The physicians at the Joslin Diabetes Center believe that a collaborative model of care is best for the patient with diabetes. Thus, patients with early diabetic nephropathy are cared for primarily by an endocrinologist in consultation with a nephrologist. When patients near end-stage renal disease, much of the care of the patient transfers to the nephrologist, but the other caregivers (eg, endocrinologist, ophthalmologist, dietitian) continue to work collaboratively to care for the patient. ACE—angiotensin-converting enzme; MAP—mean arterial pressure.

References

1. Ruggenenti P, Remuzzi G: Nephropathy of type-2 diabetes mellitus. *J Am Soc Nephrol* 1998, 9:2157–2169.

2. Ritz E, Orth SR: Nephropathy in patients with type 2 diabetes mellitus. *N Engl J Med* 1999, 341:1127–1133.

3. Agodoa LY: U.S. Renal Data System, USRDS 2001 Annual Data Report. *Am J Kidney Dis* 2001, 38(Suppl 3): S37–S52.

4. Stephenson JM, Fuller JH, Viberti GC, et al.: EURODIAB IDDM complications study group. Blood pressure, retinopathy, and urinary albumin excretion in IDDM. *Diabetologia* 1995, 38:599–603.

5. Chihara J, Takebayashi S, Takashi T, et al.: Glomerulonephritis in diabetic patients and its effect on the prognosis. *Nephron* 1986, 43:45–49.

6. Warram JH, Krolewski AS: Use of the albumin/creatinine ratio in patient care and clinical studies. In *The Kidney and Hypertension in Diabetes Mellitus.* Edited by Mogensen CE. London: Kluwer Academic Publishers; 1998:85–96

7. Tisher CC, Hostetter TH: Diabetic nephropathy. In *Renal Pathology*, edn 2. Edited by Tisher CC, Brenner BM. Philadelphia: JB Lippincott; 1994:1387–1412.

8. Parving HH, Hommel E, Mathiesen E, et al.: Prevalence of microalbuminuria, arterial hypertension, retinopathy, and neuropathy in patients with insulin dependent diabetes. *Br Med J* 1988, 296:156–160.

9. Krolewski AS, Fogarty DG, Warram JH: Hypertension and nephropathy in diabetes mellitus: what is inherited and what is acquired? *Diab Res Clin Practice* 1998, 39(suppl):S1–S14.

10. Quinn M, Angelico MC, Warram JH, et al.: Familial factors determine the development of diabetic nephropathy in patients with IDDM. *Diabetologia* 1996, 39:940–945.

11. Nelson RG, Newman JM, Knowler WC, et al.: Incidence of end stage renal disease in Type 2 (non–insulin-dependent) diabetes mellitus in Pima Indians. *Diabetologia* 1988, 31:730–736.

12. Biesenbach G, Grafinger P, Janko O, et al.: Influence of cigarette smoking on the progression of clinical diabetic nephropathy in type 2 diabetic patients. *Clin Nephrol* 1997, 48:146–150.

13. Zatz R, Rentz DB, Meyer TW, et al.: Prevention of diabetic glomerulopathy by pharmacological amelioration of glomerular capillary hypertension. *J Clin Invest* 1986, 77:1925–1930.

14. Brenner B, Mackenzie HS: Nephron mass as risk factor for the progression of renal disease. *Kidney Int* 1997, 63(Suppl):S124–S127.

15. Giugliano D, Ceriello A, Paolissa G: Oxidative stress and diabetic vascular complications. *Diabetes Care* 1996, 19:257–267.

16. Bierhaus A, Hofmann MA, Ziegler R, et al.: AGEs and their interaction with AGE-receptors in vascular disease and diabetes mellitus. I. The AGE concept. *Cardiovasc Res* 1998, 37:586–600.

17. Vlassara H, Striker LJ, Teichberg S, et al.: Advanced glycation end products induce glomerular sclerosis and albuminuria in normal rats. *Proc Natl Acad Sci U S A* 1994, 91:11704–11708.

18. Makita Z, Radoff S, Rayfield EJ, et al.: Advanced glycation end products in patients with diabetic nephropathy. *N Engl J Med* 1991, 325:836–842.

19. Koya D, King GL: Protein kinase C activation and the development of diabetic complications. *Diabetes* 1998, 47:859–866.

20. Ishii H, Jirousek MR, Koya D, et al.: Ameliorations of vascular dysfunctions in diabetic rats by an oral PKC beta inhibitor. *Science* 1996, 272:728–731.

21. Hoffman BB, Sharma K, Ziyadeh FN: Potential role of TGF-β in diabetic nephropathy. *Min Electrol Metab* 1998, 24:190–196.

22. The Diabetes Control and Complications Trial Research Group: The effect of intensive treatment of diabetes on the development and progression of long-term complications in insulin-dependent diabetes mellitus. *N Engl J Med* 1993, 329:977–986.

23. Bakris GL: Progression of diabetic nephropathy. A focus on arterial pressure level and methods of reduction. *Diab Res Clin Prac* 1998, 39(Suppl):S35–S42.

24. Wolf G, Ziyadeh FN: The role of angiotensin II in diabetic nephropathy: emphasis on nonhemodynamic mechanisms. *Am J Kidney Dis* 1997, 29:153–163.

25. Slataper R, Vicknair N, Sadler R, et al.: Comparative effects of different antihypertensive treatments on progression of diabetic renal disease. *Arch Int Med* 1993, 153:973–979.

26. Bakris GL, Weir MR, DeQuattro V, et al.: Effects of an ACE inhibitor/ calcium antagonist combination on proteinuria in diabetic nephropathy. *Kidney Int* 1998, 54:1283–1289.

27. Williams ME: The diabetic patient with end stage renal disease. In *Therapy in Nephrology and Hypertension.* Edited by Brady HR, Wilcox CS. Philadelphia: WB Saunders; 1999:249–255.

28. U. S. Renal Data System: *USRDS 1996 Annual Data Report.* Bethesda, MD: The National Institutes of Health, National Institute of Diabetes and Digestive and Kidney Diseases. April 1996.

29. Fioretto P, Steffes MW, Sutherland DER, et al.: Reversal of lesions of diabetic nephropathy after pancreas transplantation. *N Engl J Med* 1998, 339:69–75.

30. Lewis EJ, Hunsicker LG, Clarke WR, et al.: Renoprotective effect of the angiotensin-receptor antagonist irbesartan in patients with nephropathy due to type 2 diabetes. *N Engl J Med* 2001, 345(12):851–860.

31. Brenner BM, Cooper ME, de Zeeuw D, et al.: Effects of losartan on renal and cardiovascular outcomes in patients with type 2 diabetes and nephropathy. *N Engl J Med* 2001, 345(12):861–869.

32. Parving HH, Lehnert H, Brochner-Mortensen J, et al.: The effect of irbesartan on the development of diabetic nephropathy in patients with type 2 diabetes. *N Engl J Med* 2001, 345(12):870–878.

DIABETIC NEUROPATHIES

Aaron I. Vinik

13

Diabetic neuropathy is not a single entity but rather a number of different syndromes, each with a range of clinical and subclinical manifestations. According to the San Antonio Conference [1], the main groups of neurologic disturbance in diabetes mellitus include subclinical neuropathy determined by abnormalities in electrodiagnostic and quantitative sensory testing, diffuse clinical neuropathy with distal symmetric sensorimotor and autonomic syndromes, and focal syndromes. There is reason to add proximal neuropathy as a separate entity based on the nature of the pathology and response to treatment. However, we have found it more appropriate to classify neuropathy into different clinical syndromes based on their pathogenesis because this is what ultimately determines the choice of treatment. We classify neuropathies into somatic and autonomic. There are two types of autonomic neuropathy: focal and diffuse. The focal neuropathies include mononeuritis and entrapment syndromes. The diffuse neuropathies include proximal neuropathies and large- and small-fiber distal symmetric polyneuropathies.

Estimates of the prevalence of diabetic neuropathy range from 10% to 90% of the diabetic population, depending on the criteria used to define neuropathy [1–6]. Neurologic complications occur equally in patients with type 1 and type 2 diabetes mellitus, as well as various forms of acquired diabetes.

In this pictorial overview, clinical presentations and therapeutic approaches to common forms of neuropathy are presented and discussed, including distal symmetric, proximal motor, and autonomic neuropathies. Also provided are algorithms for recognition and management of common pain and entrapment syndromes. A global approach is used for recognition of syndromes requiring specialized treatments based on our improved understanding of their etiopathogenesis.

Pathogenesis

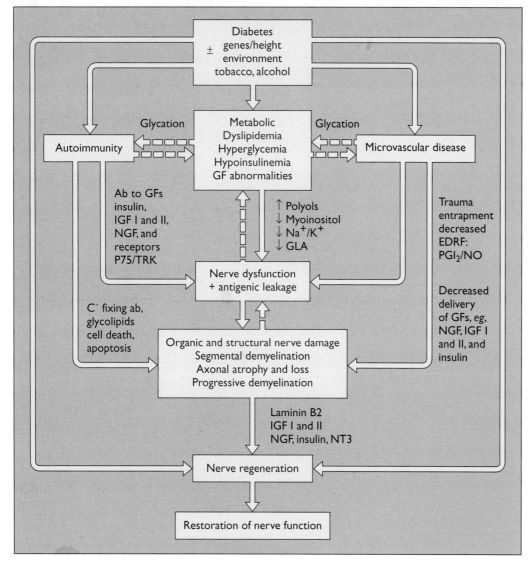

FIGURE 13-1. Current view on the pathogenesis of diabetic neuropathy. The figure depicts multiple causes, including metabolic, vascular, autoimmune, and neurohormonal growth factor deficiency. Although there is increasing evidence that the pathogenesis of diabetic neuropathy comprises several mechanisms, the prevailing theory implicates persistent hyperglycemia as the primary factor within the metabolic hypothesis [7,8]. Persistent hyperglycemia increases polyol pathway activity with accumulation of sorbitol and fructose in nerves, damaging them by an as yet unknown mechanism. This is accompanied by decreased myoinositol uptake and inhibition of the sodium-potassium ion adenosine triphosphatase pathway, resulting in sodium retention, edema, myelin swelling, axoglial dysjunction, and nerve degeneration. Deficiency of dihomo-γ-linoleic acid (GLA) as well as N-acetyl-L-carnitine also have been implicated [9]. Metabolic factors cannot account for all forms of neuropathy nor for the heterogeneity of the clinical syndromes. In a subpopulation of patients with neuropathy, immune mechanisms may be responsible for the clinical syndrome, especially in patients with the proximal variety of neuropathy and those with a more marked motor component to their neuropathy. Our data support the hypothesis that circulating antineuronal antibodies are present in diabetic serum, at least in some patients. The circulating autoantibodies directed against motor and sensory nerve structures have been detected by indirect immunofluorescence, and antibody and complement deposits in various components of sural nerves have been shown [10–12].

Microvascular insufficiency has been proposed by a number of investigators as a possible cause of diabetic neuropathy [13–15]. The interest in microvascular derangement in patients with diabetic neuropathy has arisen from studies suggesting that absolute or relative ischemia may exist in the nerves of patients with diabetes owing to altered function of the endoneurial or epineurial blood vessels, or both. Histopathologic studies show the presence of different degrees of endoneurial and epineurial microvasculopathy, mainly thickening of blood vessel wall or occlusion [16,17]. A number of functional disturbances have also been demonstrated in the microvasculature of the nerves of patients with diabetes. Studies have demonstrated decreased neural blood flow, increased vascular resistance, decreased oxygen pressure, and altered vascular permeability characteristics such as a loss of the anionic charge barrier and decreased charge selectivity [18–20]. It also has been shown that abnormalities of cutaneous blood flow correlate with neuropathy [21].

Apart from the metabolic, immunologic, and vascular factors involved in the pathogenesis of neuropathy, data exist to support a role for growth factor deficiency. Many of the neuronal changes characteristic of diabetic neuropathy are similar to those observed following either removal of target-derived growth factors by axotomy or depletion of endogenous growth factors by experimental induction of growth factor autoimmunity. Because neuronal growth factors can promote the survival, maintenance, and regeneration of neurons subject to the noxious effects of diabetes, the success of patients with diabetes in maintaining normal nerve morphology and function may ultimately depend on the expression and efficacy of these factors [9]. Ab—antibody; EDRF—endothelium-derived relaxing factor; GF—growth factor; IGF—insulin-like growth factor; NGF—neuronal growth factor; NO—nitric oxide; NT3—neurotropin 3; PGI_2—prostaglandin I_2.

Mononeuropathy and Entrapment

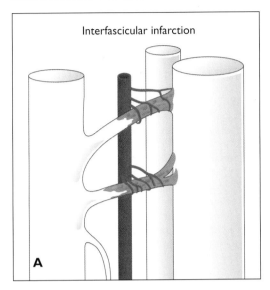

Interfascicular infarction

A

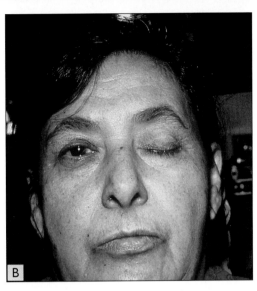

B

Medial and lateral plantar entrapments decrease sensation in the inside and outside of the foot, respectively. The entrapment neuropathies are highly prevalent in the diabetic population and should be actively sought in every patient with signs and symptoms of neuropathy because the treatment may be surgical [23].

Carpal tunnel syndrome occurs twice as frequently in a diabetic population compared with a normal healthy population. Its increased prevalence in patients with diabetes may be related to repeated undetected trauma, metabolic changes, or accumulation of fluid or edema within the confined space of the carpal tunnel [22]. If recognized, the diagnosis can be confirmed by an electrophysiologic study, and therapy is simple with surgical release. The unaware physician seldom realizes that symptoms may spread to the whole hand or arm in carpal tunnel syndrome, and the signs may extend beyond those subserved by the entrapped nerve. Thus, the very nature of the trouble goes unrecognized, and an opportunity for successful therapeutic intervention often is missed. The mainstays of nonsurgical treatment are avoidance of the use of the wrist, placement of a wrist splint in a neutral position for day and night use, and anti-inflammatory medications. Surgical treatment consists of sectioning the volar carpal ligament. The decision to proceed with surgery should be based on several considerations, including severity of symptoms, appearance of motor weakness, and failure of nonsurgical treatment.

FIGURE 13-2. Focal neuropathies: mononeuritis and entrapment syndromes. Mononeuropathies are caused by vasculitis and subsequent ischemia or infarction of nerves (**A**) [22]. Mononeuropathies heal spontaneously, usually within 6 to 8 weeks. The isolated peripheral nerve lesions involve particularly ulnar, median, radial, femoral, and lateral cutaneous nerves of the thigh. In mononeuropathies in which weakness is a prominent feature, such as peroneal palsy, physical therapy may be necessary to maintain good muscle tone and prevent contractures.

The common mononeuropathies (**B**) involve cranial nerves 3, 4, 6, and 7; and thoracic and peripheral nerves including peroneal, sural, sciatic, femoral, ulnar, and median. Their onset is acute and associated with pain, and their course is self-limiting, resolving over a period of 6 weeks. The common mononeuropathies must be distinguished from entrapment syndromes, which start slowly, progress, and persist without intervention. Common entrapments involve the median nerve with impaired sensation in the first three fingers and a positive Tinel sign. Ulnar entrapment decreases sensory perception in the little and ring fingers.

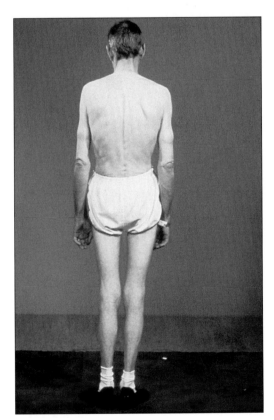

FIGURE 13-3. Proximal motor neuropathy can be identified clinically based on proximal muscle weakness and muscle wasting. This neuropathy may be symmetric or asymmetric in distribution and is sometimes associated with pain in the lateral aspect of the thighs [24,25]. The condition is readily recognizable clinically. Prevailing weakness of the iliopsoas, obturator, and adductor muscles is observed together with relative preservation of the gluteus maximus and minimus, and hamstrings [24,25]. Those affected have great difficulty rising out of a chair unaided and often climb up their bodies. Heel or toe standing is surprisingly good. In the classic form of diabetic amyotrophy, axonal loss is the predominant process, and the condition coexists with distal sensory polyneuropathy [10]. Electrophysiologic evaluation reveals lumbosacral plexopathy [11]. In contrast, if demyelination predominates and the motor deficit affects proximal and distal muscle groups, the diagnosis of chronic inflammatory demyelinating polyneuropathy (CIDP) should be considered [11,12]. It is important to divide proximal syndromes into these two subcategories because the CIDP variant responds dramatically to intervention [12], whereas amyotrophy runs its own course over months to years. Until more evidence is available, we consider them to be separate syndromes. Another frequently seen focal syndrome is multifocal, predominantly sensory neuropathy, which easily can be identified based on clinical evaluation. (*From* Chia et al. [26]; with permission.)

Distal Neuropathy

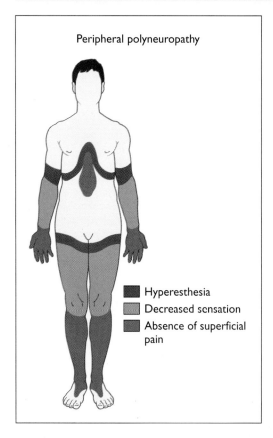

Peripheral polyneuropathy

■ Hyperesthesia
□ Decreased sensation
■ Absence of superficial
pain

FIGURE 13-4. Peripheral polyneuropathy. The spectra of clinical neuropathic syndromes described in patients with diabetes mellitus include dysfunction of almost every segment of the somatic peripheral and autonomic nervous systems [22]. Each syndrome can be distinguished by its pathophysiologic, therapeutic, and prognostic features. Initial neurologic evaluation should be directed toward detection of the specific part of the nervous system affected by diabetes. Diabetes may damage small fibers, large fibers, or both. Small nerve fiber dysfunction usually, but not always, occurs early and often is present before objective signs or electrophysiologic evidence of nerve damage is found [27–29]. Small nerve fiber dysfunction is manifested first in the lower limbs by pain and hyperalgesia. Loss of thermal sensitivity follows, with reduced light touch and pinprick sensation. Large fiber neuropathies may involve sensory or motor nerves, or both. The neuropathies are manifested by reduced vibration (often the first objective evidence of neuropathy) and position sense, weakness, muscle wasting, and depressed tendon reflexes. Most patients with distal sensory polyneuropathy have a mixed variety, with both large and small nerve fiber involvement. In the case of distal sensory polyneuropathy, a "glove and stocking" distribution of sensory loss is almost universal [22]. Early in the course of the neuropathic process, multifocal sensory loss may also be found.

Diabetic peripheral symmetric polyneuropathy is thought to be a dying-back disorder, with prevailing effects on the axons and consequent demyelination. There is an early functional phase in which metabolic abnormalities are responsible for the clinical symptoms and signs. Later structural changes occur in the nerves so that treatment strategies have been to arrest or slow the rate of progression. When neuronal cell death occurs, little can be done to induce recovery. Clearly, all attempts at treating neuropathy should be oriented toward the reversible phase of the disorder.

Cutaneous Nerve Components

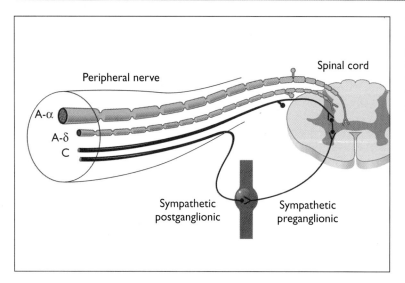

Spinal cord

Peripheral nerve

A-α
A-δ
C

Sympathetic
postganglionic

Sympathetic
preganglionic

FIGURE 13-5. Cutaneous nerve components. Peripheral nerves are composed of several different types of nerve fibers, each with their own function. The large myelinated α fibers conduct rapidly and subserve motor power and proprioception and coordination. The thinner yet myelinated A-δ fibers subserve cold thermal detection and deep-seated pain. The thin unmyelinated fibers are responsible for warm detection threshold, heat pain, part of touch sensation, and sympathetic nerve supply to the skin.

Large Fiber Neuropathy

CLINICAL PRESENTATION AND MANAGEMENT OF LARGE FIBER NEUROPATHY

Presentation
Impaired vibration perception
Pain of A-δ type: deep-seated, gnawing
Ataxia
Wasting of small muscles, intrinsic minus feet with hammer toes
Weakness
Increased blood flow (the hot foot)
  Risk of Charcot neuroarthropathy
Management
  Proper shoes
  Orthotics
  Tendon lengthening
  Foot reconstruction

FIGURE 13-6. Clinical presentation and management of large fiber neuropathy.

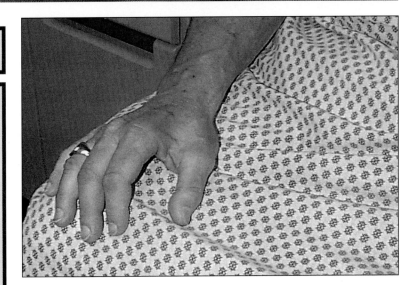

FIGURE 13-7. Wasting of the small muscle of the hand in large fiber neuropathies. This must not be mistaken for ulnar entrapment, which is amenable to treatment. In large fiber neuropathies all peripheral nerves are affected equally and the sensory disturbance is of the "glove and stocking" variety not confined to the nerve distribution. In ulnar entrapment the sensory loss involves the ring and little fingers.

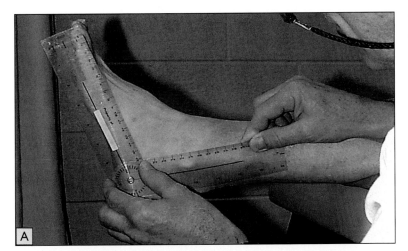

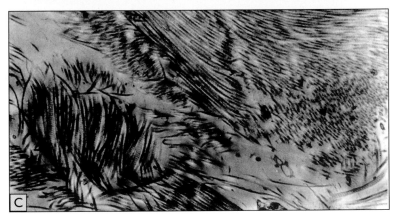

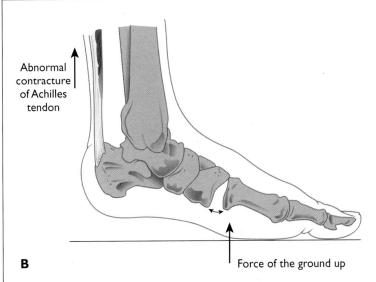

Abnormal contracture of Achilles tendon

Force of the ground up

FIGURE 13-8. In large fiber neuropathies there is wasting of the small muscles of the feet: intrinsic minus feet as well as talipes equinovarus owing to shortening of the Achilles tendon. **A,** Measurement of the angle of the ankle in full flexion. Using a goniometer, the flexion should be at least 90°. **B,** Greater than 100° indicates tendo-achilles shortening, with its impact on increasing midfoot pressure and breakdown of Lisfranc's joint in the midfoot. **C,** Electron micrograph of disrupted collagen fibers in the Achilles tendon in a patient with large nerve neuropathy.

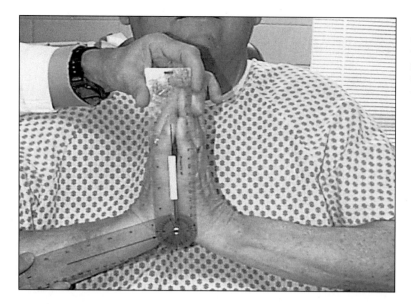

FIGURE 13-9. Upper extremity features of large fiber neuropathies. This patient is unable to extend his hands at the wrist to beyond 90°, as shown using the goniometer. Note the separation of the small fingers, creating a diamond-shaped open space indicative of cheiroarthropathy. These features accompany large fiber neuropathies as well as entrapment syndromes. This is not universal, and the two conditions may well have different causes.

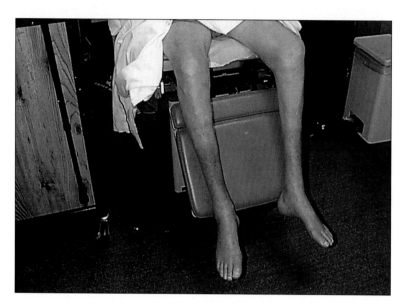

FIGURE 13-10. Lower extremity features of large fiber neuropathies. This patient shows a combination of severe muscle wasting of the lower limbs resembling that seen in Charcot-Marie-Tooth disease, the equinus of the feet owing to shortening of the Achilles tendon, and wasting of the proximal muscles of the thigh owing to a combination of a proximal neuropathy and a distal large fiber neuropathy.

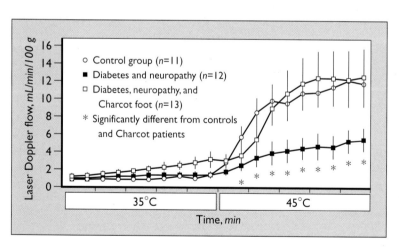

FIGURE 13-11. Neurovascular dysfunction in neuropathy. (*Adapted from Shapiro et al.* [30].)

C-Fiber Dysfunction in Small Fiber Neuropathy

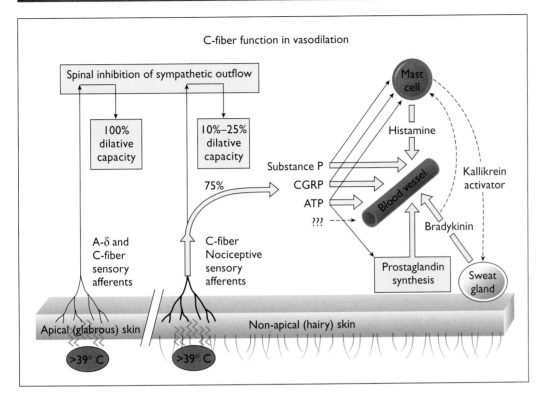

FIGURE 13-12. Vasodilation and C-fiber function. Factors controlling vasodilation in glabrous skin such as that found on the pads and soles and hairy skin found on the dorsum of the feet and hands. In glabrous skin, vasodilation is for the most part a consequence of relaxation of the sympathetic tone. In hairy skin, C fibers are essential for vasodilation, a process mediated by a variety of neurotransmitters including the neuropeptides, substance P, and calcitonin gene-related peptide (CGRP) as well as bradykinin. Defective trophic support for skin with reduced levels of neuronal growth factor results in decreased substance P and CGRP, thereby impairing the ability to dilate in response to noxious stimuli and heat. Thus nutrient delivery is compromised and there is susceptibility to ulceration. ATP—adenosine triphosphate. (*Adapted from* Burnstock and Ralevic [31].)

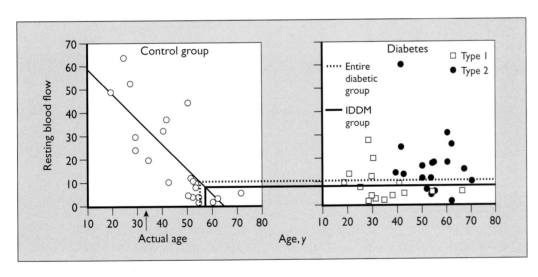

FIGURE 13-13. Age and resting blood flow. IDDM—insulin-dependent diabetes mellitus. (*Adapted from* Stansberry *et al.* [32].)

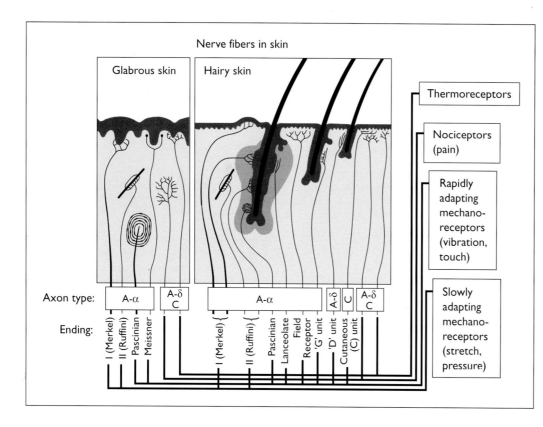

Nerve fibers in skin

FIGURE 13-14. Different nerve fibers in skin and their different roles in sensory perception and mechanoreceptor function. C-fiber type pain generally is described as throbbing, shooting, stabbing, sharp, hot, burning, and tender. Touch is misinterpreted as pain, ie, allodynia, and patients cannot bear contact with bedclothes or other objects. In contrast, A-δ pain often is described as cramping, gnawing, aching, heavy, splitting, tiring and exhausting, sickening, fearful, and punishing and cruel. A patient may say, "I have toothache in my foot," "there is a dog gnawing at the bones of my feet," or "my feet feel as if they are encased in concrete." These pains derive from different fibers and have a different mechanism of production. The scheme is based on this information, which proves helpful in the management of patients with neuropathic pain.

Pain disappears when a loss of C-fibers occurs, and the loss heralds the phase of hypoalgesia, and hypesthesia, with impairment of warm thermal perception and insensitivity to heat pain. These symptoms are particularly dangerous and are the forerunners of repeated minor injury and subsequent loss of toes and feet.

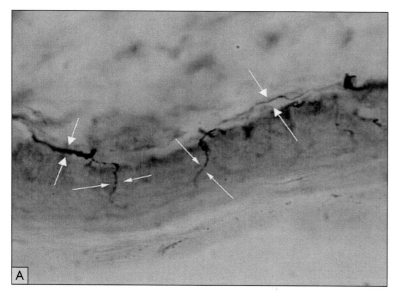

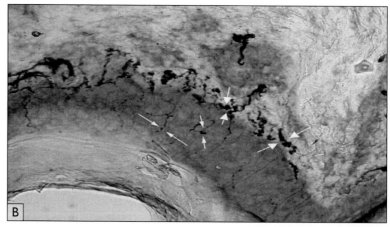

FIGURE 13-15. Photomicrographs of 50-µm sections from skin biopsy specimens taken from the upper thigh of a control subject (**A**) and a neuropathic patient (**B**). The sections were stained with antibody to PCP 9.5 and neuronal antigen and were evaluated by immunocytochemistry to reveal peripheral small unmyelinated neurons. **A** shows straight, uninterrupted unmyelinated nerve fibers running between the dermis and epidermis in normal skin (*broad arrows*). In addition, there are numerous single, relatively straight fibers projecting into the epidermis (*narrow arrows*) of normal skin. **B** demonstrates the changes observed in neuropathic skin, including malformation of the fibers running between dermis and epidermis, with multiple, irregular swelling (*broad arrows*). The fibers in the epidermis of neuropathic skin are reduced in number compared with normal skin. These changes in skin are characteristic of small fiber neuropathies and may occur in the absence of any other clinical or laboratory evidence of neuropathy.

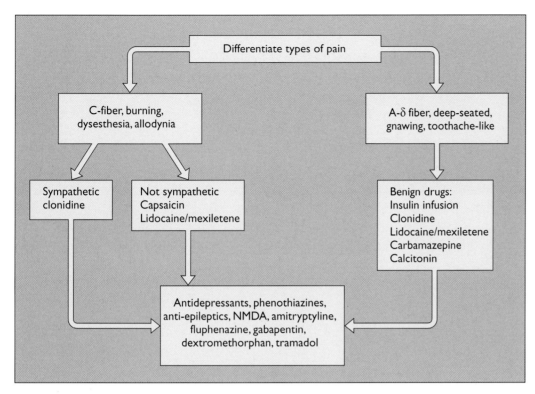

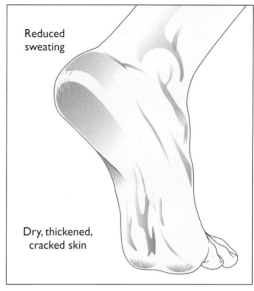

FIGURE 13-17. Clinical presentation of small fiber neuropathy. The signs of this disorder include pain (C-fiber type, burning and superficial), late hypoalgesia, hypoesthesia, impaired warm thermal perception, decreased sweating, and impaired cutaneous blood flow (the cold foot). The risks are foot ulcers, gangrene, and amputations.

FIGURE 13-16. Managing painful diabetic neuropathy. NMDA—N-methyl-D-aspartate.

FIGURE 13-18. Management of C-fiber dysfunction.

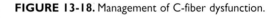

MANAGEMENT OF C-FIBER DYSFUNCTION

Patients must be instructed on foot care with daily foot inspection (they must have a mirror in the bathroom for inspection of the soles of the feet)

Patients should be provided with a monofilament for self-testing

All diabetic patients should wear padded socks

Shoes must fit well with adequate support and must be inspected for the presence of foreign bodies (eg, nails, pins, teeth) before wearing

Patients must exercise care with exposure to heat (eg, avoid falling asleep in front of the fireplace)

Emollient creams should be used for the drying and cracking of skin

After bathing, feet should be thoroughly dried and powdered between the toes

Nails should be cut transversely, preferably by a podiatrist

FIGURE 13-19. Management of small fiber neuropathies. In the United States, 65,000 amputations are performed each year. Half of these are attributable to diabetes, and small fiber neuropathy is implicated in 87% of cases. The combination of decreased pain perception with decreased warm thermal perception and the resulting hammer toe deformity that follows intrinsic minus feet leads to blisters on the top of the knuckles of the toes or ulcers over the heads of the metatarsals. These high-pressure points are easily recognized by forced gate analysis scans of the feet. With correct shoes, padded socks and orthotics, the likelihood of amputation can be reduced by half. Patients should be instructed to protect their feet with padded socks, wear shoes that have adequate support, regularly inspect their feet and shoes, be careful of exposure to heat, and use emollient creams for sympathetic dysfunction.

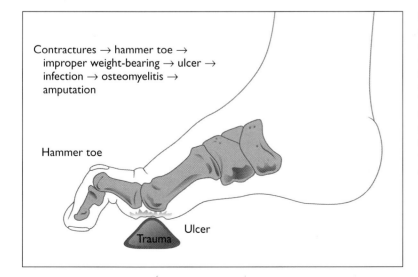

Contractures → hammer toe → improper weight-bearing → ulcer → infection → osteomyelitis → amputation

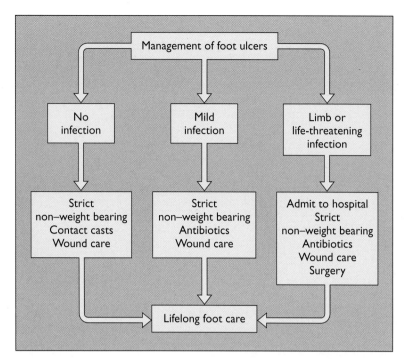

FIGURE 13-20. Management of foot ulcers.

Neuroarthropathy

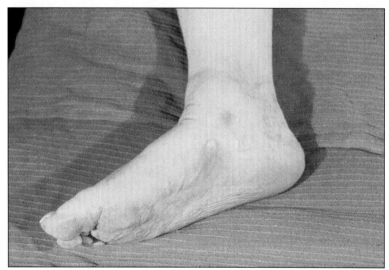

FIGURE 13-21. (See Color Plate) The hot foot of Charcot neuroarthropathy showing the end result of large fiber neuropathy. Note the red inflamed foot that is easily mistaken for infection and the collapse of the midfoot.

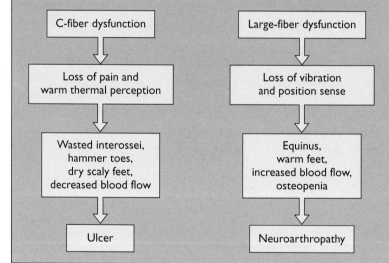

FIGURE 13-22. Prediction of foot ulcers versus neuroarthropathy.

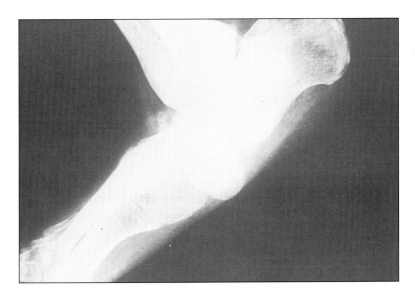

FIGURE 13-23. Radiograph of the foot shown in Figure 13-21. Note the rarefaction and osteopenia of the calcaneus with collapse of the midfoot and loss of architecture of the foot. These results of large fiber neuropathy and increased blood flow could have been prevented if recognized early.

Autonomic Neuropathy

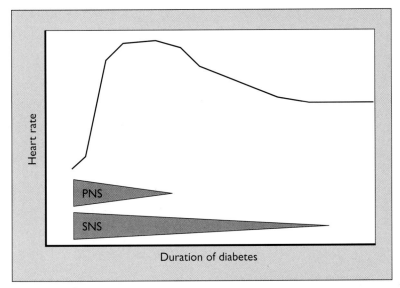

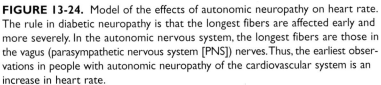

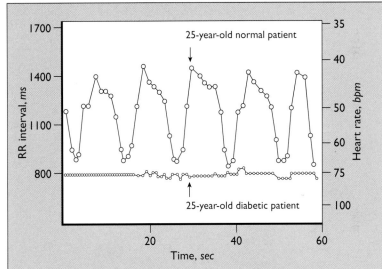

FIGURE 13-24. Model of the effects of autonomic neuropathy on heart rate. The rule in diabetic neuropathy is that the longest fibers are affected early and more severely. In the autonomic nervous system, the longest fibers are those in the vagus (parasympathetic nervous system [PNS]) nerves. Thus, the earliest observations in people with autonomic neuropathy of the cardiovascular system is an increase in heart rate.

Later, as the short efferent fibers of the sympathetic nervous system (SNS) become involved, the heart rate slows down but not to normal. It is indeed a denervated heart. With loss of the afferent fibers there also is loss of pain perception, accounting for the high incidence of painless myocardial infarctions in patients with diabetic neuropathy. (*Adapted from* Ewing *et al.* [33].)

FIGURE 13-25. Respiratory rate (RR) intervals and effects of cardiac autonomic dysfunction. The most sensitive indicator of cardiac autonomic neuropathy is the loss of the normal sinus arrhythmia with breathing. This loss can be measured on an electrocardiogram as loss of the change in the RR interval with deep breathing at six breaths per minute and reflects almost entirely damage to the parasympathetic nervous system. With more sophisticated approaches, computerized spectral analysis of the electrocardiogram tracing allows one to infer the status of the sympathetic nervous system as well. Late in the course of cardiac autonomic neuropathy the advent of *orthostasis* (a decrease in blood pressure of > 30 mm Hg when arising from a lying position) reflects sympathetic nerve damage. Peripheral measures of autonomic function are described in Figures 13-11 to 13-13 on blood flow in the diabetic foot.

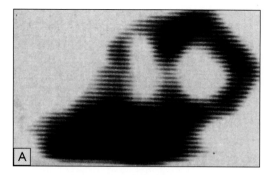 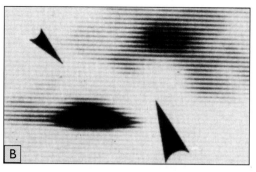 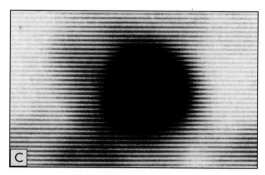

FIGURE 13-26. Segmental loss of sympathetic nerve fibers in the heart, demonstrable using multiple gated acquisition (MUGA) (**A**), meta-iodobenzyl-guanidine (**B**), and thallium scans (**C**), does not demonstrate ventricular wall defects. It is now thought that this imbalance in the sympathetic nerve supply of the myocardium is what leads to the irritable foci, leading to arrhythmia and possibly accounting for sudden death in diabetic patients with autonomic neuropathy. This mechanism also is thought to operate in people who have had a myocardial infarction and may be the reason for the effectiveness of β-blockade in reducing mortality in patients who have had a myocardial infarction. (*From* Kahn *et al.* [34]; with permission.)

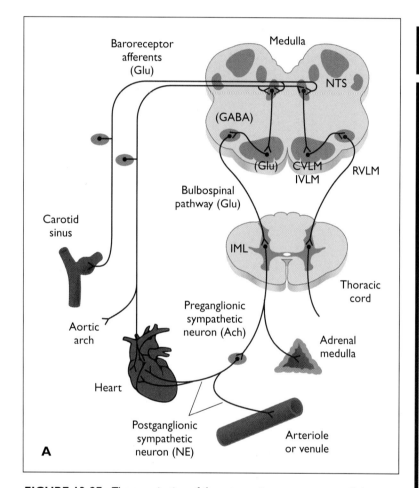

B. ORGANIZATION OF THE AUTONOMIC NERVOUS SYSTEM OF THE HEART

Eye
  Abnormal pupillary reaction, with night blindness
Cardiovascular
  Sudden death, silent myocardial infarction
  Orthostasis
  Impaired peripheral vascular reflexes
Respiratory
  Failure of hypoxia-induced respiration
Gut
  Gustatory sweating
  Gastroparesis
  Diarrhea
  Constipation
  Loss of anal sphincter tone and incontinence
Metabolic
  Hypoglycemia unawareness
  Hypoglycemia unresponsiveness
  Hypoglycemia-associated autonomic failure
Genitourinary
  Overflow incontinence
Sexual
  Males, erectile dysfunction
  Females, decreased vaginal lubrication

FIGURE 13-27. The organization of the autonomic nervous system of the heart (**A**). Note that diabetes affects the afferent and efferent components of the sympathetic and parasympathetic nervous systems and has diffuse effects throughout the body (**B**). CVLM and IVLM—paraventricular nuclei of vaso-motor center; GABA—γ-aminobutyric acid; IML—intermediolateral nucleus; NTS—solitary tract nucleus; RVLM—motor nucleus of vagus.

Gastropathy

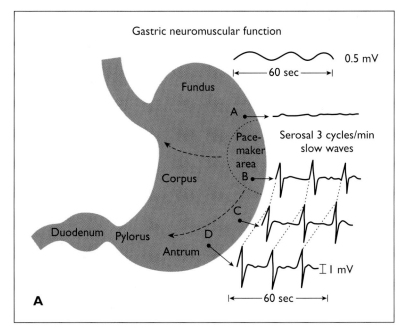

A

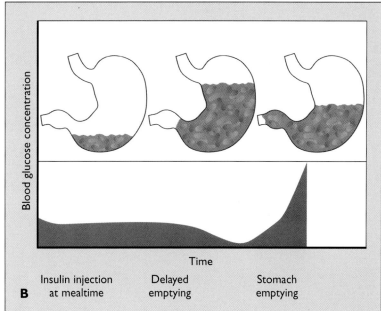

B

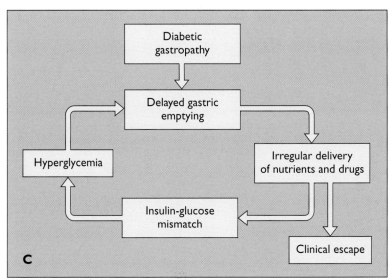

C

FIGURE 13-28. Gastropathy. **A** and **B,** Gastric neuromuscular function. The stomach is a complex neuromuscular organ. It has a pacemaker that discharges rhythmic electrical impulses that initiate propulsive contractions. It is sensitive to volume, viscosity, osmolarity, caloric density, and the nature of the fuel within.

Functional disturbances may occur such as arrhythmias, tachygastria and bradygastria, pylorospasm, and hypomotility. Organic lesions include gastroparesis, antral dilation and obstruction, inflammation, ulceration, and bezoar formation. Gastric dysfunction should be suspected in patients with type I and type II diabetes; who have had diabetes for over 20 years; who display evidence of distal symmetric polyneuropathy and autonomic neuropathy; observations of brittle diabetes in patients with previously well-controlled symptoms; and symptoms of early satiety, bloating, and a succussion splash. Anorexia, nausea, vomiting, and dyspepsia are nonspecific and herald other conditions.

C, Clinical presentation of gastropathy. Many more patients with gastropathy present with brittle diabetes than do those who present with gastric symptoms. In fact, it has been shown that many of the gastrointestinal symptoms of gastropathy can be nonspecific and do not reflect an abnormality in gastric emptying. The most fertile soil for discovery of those with gastric dysfunction are patients with "difficult to control diabetes." The stomach can be regarded as the coarse regulator of blood glucose concentrations, releasing fuel to the small bowel at its own predetermined rate. Any dysfunction in the bowel therefore would result in a mismatch of fuel delivery and either endogenous or exogenous insulin, thereby creating the apparent pattern of insulin resistance or brittle diabetes. Of interest is that the irregular pattern of delivery applies to drugs used in the treatment of diabetes and may confound the problem. Similar concern applies to other drugs that may fail to reach their absorptive site in the small bowel leading to clinical escape from the condition being treated. Overzealous adjustment of the insulin dose may result because the real cause may be easily overlooked.

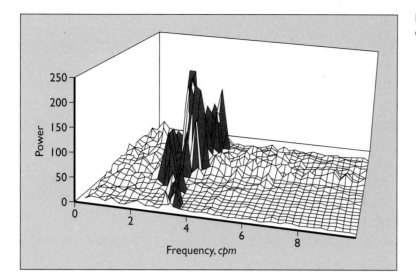

FIGURE 13-29. Normal electrogastrogram. This electrogastrogram was obtained in a normal patient. Note the predominant frequency of 3 to 6 cpm.

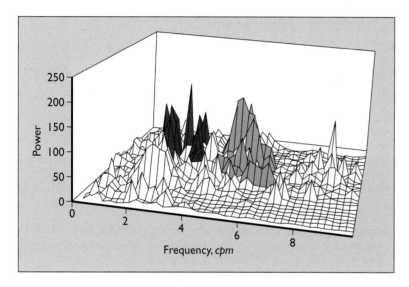

FIGURE 13-30. Electrogastrogram showing hyperglycemia-induced tachygastria. Note two peaks of activity, one at the usual frequency of 3 to 6 cpm and the major peak at over 6 cpm. Thus, hyperglycemia *per se* can markedly affect gastric function; many have made the costly error of carrying out gastric-emptying studies when the blood glucose is over 400 mg/dL. Not only does this induce tachygastria, but it may inhibit the interdigestive myoelectric complex and thus give the erroneous impression of gastroparesis.

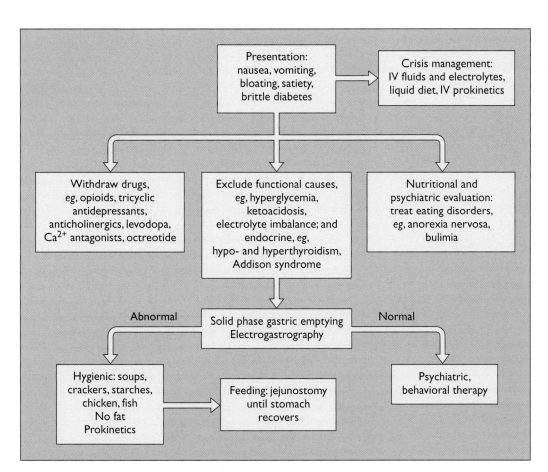

FIGURE 13-31. Algorithm for the management of gastropathy in patients with diabetes. IV—intravenous.

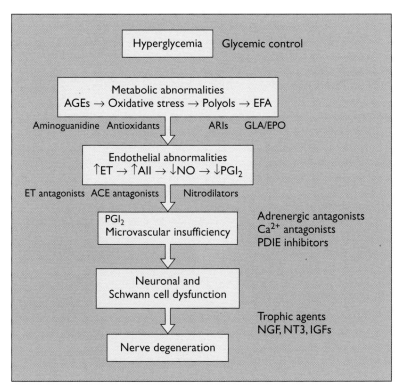

FIGURE 13-32. Specific interventions in diabetic neuropathy designed to target the major defect. Many of these interventions already have been tested in animal models and currently are in phase 2 and 3 clinical trials in the United States. Some of these interventions are further along and may well be in clinical trials shortly. ACE—angiotensin-converting enzyme; AGEs—advanced glycation end products; AII—angiotensin II; ARIs—aldose-reductose inhibitors; Ca²⁺—calcium ion; EFA—essential fatty acid; EPO—evening primrose oil; ET—endothelin; GLA—γ-linolenic acid; IGF—insulin-like growth factor; NGF—neuronal growth factor; NO—nitric oxide; NT3—neurotropin 3; PDIE—phosphodiesterase; PGI₂—prostaglandin I₂.

References

1. American Diabetes Association, American Academy of Neurology: Consensus statement: report and recommendations of the San Antonio Conference on Diabetic Neuropathy. *Diabetes Care* 1988, 11:592–597.

2. Vinik AI, Mitchell BD, Leichter SB, *et al.*: Epidemiology of the complications of diabetes. In *Diabetes: Clinical Science and Practice,* Edited by Leslie RDG, Robbins DC. Cambridge: Cambridge University Press; 1995:15,221.

3. Kjiturnan M, Welborn T, McCann V, *et al.*: Prevalence of diabetic complications in relation to risk factors. *Diabetes* 1986, 35:1332–1339.

4. Young MJ, Boulton AJ, MacLeod AF, *et al.*: A multicenter study of the prevalence of diabetic neuropathy in the United Kingdom hospital clinic population. *Diabetologia* 1993, 36:150–154.

5. Feldman JN, Hirsch SR, Bever BS, *et al.*: Prevalence of diabetic nephropathy at time of treatment for diabetic retinopathy. In *Diabetic Renal-Retinal Syndrome.* Edited by Friedman L'Esperance FA. London: Grune & Stratton; 1982:9.

6. Dyck PJ, Kratz KM, Karnes MS, *et al.*: The prevalence by staged severity of various types of diabetic neuropathy, retinopathy, and nephropathy in a population based cohort: The Rochester Diabetic Neuropathy Study. *Neurology* 1993, 43:817–824.

7. Brownlee M: Advanced products of nonenzymatic glycosylation and the pathogenesis of diabetic complications. In *Diabetes Mellitus. Theory and Practice.* Edited by Rifkin H, Porte D. New York: Elsevier, 1990:279.

8. Diabetes Control and Complications Trial Research Group: Effect of intensive diabetes treatment on nerve conduction in the Diabetes Control and Complications Trial. *Ann Neurol* 1995, 38:869–880.

9. Vinik AI, Newlon PG, Lauterio TJ, *et al.*: Nerve survival and regeneration in diabetes. *Diabetes Rev* 1995, 3:139–157.

10. Said G, Goulon-Gorcau C, Lacroix C, Moulonguet A: Nerve biopsy findings in different patterns of proximal diabetic neuropathy. *Ann Neurol* 1994, 35:559–569.

11. Krendel DA, Costigan DA, Hopkins LC: Successful treatment of neuropathies in patients with diabetes mellitus. *Arch Neurol* 1995, 52:1053–1061.

12. Vinik AI, Milicevic Z, Colen LB, *et al.*: Histopathological and electro-physiologic heterogeneity in patients with proximal diabetic neuropathy (PDN) [abstract]. *Diabetes* 1996, 769:209.

13. Malik RA, Tesfaye S. Thompson SD, *et al.*: Transperineurial capillary abnormalities in the sural nerve of patients with diabetic neuropathy. *Microvasc Res* 1994, 48:236–245.

14. Dyck P, Hansen S, Karnes J: Capillary number and percentage closed in human diabetic sural nerve. *Proc Natl Acad Sci USA* 1985, 82:2513–2517.

15. Low PA, Lagerlund TD, McManis PG: Nerve blood flow and oxygen delivery in normal, diabetic, and ischemic neuropathy. *Int Rev Neurobiol* 1989, 31:355–438.

16. Yasuda H, Dyck P: Abnormalities of endoneurial microvessels and sural nerve pathology in diabetic neuropathy. *New Urology* 1987, 37:20–28.

17. Malik RA, Veves A, Masson EA, *et al.*: Endoneurial capillary abnormalities in human diabetic neuropathy. *J Neurol Neurosurg Psychiatry* 1992, 55:557–561.

18. Tuck RR, Schinelzer JD, Low PA: Endoneurial blood flow and oxygen tension in the sciatic nerves of rats with experimental diabetic neuropathy. *Brain* 1984, 107:935–950.

19. Newrick PG, Wilson AJ, Jakubowski J, *et al.*: Sural nerve oxygen tension in diabetes. *Br Med J* 1986, 293:1053–1054.

20. Zachodne DW, Ho LT: Normal blood flow but lower oxygen tension in diabetes of young rats: microenvironment and the influence of sympathectomy. *Can J Physiol Pharmacol* 1992, 70:651–659.

21. Hotta N, Koh N, Sakakibara F, *et al.*: Effect of proplionyl-L-carnitine on motor nerve conduction, autonomic cardiac function, and nerve blood flow in rats with streptozotocin-induced diabetes: comparison with an aldose reductase inhibitor. *Diabetes* 1992, 41:587–591.

22. Vinik AI, Holland MT, LeBeau JM, *et al.*: Diabetic neuropathies. *Diabetes Care* 1992, 15:1926–1975.

23. Dawson DM: Entrapment neuropathies of the upper extremities. *N Engl J Med* 1993, 329:2013–2018.

24. Leedman PJ, Davis S, Harrison LS: Diabetic amyotrophy-reassessment of the clinical spectrum. *Aust N Z J Med* 1988, 18:768–773.

25. Barohn RJ, Salienk Z, Warmolts JR, Mendell JR: The Bruns Garland syndrome (diabetic amyotrophy). *Arch Neurol* 1991, 48:1130–1135.

26. Chia L, Fernandez A, Lacroix C: Contribution of nerve biopsy findings to the diagnosis of disabling neuropathy in the elderly: a retrospective review of 100 consecutive patients. *Brain* 1996, 119:1091–1098.

27. Hanson PH, Schumaker P, Debugne T, Clerin M: Evaluation of somatic and autonomic small fibers neuropathy in diabetes. *Am J Phys Med Rehabil* 1992, 71:44–47.

28. Dyck PJ: Small-fiber neuropathy determination. *Muscle Nerve* 1988, 11:998–999.

29. Jarnal GA, Hansen S, Weir AI, Ballantyne JP: The neurophysiologic investigation of small fiber neuropathies. *Muscle Nerve* 1987, 10:537–545.

30. Shapiro SA, Stansberry KB, Hill MA, *et al.*: Normal blood flow response and vasomotion in the diabetic Charcot foot. *J Diabetes Complications* 1998, 12:147–153.

31. Burnstock G, Ralevic V: New insights into the local regulation of blood flow by perivascular nerves and endothelium. *Br J Plastic Surg* 1994, 47:527–543.

32. Stansberry KB, Hill MA, Shapiro SA, *et al.*: Impairment of peripheral blood flow responses in diabetes resembles an enhanced aging effect. *Diabetes Care* 1997, 20:1711–1716.

33. Ewing J, Campbell IW, Clarke BF, *et al.*: Heart rate changes in diabetes mellitus. *Lancet* 1981, 1:183–186.

34. Kahn J, Ida B, Vinik A: Stress and cardiovascular function in diabetes. *Diabetes Care* 1985, 12:3–5.

SECONDARY FORMS OF DIABETES

Veronica M. Catanese

14

Primary forms of diabetes mellitus include type 1, or insulin-dependent diabetes mellitus, and type 2, or non–insulin-dependent diabetes mellitus. Secondary forms of diabetes and glucose intolerance may occur in association with a variety of disorders of both endocrinologic and nonendocrinologic origin [1].

Most endocrine diseases associated with glucose intolerance produce the metabolic abnormality through excessive production of insulin counterregulatory hormones, such as growth hormone, glucocorticoids, glucagon, and catecholamines. These hormones affect both glucose production (through glycogenolysis and gluconeogenesis) and glucose utilization (through insulin secretion and insulin action) to varying degrees. In these diseases, the secondary diabetes is usually reversible with successful treatment of the underlying disorder, and the risk for ketoacidosis is low.

Nonendocrine conditions associated with abnormal glucose tolerance may be grouped into three major categories: diseases affecting pancreatic function (pancreatoprivic); drug-induced glucose intolerance; and complex genetic syndromes that affect multiple aspects of hepatic, renal, and musculoskeletal function. Pancreatitis, pancreatectomy, and hemochromatosis are the main components of the pancreatoprivic group. As expected, these conditions are associated with variable amounts of insulin deficiency and at least the potential for ketoacidosis. Pharmacologic agents can alter glucose tolerance by affecting insulin secretion, insulin action, or both. Genetic syndromes producing diabetes have multiple mechanisms, but in most cases, the exact cause still remains poorly understood.

Microangiopathic complications of diabetes are uncommon in patients with glucose intolerance secondary to diseases of hormonal overproduction. This is because these diseases rarely persist in an untreated state for many years. Retinal, renal, and neurologic sequelae do occur, however, in patients whose disease has lasted a decade or more. Because duration of hyperglycemia is a critical factor in the development of microvascular complications, it is not surprising that patients with long-standing pancreatitis, exocrine, and endocrine pancreatic dysfunction secondary to pancreatic reductive surgery, hemochromatosis, and genetic syndromes that include glucose intolerance are at risk for the development of classic diabetic complications.

Therapy for all types of secondary diabetes should center on correction of the underlying disturbance when possible. If this cannot be accomplished or until this is accomplished, treatment should reflect an understanding of the pathophysiologic basis of the diabetes. If insulin secretion is impaired (for example, in patients with pheochromocytoma), then exogenous insulin therapy should be instituted promptly until the underlying source of the problem has been eliminated. Patients with preserved insulin secretion should be treated with diet or oral hypoglycemic agents given as single drugs or in combination. In these cases, insulin should also be used if necessary to achieve glycemic goals. In all cases, little evidence suggests a correlation between the need for insulin therapy during a period of secondary diabetes and the risk for permanently altered glucose tolerance after successful treatment of the underlying primary disease.

FIGURE 14-1. Secondary forms of diabetes mellitus.

SECONDARY FORMS OF DIABETES

Endocrine diseases
  Changes in balance of insulin counterregulatory hormones disrupt
    glucose homeostasis
Nonendocrine conditions
  Pancreatic functional defects
  Drug-induced glucose intolerance
  Genetic syndromes

Abnormal Glucose Homeostasis Secondary to Endocrinologic Disorders: Acromegaly

ACUTE AND DELAYED EFFECTS OF SUPRAPHYSIOLOGIC GROWTH HORMONE ON CARBOHYDRATE METABOLISM

Metabolic Variable	Short-Term GH Administration	Chronic GH Excess
Glucose uptake	↑	↓
Glucose utilization	↑	↓

FIGURE 14-2. Acute and delayed effects of supraphysiologic growth hormone (GH) on carbohydrate metabolism. Intravenous administration of GH produces insulinomimetic effects during the first 4 hours after infusion. Glucose uptake and glucose utilization by insulin-sensitive tissues are increased, and plasma glucose and free fatty acid levels decrease. These effects may result from a rapid, direct effect of GH on insulin secretion; GH-mediated increase in hepatic production of insulin-like growth factor-I; or GH-induced activation of some of the early steps in insulin receptor intracellular signaling pathways [2]. The delayed effects of GH administration, however, counter insulin action. Glucose uptake and use by insulin-sensitive tissues are impaired, resulting in hyperinsulinism and varying patterns of glucose tolerance. Free fatty acid levels increase only with concomitant fasting; this supports the concept that excess GH does not promote significant lipolysis in the presence of adequate insulin.

A. RESPONSES TO ORAL GLUCOSE TOLERANCE TESTING IN ACROMEGALY

Abnormal OGTT	Normal OGTT
↑ Glucose	→ Glucose
↑ Insulin	↑ Insulin
↑ Glucose	→ Glucose
↓ Insulin	→ Insulin

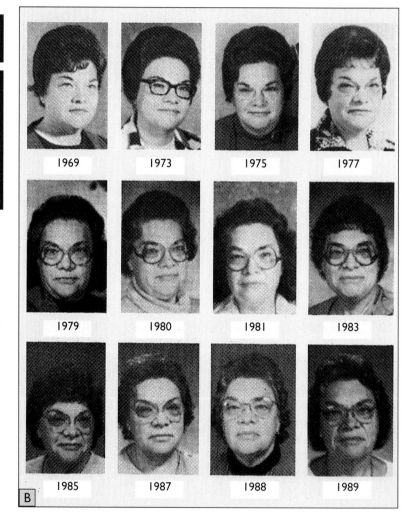

FIGURE 14-3. Spectrum of response to oral glucose tolerance testing in acromegaly. **A,** The spectrum of abnormalities in glucose homeostasis. The prevalence of glucose intolerance in patients with acromegaly is approximately 60%. Most acromegalic patients with abnormal results on oral glucose tolerance tests (OGTTs) have normal fasting plasma glucose levels but impaired handling of a glucose load associated with elevated basal or stimulated insulin levels. A small subset have low basal insulin levels and profoundly impaired insulin responses to glucose loading, and they clinically manifest severe hyperglycemia. It is not clear whether these patients represent a distinct subgroup with coincident insulin-dependent diabetes or β-cell desensitization as a consequence of prolonged hyperglycemia. Acromegalic patients with normal glucose tolerance, however, often exhibit insulin resistance as defined by elevated plasma insulin levels under basal or glucose-stimulated conditions. In these patients, glucose uptake in skeletal muscle and nonoxidative glucose metabolism are impaired in the postabsorptive state [3]. Therefore, oral glucose tolerance testing underestimates the prevalence of insulin resistance in patients with acromegaly. It is not clear, however, that progression from hyperinsulinemic euglycemia to a more severe defect manifested by hyperglycemia occurs with progressive acromegaly, such as that seen in the patient photographed over time in **B**. (Panel B from Thorner et al. [4]; with permission.)

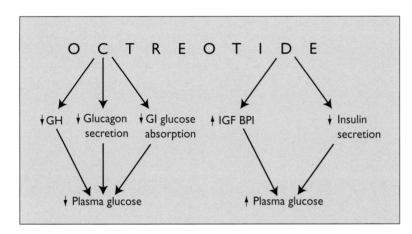

FIGURE 14-4. Growth hormone (GH)–induced hepatic and peripheral insulin resistance. Continuous administration of recombinant human GH to normal rats reduces insulin-mediated suppression of hepatic glucose output (HGO) and produces significant decreases in steady-state glucose infusion rate (GIR) and glucose disposal rate (GDR) during hyperinsulinemic glucose clamping. Similar results have been obtained in normal human patients studied under conditions of continuous GH infusion [5]. In both rats and humans, fasting plasma glucose and insulin levels during GH treatment did not differ from those in controls, providing an experimental correlate of patients with acromegaly who have evidence of impaired insulin action in the postabsorptive state. The mechanisms responsible for this insulin resistance, however, remain unclear. Impairment of early events in insulin signal transduction in liver and muscle is a likely contributing factor. Insulin receptor substrate (IRS)-1 and IRS-2 tyrosine phosphorylation and association of these substrates with phosphatidylinositol 3-kinase are reduced in the livers and muscle of rats receiving long-term GH therapy [6]. It is not known whether troglitazone, which alleviates the GH-induced alterations in HGO, GIR, and GDR [5], affects the changes in IRS-1 and IRS-2 phosphorylation and phosphatidylinositol 3-kinase association or activity observed in liver or muscle of GH-treated rats. (*Adapted from* Sugimoto *et al.* [7].)

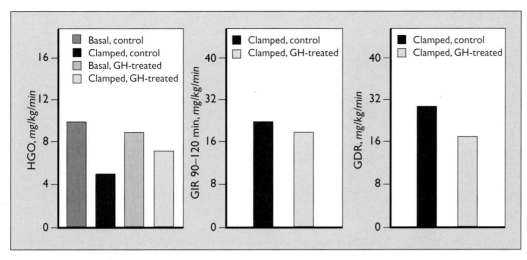

FIGURE 14-5. Effects of octreotide on glucose homeostasis in acromegaly. Unlike other effective treatment options for acromegaly, octreotide (the synthetic, long-acting somatostatin analogue) has complex effects on several hormonal factors that affect carbohydrate metabolism. In addition to inhibiting growth hormone (GH) and insulin-like growth factor-I (IGF-I) hypersecretion, octreotide inhibits insulin and glucagon secretion, delays gastrointestinal glucose absorption, and increases production of insulin-antagonistic IGF-binding protein I (BPI) [8]. The interplay of these pharmacologic effects may lead to concomitant improvement in glucose tolerance with control of the GH hypersecretion; however, it may also cause worsened glucose tolerance upon institution of octreotide therapy, particularly if GH secretory profiles remain abnormal [9].

Cushing Syndrome

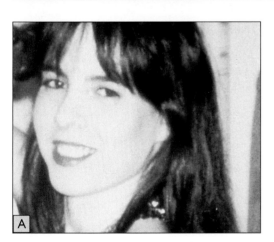 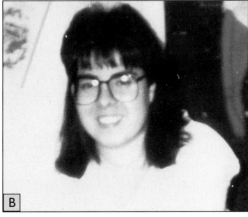

coids due to pituitary hypersecretion of adrenocorticotropic hormone (ACTH), paraneoplastic production of ACTH by tumor cells, or autonomous adrenal cortical hyperfunction. The latter affected this patient, photographed (**A**) before and (**B**) after presentation with phenotypic Cushing syndrome. The patient was found to have an adrenal cortical adenoma.

Although fasting hyperglycemia occurs in approximately 5% of patients with Cushing syndrome, insulin resistance with basal or stimulated hyperinsulinemia occurs in up to 90% of patients. Patients with Cushing syndrome may present in a hyperosmolar, nonketotic state [1]. This presentation is extremely unusual in patients with acromegaly, who otherwise display a spectrum of abnormal glucose and insulin profiles similar to those of patients with Cushing syndrome. (*Courtesy of* Jaishree Jagirdar, New York University School of Medicine, New York.)

FIGURE 14-6. Cushing syndrome. Cushing syndrome is a common endocrine cause of secondary glucose intolerance and diabetes. Abnormal glucose homeostasis may result from exogenous daily or alternate-day administration of glucocorticoids or as a consequence of chronic endogenous excess of glucocorti-

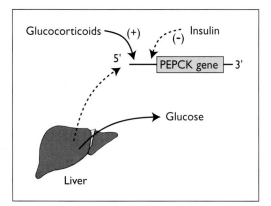

FIGURE 14-7. Glucocorticoid excess promotes hepatic glucose production. Several key enzymes controlling the production and utilization of metabolic fuels are directly regulated by glucocorticoids at the level of gene transcription. Phosphoenolpyruvate carboxykinase (PEPCK), a critical enzyme in gluconeogenesis, is positively regulated by glucocorticoids [10]. Transgenic mice overexpressing PEPCK, in fact, exhibit impaired glucose tolerance [11]. In addition, exposure of pregnant rats during late gestation to glucocorticoid excess permanently increases hepatic expression of PEPCK and glucocorticoid receptor and causes glucose intolerance in adult offspring [12]. Under normal physiologic conditions, however, insulin regulates PEPCK even more potently and dominantly in a negative manner [13]. Thus, replete insulin prevents the enhanced gluconeogenesis that would be caused by glucocorticoid excess. In the presence of insulin deficiency or impaired insulin action, however, the stimulatory effects of glucocorticoids on glucose production become apparent. Because patients with Cushing syndrome almost always have insulin resistance, the stage is set for glucocorticoid-enhanced gluconeogenesis, which contributes to glucose intolerance.

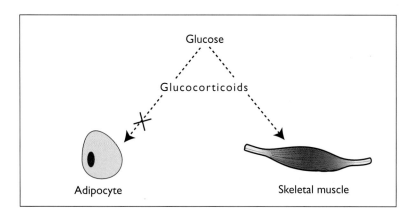

FIGURE 14-8. Glucocorticoid excess diminishes peripheral glucose utilization. Glucocorticoids induce resistance to insulin-stimulated glucose uptake in rat adipocytes [14]. This effect may be at least partly mediated by direct glucocorticoid-mediated inhibition of insulin-induced protein kinase C translocation from cytosol to plasma membrane. Glucocorticoids also inhibit activation of glucose transport in rat skeletal muscle by insulin, insulin-like growth factor-I, and hypoxia [15]. In rat soleus muscle, this effect is associated with preservation of total content of GLUT4 glucose transporters but also reduced translocation of GLUT4 transporter units to the plasma membrane [16]. In addition to these effects on GLUT4 subcellular trafficking, glucocorticoids affect early steps in insulin receptor signaling in skeletal muscle and in the liver [17]. As a result, both basal and insulin-stimulated glucose uptake and utilization are subject to modulation by excess glucocorticoids.

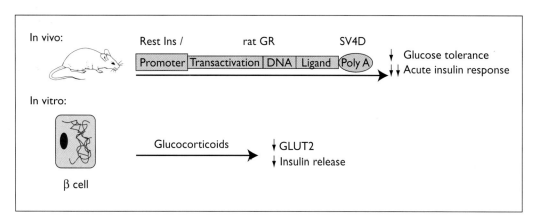

FIGURE 14-9. Glucocorticoids inhibit insulin secretion from pancreatic β cells. Insulin resistance has long been a recognized consequence of glucocorticoid excess. Effects of glucocorticoids on insulin secretion in vivo and in vitro, however, have only recently been described. Transgenic mice overexpressing the glucocorticoid receptor (GR) under the control of the insulin promoter have increased glucocorticoid sensitivity that is restricted to pancreatic β cells [18]. These animals have normal fasting and postabsorptive blood glucose levels but also have a markedly reduced insulin response and impaired glucose tolerance during intravenous glucose loading. This in vivo evidence suggesting a diabetogenic effect of glucocorticoids on pancreatic β cells is supported by in vitro evidence for dexamethasone-induced, posttranslational degradation of β cell GLUT2 glucose transporters [19] and by dexamethasone-induced inhibition of exocytotic insulin release from rodent islets in culture [20]. Diminished glucose utilization in Cushing syndrome may therefore be a composite result of deficient insulin secretion and impaired insulin action.

Glucagonoma

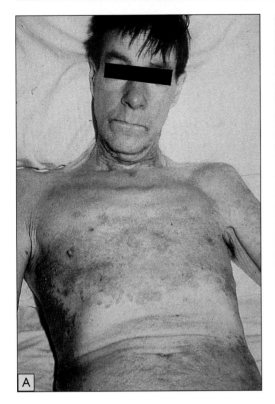

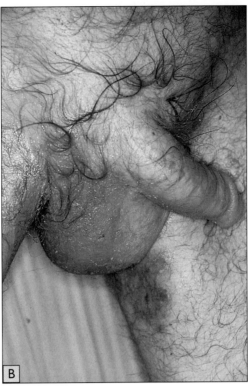

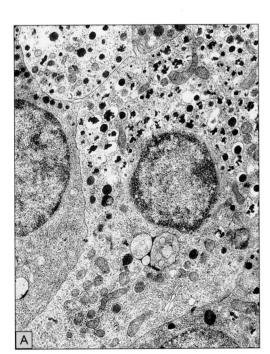

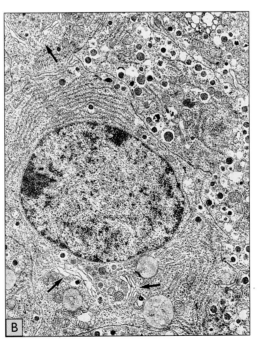

FIGURE 14-10. (See Color Plate) Glucose intolerance in the "glucagonoma syndrome." Although hyperglucagonemia may be associated with a variety of secretory islet-cell tumors and is rarely associated with multiple endocrine neoplasia type I (MEN I), the characteristic glucagonoma syndrome is most frequently seen in patients with clinically malignant, glucagon-producing tumors of pancreatic α cells. Central to the classic glucagonoma syndrome is necrolytic migratory erythema—the pathognomonic erythematous rash involving the perineum, extremities, trunk, or perioral region. This rash may be reproduced by infusion of glucagon into normal individuals and can be alleviated by infusion of parenteral amino acids, despite continued hyperglucagonemia. Thus, it is likely that amino acid deficiency produced by glucagon-induced muscle proteolysis is responsible for the rash. The incidence of glucose intolerance in patients with glucagonoma approaches 100%, with metabolic defects ranging from mild to very severe. Despite the excess production of glucagon and its potent effects on glycogenolysis and gluconeogenesis, ketoacidosis is rare. This probably reflects the stimulatory effect of glucagon on insulin secretion and the importance of the relative concentrations of both insulin and glucagon to hepatic glucose production and ketogenesis. In addition, functional heterogeneity of the various circulating species of immunoreactive glucagon may titrate glucagon's biological effects. (*Courtesy of* Dr. C.R. Kahn, Joslin Diabetes Center, Boston.)

ished glucose utilization. Insulin resistance has not been described clinically in patients with glucagonoma. Glucagon is a potent stimulus of epinephrine release; thus, α-adrenergic receptor–mediated inhibition of insulin secretion may diminish glucose disposal in patients with glucagonoma syndrome. Excess glucagon also has direct paracrine stimulatory effects on β-cell insulin secretion. β cells in the nontumoral endocrine pancreatic tissue of patients with glucagonoma have reduced immunoreactive insulin content and have ultrastructural features suggestive of accelerated insulin synthesis and secretion.

A, β cell from a control human pancreas, with moderate amounts of rough endoplasmic reticulum, a small Golgi apparatus, and numerous mature granules with crystal-like cores. **B,** β cell from a glucagonoma-associated pancreas. This cell contains several elongated rough endoplasmic reticulum cisternae, stacks of Golgi with adjacent progranules (*arrows*), and fewer secretory granules, which primarily contain immature rounded cores. It is therefore possible that the balance of multiple effects of hyperglucagonemia on insulin secretion may determine the degree of impairment in glucose utilization rate. (*From* Bani et al. [21]; with permission.)

FIGURE 14-11. Effects of endogenous hyperglucagonemia on pancreatic β cells. It is unlikely that an increased glucose production rate alone could produce glucose intolerance in the absence of an absolute or relative decrease in glucose disposal rate. Decreased insulin secretion or insulin resistance could result in dimin-

Pheochromocytoma

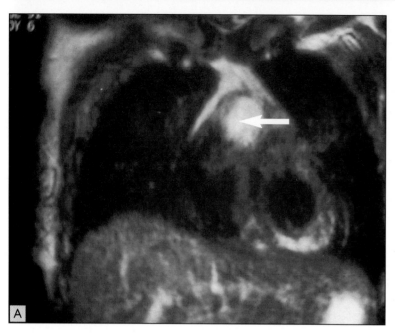

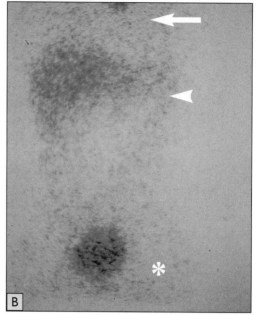

FIGURE 14-12. Glucose intolerance is a prominent feature in pheochromo-cytoma. Continuous or intermittent overproduction of the insulin counterreg-ulatory hormones epinephrine or norepinephrine by pheochromocytomas results in glucose intolerance in up to 75% of patients. Ninety percent of tumors are located within the adrenal medulla, but tumors may occur in several other sites, including along the abdominal aorta, in the organ of Zuckerkandl, in the urinary bladder, or in the mediastinum. As an adjunct to biochemical diagnosis, the tumor may be localized before surgery by many techniques, including CT and MRI. Multiple tumor foci, as well as metastatic sites, are best visualized by ^{131}I-labeled metaiodobenzylguanidine (mIBG) scanning. This nuclear medicine technique is accurate in 80% to 95% of pheochromocytomas, but its specificity is reduced by its capacity to detect neuroblastomas, medullary carcinomas of the thyroid, and carcinoid tumors [22]. In this figure, mediastinal metastases in a patient with a previously resected adrenal medullary pheochromocytoma are demonstrated by MRI (**A**, *arrow*) and by ^{131}I-mIBG (**B**; *arrow* points to the pheochromocytoma, *arrowhead* to the liver, *asterisk* to the bladder). (*Courtesy of* Dr. Elissa Kramer, New York University School of Medicine, New York.)

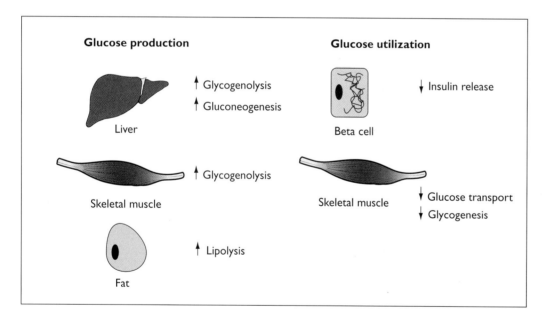

FIGURE 14-13. Excess catecholamines affect both glucose production and glucose utilization. Under pathologic conditions, the effects of cate-cholamines on glucose disposal are more profound than the effects on glucose production. Epinephrine directly interferes with exocytosis of insulin from pancreatic β cells [23] and does so at a step distal to the membrane depolarization-induced increase in intracellular calcium [24]. Catecholamines also impair insulin sensitivity, particularly in skeletal muscle [25], by inhibiting both insulin-stimulated glucose transport [26] and insulin-mediated muscle glycogenesis [27]. Catecholamines, especially epinephrine, increase net glucose production rate by directly affecting liver glycogenolysis and gluco-neogenesis, muscle glycogenolysis, and fat lipolysis. The effects of catecholamines on pancreatic insulin secretion are mediated mainly through α-adren-ergic receptors, whereas the effects on insulin target tissues are mediated primarily through β-adren-ergic receptor activation. Glucose tolerance in patients with pheochromocytoma is often restored by administration of α-adrenergic blockers, such as phentolamine; this supports the notion that the effects of excess catecholamines on glucose utilization outweigh the effects on glucose production.

Thyrotoxicosis

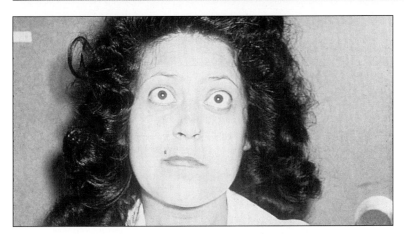

FIGURE 14-14. Glucose production and glucose utilization are altered in the thyrotoxic state. Hyperthyroidism of any cause, including thyrotoxic Graves disease—as manifested by this patient—alters glucose homeostasis. Thyroid hormones directly affect the activity of several glycometabolic enzymes, such as hepatic [28] and muscle [29] glycogen synthase, and also impair insulin-mediated suppression of hepatic glycogenolysis and gluconeogenesis [30]. In addition to their direct effects on glucose production, thyroid hormones in excess may also impair glucose-induced growth hormone suppression [31]; this adds another factor favoring the development of glucose intolerance. Glucose disposal, particularly in adipocytes, also is affected by thyrotoxicosis. Insulin-stimulated glucose transport is increased minimally [32], and this effect is associated with an increase in appearance of GLUT4 glucose transporters in the plasma membrane of adipocytes [33]. More important, hyperthyroidism increases basal rates of lipolysis, augments the maximal response of lipolysis to norepinephrine stimulation, and blunts the sensitivity of norepinephrine-stimulated lipolysis to suppression by insulin [32]. Clinically, these effects on glucose tolerance and insulin sensitivity appear more pronounced in obese than nonobese hyperthyroid women [34], perhaps because the decrease in nonoxidative glucose metabolism caused by hyperthyroidism cannot be adequately compensated for in the presence of the impaired oxidative glucose metabolism of obesity [35]. (*Courtesy of* Dr. Herbert Samuels, New York University School of Medicine, New York.)

Hyperprolactinemia

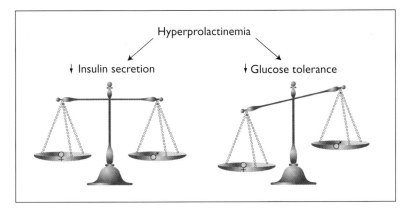

FIGURE 14-15. Sexual dimorphism of the diabetogenic effects of hyperprolactinemia. Moderate chronic hyperprolactinemia is associated with reduced thresholds for basal and glucose-induced insulin release [36] and pancreatic β-cell proliferation [37], mediated largely by altered expression of glucokinase, hexokinase, and GLUT2 glucose transporter in islet cells [38]. However, prolactin also affects insulin resistance in extramammary tissue and glucose tolerance [39]. Studies in hyperprolactinemic, pituitary-grafted mice [40] and rats [41], however, suggest that prolactin's effects on hepatic insulin action, unlike its sex-neutral effects on insulin secretion, may require estrogen for full expression. The molecular basis for prolactin's effects on insulin action in the presence and absence of estrogen has not been elucidated, and well-controlled studies testing this hypothesis in hyperprolactinemic men and women have not yet been performed.

Pancreatoprivic Diabetes: Pancreatectomy and Chronic Pancreatitis

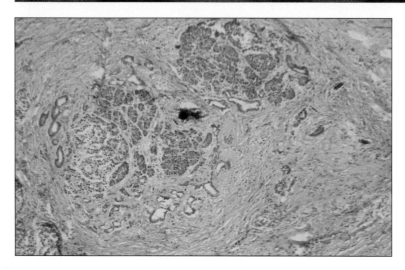

FIGURE 14-16. (See Color Plate) Reductions in pancreatic functional mass impair glucose tolerance by affecting multihormonal islet cell activity. Pancreatic exocrine and endocrine deficiency develop predictably with removal or destruction of more than 75% of pancreatic tissue. Glucose intolerance after pancreatectomy,

fibrocalcific or "J-type" tropical diabetes, and chronic pancreatitis, particularly as a result of alcoholism, share several features that distinguish them from other types of primary and secondary diabetes. Endocrine secretion from all islet cell types is reduced, resulting not only in insulin deficiency under basal or stimulated conditions, but also diminished pancreatic glucagon, somatostatin, and pancreatic polypeptide secretion. Despite preserved secretion of glucagon-like substances of duodenal origin in patients who have not undergone pancreaticoduodenectomy, reduced levels of pancreatic glucagon account for the relative resistance of these patients to ketoacidosis under conditions of insulin deficiency. In addition, iatrogenic hypoglycemia is common, and the response to spontaneous or induced hypoglycemia is delayed compared to that observed in both insulin-dependent and non–insulin-dependent diabetics. Although carbohydrate intolerance in these patients is usually attributed to reduced insulin secretion, insulin deficiency alone may not be the only factor responsible for secondary diabetes under these conditions. Hepatic resistance to insulin, accompanied by loss of sensitivity to insulin-induced hepatic glucose suppression, is a prominent feature of canine chronic pancreatitis. Deficiency of pancreatic polypeptide has been implicated as a factor in this resistance. Infusion of bovine pancreatic polypeptide improves glucose tolerance and restores suppression of hepatic glucose output by insulin in pancreatic polypeptide–deficient animals [42] and patients with chronic pancreatitis [43] (hematoxylin-eosin stain). (*Courtesy of* Dr. Howard Mizrachi, St. Luke's–Roosevelt Hospital Center, New York.)

Hemochromatosis

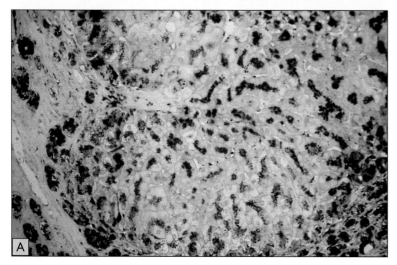

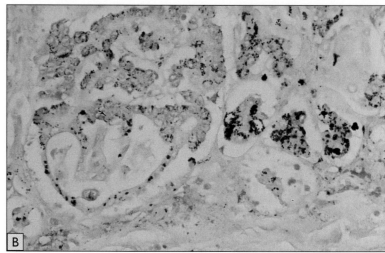

FIGURE 14-17. (See Color Plate) Hemochromatosis. Whether hereditary or secondary to iron overload, hemochromatosis is associated with abnormal glucose tolerance. Clinical diabetes or impaired glucose tolerance occurs in 75% to 90% of patients with primary hemochromatosis and in up to 65% of patients with hemochromatosis as a consequence of hemolytic anemia, multiple transfusion, or iron ingestion. Although the presence of cirrhosis increases the likelihood of abnormal glucose metabolism, hepatic iron content (shown by Prussian blue staining in **A**), serum ferritin levels, or extent of liver damage correlate poorly with the presence of impaired glucose homeostasis. A positive family history of diabetes may be the best predictor of glucose intolerance, at

least among patients with hereditary hemochromatosis [44]. Hepatic insulin resistance clearly plays an important role in patients with both varieties of hemochromatosis [45,46]. Defective first-phase insulin secretion, however, is also observed, even in the absence of significant degrees of islet iron deposition, such as that shown in **B**. Taken together, these physiologic abnormalities resemble those seen during the natural history of non–insulin-dependent diabetes. The relative importance of genetic factors versus iron overload in the pathophysiology of diabetes secondary to hemochromatosis, however, is not yet clear. (*Courtesy of* Dr. Howard Mizrachi, St. Luke's–Roosevelt Hospital Center, New York.)

Pharmacologic Effects on Glucose Homeostasis

DRUGS CAUSING DIABETES

Drugs That Affect Insulin Secretion

Anticonvulsants	Cations	Hormones	Anthelmintics
Phenytoin	Barium	Somatostatin	Pentamidine
Diuretics	Cadmium	Pesticides	Antineoplastics
Thiazides	Lithium	DDT	L-Asparaginase
Furosemide	Potassium	Fluoride	Mithramycin
Ethacrynic acid	Zinc	Pyriminil (Vacor)	

Drugs That Affect Insulin Action

Hormones
  Growth hormone

Drugs That Affect Both Insulin Secretion and Insulin Action

Hormones/hormone antagonists	Antihypertensives	Blocking agents	Psychopharmacologic agents
Glucagon	Clonidine	β-Adrenergic blockers	Benzodiazepines
Glucocorticoids	Diazoxide	Calcium-channel blockers	Ethanol
Octreotide	Prazosin	Histaminergic blockers	Opiates
Adrenergic compounds			Phenothiazines
Epinephrine			
Norepinephrine			

FIGURE 14-18. Drug-induced diabetes. The list of pharmacologic agents that can induce diabetes is long. Individual drugs may affect glucose homeostasis by interfering with insulin secretion, insulin action, or both. Whether its effect is primarily on insulin secretion or insulin action, a drug itself may mediate the effect directly, or indirectly through hormones or cations critical to the mechanisms that control insulin release or biologic effect. Glucohomeostatic effects of supraphysiologic levels of growth hormone, glucocorticoids, and catecholamines best illustrate the direct and indirect consequences of "pharmacologically" altered insulin action. As the links between altered insulin sensitivity and altered insulin secretion tighten, it becomes more and more difficult to assign an effect to a drug solely on the basis of insulin action. Clinically, these agents may uncover previously silent insulin secretory defects or insulin resistance and consequently induce glucose intolerance in a previously undiagnosed patient or worsen the diabetic state when administered to patients with antecedent diabetes mellitus. (*Adapted from* Argetsinger and Carter-Su [2].)

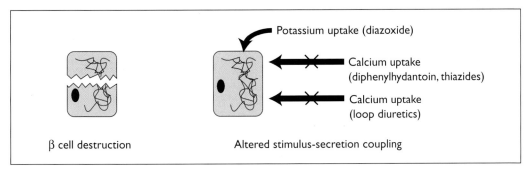

β cell destruction   Altered stimulus-secretion coupling

Potassium uptake (diazoxide)
Calcium uptake (diphenylhydantoin, thiazides)
Calcium uptake (loop diuretics)

FIGURE 14-19. Prototypical pharmacologic impairment of insulin secretion: direct and indirect effects. Insulin secretion by pancreatic β cells may be impaired directly by destruction of the β cells themselves or by interference with the normal mechanism of stimulated insulin secretion. Pentamidine, a widely used anthelmintic agent active against *Pneumocystis carinii*, produces β–cell-selective necrosis and irreversibly reduces β-cell responses to glucose and nonglucose secretagogues after initially causing cytolytic release of insulin [47]. In contrast, diphenylhydantoin, at therapeutic blood levels, reversibly reduces both first and second phases of insulin release by inhibiting calcium inflow into the β cell through voltage-dependent Ca^{2+} channels [48]. Unlike diphenylhydantoin, thiazide diuretics were thought to adversely affect insulin secretion and promote glucose intolerance indirectly through production of hypokalemia [49], in a manner similar to that proposed for primary hyperaldosteronism. Although prevention or correction of hypokalemia does alleviate thiazide-induced glucose intolerance, direct effects of thiazides themselves on the β cell secretion have been described. Unlike the structurally related compound diazoxide, thiazides do not hyperpolarize β cells by opening the adenosine triphosphate–sensitive potassium channels closed by the sulfonlyureas [50]. Instead, they, like diphenylhydantoin, may affect stimulus-secretion coupling in the β cell by inhibiting calcium uptake [51]. Similarly, the loop diuretics, thought to share with the thiazides an indirect effect on β-cell secretion mediated through hypokalemia, also directly affect insulin secretion by inhibiting chloride pump function in the β-cell membrane [52].

Genetic Syndromes Associated with Impaired Glucose Tolerance

GENETIC SYNDROMES ASSOCIATED WITH IMPAIRED GLUCOSE TOLERANCE

Acute intermittent porphyria

Alström syndrome (obesity, deafness, retinitis pigmentosa)

Ataxia-telangiectasia

Cockayne's syndrome

Cystic fibrosis

Friedreich's ataxia (spinocerebellar ataxia)

Glycogen storage disease type I

Herrmann's syndrome (photomyoclonus, nerve deafness, nephropathy, cerebral dysfunction)

Huntington's chorea

Isolated growth hormone deficiency

Klinefelter's syndrome

Laurence-Moon-Biedl syndrome

Leprechaunism

Lipoatrophic diabetes

Machado-Joseph disease (ataxia, nystagmus, dysarthria, depressed tendon reflexes, distal muscle atrophy)

Myotonic dystrophy

Panhypopituitary dwarfism

Prader-Willi syndrome

Trisomy 21

Turner's syndrome

Werner's syndrome

Wolfram syndrome (hereditary optic atrophy, visual loss, neurosensory deafness)

FIGURE 14-20. Genetic syndromes associated with impaired glucose tolerance. The list of genetic syndromes that include glucose intolerance as part of their profile is extensive and growing. Among members of this list, relatively "pure" defects in insulin secretion are represented by diseases such as cystic fibrosis; leprechaunism, on the other hand, may be regarded as a prototypical syndrome of insulin resistance. It is clear, however, that multiple pathophysiologic mechanisms that affect both glucose production and glucose utilization coalesce, in most cases, to produce the full-blown syndromes and the glucose intolerance that characterize them. It is likely that advances in the molecular genetics and molecular pathophysiology of these syndromes will shed light not only on the dysregulated glucose handling in these syndromes, but also on mechanisms of altered glucose homeostasis common both to secondary and primary forms of diabetes.

References

1. Catanese VM, Kahn DR: Secondary forms of diabetes. In *Principles and Practice of Endocrinology and Metabolism*. Edited by Becker KL, Bremner WJ, Hung W, et al. Philadelphia: JB Lippincott; 1995:1220–1228.

2. Argetsinger L, Carter-Su C: Mechanism of signaling by growth hormone receptor. *Physiol Rev* 1996, 76:1089–1107.

3. Foss MC, Saad MJ, Paccola GM, et al.: Peripheral glucose metabolism in acromegaly. *J Clin Endocrinol Metab* 1991, 72:1048–1053.

4. Thorner MO, Vance ML, Laws ER, et al.: The anterior pituitary. In *Williams Textbook of Endocrinology*, edn 9. Edited by Wilson JD, Foster DW, Kronenberg HM, Larsen PR. Philadelphia: WB Saunders; 1998: 296.

5. Orskov L, Schmitz O, Jorgensen JOL, et al.: Influence of growth hormone on glucose-induced glucose uptake in normal men as assessed by the hyperglycemic clamp technique. *J Clin Endocrinol Metab* 1989, 68:276–282.

6. Thirone ACP, Carvalho CRO, Brenelli SL, et al.: Effect of chronic growth hormone treatment on insulin signal transduction in rat tissues. *Mol Cell Endocrinol* 1997, 130:33–42.

7. Sugimoto M, Takeda N, Nakashima K, et al.: Effects of troglitazone on hepatic and peripheral insulin resistance induced by growth hormone excess in rats. *Metabolism* 1998, 47:783–787.

8. Ezzat S, Ren SG, Braunstein GD, et al.: Octreotide stimulates insulin-like growth factor-binding protein-1: a potential pituitary-independent mechanism for drug action. *J Clin Endocrinol Metab* 1992, 75:1459–1463.

9. Koop BL, Harris AG, Ezzat S: Effect of octreotide on glucose tolerance in acromegaly. *Eur J Endocrinol* 1994, 130:581–586.

10. Imai E, Stromstedt PE, Quinn PG, et al.: Characterization of a complex glucocorticoid response unit in the phosphoenolpyruvate carboxykinase gene. *Mol Cell Biol* 1990, 10:4712–4719.

11. Valera A, Pujol A, Pelegrin M, et al.: Transgenic mice overexpressing phosphoenolpyruvate carboxykinase develop non-insulin-dependent diabetes. *Proc Natl Acad Sci U S A* 1994, 91:9151–9154.

12. Nyirenda MJ, Lindsay RS, Kenyon CJ, et al.: Glucocorticoid exposure in late gestation permanently programs rat hepatic phosphoenolpyruvate carboxykinase and glucocorticoid receptor expression and causes glucose intolerance in adult offspring. *J Clin Invest* 1998, 101:2174–2181.

13. O'Brien RM, Granner DK: Regulation of gene expression by insulin. *Biochem J* 1991, 278:609–619.

14. Ishizuka T, Nagashima T, Kajita K, et al.: Effect of glucocorticoid receptor antagonist RU 38486 on acute glucocorticoid-induced insulin resistance in rat adipocytes. *Metabolism* 1997, 46:997–1002.

15. Weinstein SP, Paquin T, Pritsker A, et al.: Glucocorticoid-induced insulin resistance: dexamethasone inhibits the activation of glucose transport in rat skeletal muscle by both insulin- and non–insulin-related stimuli. Diabetes 1995, 44:441–445.

16. Dimitriadis G, Leighton B, Parry-Billings M, et al.: Effects of glucocorticoid excess on the sensitivity of glucose transport and metabolism to insulin in rat skeletal muscle. Biochem J 1997, 321:707–712.

17. Saad MJA, Folli F, Kahn JA, et al.: Modulation of insulin receptor, insulin receptor substrate-1, and phosphatidylinositol 3-kinase in liver and muscle of dexamethasone-treated rats. J Clin Invest 1993, 92:2065–2072.

18. Delaunay F, Khan A, Cintra A, et al.: Pancreatic beta cells are important targets for the diabetogenic effects of glucocorticoids. J Clin Invest 1997, 100:2094–2098.

19. Gremlich S, Roduit R, Thorens B: Dexamethasone induces posttranslational degradation of GLUT2 and inhibition of insulin secretion in isolated pancreatic beta cells. J Biol Chem 1997, 272:3216–3222.

20. Lambillotte C, Gilon P, Henquin JC: Direct glucocorticoid inhibition of insulin secretion. J Clin Invest 1997, 99:414–423.

21. Bani D, Biliotti G, Sacchi TB: Morphological changes in the human endocrine pancreas induced by chronic excess of endogenous glucagon. Virchows Archiv B Cell Pathol 1991, 60:199–206.

22. Keiser HR: Pheochromocytoma and other diseases of the sympathetic nervous system. In Principles and Practice of Endocrinology and Metabolism. Edited by Becker KL, Bremner WJ, Hung W, et al. Philadelphia: JB Lippincott; 1995:762–770.

23. Lehr S, Herbst M, Kampermann J, et al.: Adrenaline inhibits depolarization-induced increases in capacitance in the presence of elevated intracellular calcium concentration in insulin secreting cells. FEBS Lett 1997, 415:1–5.

24. Renstrom E, Ding WG, Bokvist K, et al.: Neurotransmitter-induced inhibition of exocytosis in insulin-secreting beta cells by activation of calcineurin. Neuron 1996, 17:513–522.

25. Capaldo B, Napoli R, Di Marino L, et al.: Epinephrine directly antagonizes insulin-mediated activation of glucose uptake and inhibition of free fatty acid release in forearm tissues. Metab Clin Exp 1992, 41:1146–1149.

26. Laakso M, Edelman SV, Brechtel G, et al.: Effects of epinephrine on insulin-mediated glucose uptake in whole body and leg muscle in humans: role of blood flow. Am J Physiol 1992, 263:E199–204.

27. Raz I, Katz A, Spencer MK: Epinephrine inhibits insulin-mediated glycogenesis but enhances glycolysis in human skeletal muscle. Am J Physiol 1991, 260:E430–435.

28. Malbon CC, Campbell R: Thyroid hormones regulate hepatic glycogen synthase. Endocrinology 1984, 115:681–686.

29. Dimitriadis GD, Leighton B, Vlachonikolis IG, et al.: Effects of hyperthyroidism on the sensitivity of glycolysis and glycogen synthesis to insulin in the soleus muscle of the rat. Biochem J 1988, 253:87–92.

30. Holness MJ, Sugden MC: Hepatic carbon flux after re-feeding: hyperthyroidism blocks glycogen synthesis and the suppression of glucose output observed in response to carbohydrate re-feeding. Biochem J 1987, 247:627–634.

31. Tosi F, Moghetti P, Castello R, et al.: Early changes in plasma glucagon and growth hormone response to oral glucose in experimental hyperthyroidism. Metabolism 1996, 45:1029–1033.

32. Fryer LG, Holness MJ, Sugden MC: Selective modification of insulin action in adipose tissue by hyperthyroidism. J Endocrinol 1997, 154:513–522.

33. Matthei S, Trost B, Hamann A, et al.: Effect of in vivo thyroid hormone status on insulin signalling and GLUT1 and GLUT4 glucose transport systems in rat adipocytes. J Endocrinol 1995, 144:347–357.

34. Gonzalo MA, Grant C, Moreno I, et al.: Glucose tolerance, insulin secretion, insulin sensitivity and glucose effectiveness in normal and overweight hyperthyroid women. Clin Endocrinol 1996, 45:689–697.

35. Bonadonna RC, DeFronzo RA: Glucose metabolism in obesity and type II diabetes. In Obesity. Edited by Bjorntorp P, Brodoff BN. Philadelphia: JB Lippincott; 1992:474–501.

36. Sorenson RL, Brejle TC, Hegre OD, et al.: Prolactin (in vitro) decreases the glucose stimulation threshold, enhances insulin secretion, and increases dye coupling among islet B cells. Endocrinology 1987, 121:1447–1453.

37. Brejle TC, Parsons JA, Sorenson RL: Regulation of islet beta-cell proliferation by prolactin in rat islets. Endocrinology 1994, 43:263–273.

38. Weinhaus AJ, Stout LE, Sorenson RL: Glucokinase, hexokinase, glucose transporter 2, and glucose metabolism in islets during pregnancy and prolactin-treated islets in vitro: mechanisms for long term up-regulation of islets. Endocrinology 1996, 137:1640–1649.

39. Wade GN, Schneider JE: Metabolic fuels and reproduction in female mammals. Neurosci Biobehav Rev 1992, 16:235–272.

40. Matsuda M, Mori T: Effect of estrogen on hyperprolactinemia-induced glucose intolerance in SHN mice. Proc Soc Exp Biol Med 1996, 212:243–247.

41. Reis FM, Reis AM, Coimbra CC: Effects of hyperprolactinaemia on glucose tolerance and insulin release in male and female rats. J Endocrinol 1997, 153:423–428.

42. Sun YS, Brunicardi FC, Druck P, et al.: Reversal of abnormal glucose metabolism in chronic pancreatitis by administration of pancreatic polypeptide. Am J Surg 1986, 151:130–140.

43. Brunicardi FC, Chaiken RL, Ryan AS, et al.: Pancreatic polypeptide administration improves abnormal glucose metabolism in patients with chronic pancreatitis. J Clin Endocrinol Metab 1996, 81:3566–3572.

44. Hramiak IM, Finegood DT, Adams PC: Factors affecting glucose tolerance in hereditary hemochromatosis 1. Clin Invest Med 1997, 20:110–118.

45. Stremmel W, Niederau C, Berger M, et al.: Abnormalities in estrogen, androgen, and insulin metabolism in hereditary hemochromatosis. Ann N Y Acad Sci 1988, 526:209–223.

46. Merkel PA, Simonson DC, Amiel SA, et al.: Insulin resistance and hyperinsulinemia in patients with thalassemia major treated by hypertransfusion. N Engl J Med 1988, 318:809–814.

47. Shen M, Orwoll ES, Conte JE Jr, et al.: Pentamidine-induced pancreatic beta-cell dysfunction. Am J Med 1989, 86:726–728.

48. Siegel EG, Janjic D, Wollheim CB: Phenytoin inhibition of insulin release. Studies on the involvement of Ca^{2+} fluxes in rat pancreatic islets. Diabetes 1982, 31:265–269.

49. Helderman JH, Elahi D, Andersen DK, et al.: Prevention of the glucose intolerance of thiazide diuretics by maintenance of body potassium. Diabetes 1983, 32:106–111.

50. Tucker SJ, Gribble FM, Zhao C, et al.: Truncation of Kir6.2 produces ATP-sensitive K^+ channels in the absence of the sulphonylurea receptor. Nature 1997, 387:179–183.

51. Sandstrom PE: Inhibition by hydrochlorothiazide of insulin release and calcium influx in mouse pancreatic beta cells. Br J Pharmacol 1993, 110:1359–1362.

52. Sandstrom PE: Bumetanide reduces insulin release by a direct effect on the pancreatic beta cells. Eur J Pharmacol 1990, 187:377–383.

OBESITY

Eleftheria Maratos-Flier

15

Obesity, generally defined as weight exceeding 20% of ideal body weight or a body mass index (BMI) greater than 30, is a complex problem. In the United States, the prevalence of clinically significant obesity is more than 25%. Obesity is associated with excess mortality because of the elevated risk for such diseases as diabetes, hypertension, lipid disorders, and coronary artery disease, and increased rates of endometrial and colon carcinoma. Despite the magnitude of the problem, the cause of obesity is poorly understood and effective weight loss is difficult to achieve.

Recent work in mouse models has increased our understanding of the molecular mechanisms that may lead to obesity. The identification of leptin has provided insight into peripheral signals important in mediating eating behavior. Leptin, the product of the obese gene, is predominantly expressed in white fat tissue and signals information about peripheral energy stores to the central nervous system. In ob/ob mice, a premature stop codon prevents transcription of the mature leptin peptide and leads to a severe obesity syndrome. Leptin interacts with two leptin receptor variants, the long form and the short form. Severe obesity is seen in db/db mice, which do not make the long form of the leptin receptor, are leptin-resistant, and have high circulating leptin levels. In ob/ob animals, exogenous leptin leads to weight reduction, restoration of fertility, and correction of abnormal physiologic measures, including hyperglycemia, hyperinsulinemia, and hypercortisolemia. Leptin administration also reduces hypothalamic neuropeptide Y messenger RNA (mRNA).

Attention has recently focused on a number of neuropeptides known to affect feeding behavior in mice. For example, ablation of the melanocortin-4 receptor leads to rodent obesity and has brought to the fore the importance of the melanocortin pathway. Similarly, ablation of melanin-concentrating hormone (MCH) leads to a model of rodent leanness, indicating that MCH is a significant contributor to feeding.

The findings of single gene defects in rodents focused attention on certain peptides and receptors, and led to a search for single gene defects in humans. Thus far, humans with obesity secondary to leptin deficiency, leptin-receptor deficiency, preproopiomelanocortin abnormalities, melanocortin-4 receptor abnormalities, prohormone convertase-1 abnormalities, and abnormalities of peroxisome proliferator-activated receptor-gamma have been identified.

The neuropeptides regulating body weight and eating probably interact at several levels in the central nervous system; however, the anatomic and functional basis for this interaction has not been defined. In addition, the molecular basis by which signals from the lateral hypothalamus might be integrated into systems involved in weight regulation has only recently been explored.

Understanding of the molecular mechanisms of obesity in the general population will improve as our understanding of the regulators of eating behavior improves. Most human obesity is likely caused by dysregulation of several factors. Although current treatments are limited, the potential for new specific treatments based on the identification of specific molecular targets has increased.

Prevalence of Obesity

PREVALENCE OF OBESITY IN THE US POPULATION

Preobesity: BMI 25.0–25.9

Constant rate over last 3–4 decades; prevalence has remained constant at 32%

Obesity: BMI > 30

Prevalence is increasing

≈ 13% in 1960

≈ 23% in 1994

More than half the adult US population has a BMI that exceeds the healthy range

FIGURE 15-1. Prevalence of obesity. In the United States, the prevalence of obesity has increased over the past four decades. In some populations, such as non-Hispanic white men 50 to 59 years of age, the prevalence of overweight and obesity (body mass index [BMI] greater than 25) is 72.9%. The prevalence in non-Hispanic black women of the same age is 78.1% [1].

Obesity and the Risk for Other Diseases

DISEASES FOR WHICH OBESITY IS A RISK FACTOR

Diabetes

Cardiovascular disease

Hypertension

Sleep apnea

Endometrial cancer

Breast cancer

Colon cancer

Gallbladder disease

FIGURE 15-2. Obesity increases the risk for many diseases [2].

EXAMPLES OF INCREASED RISK RELATED TO OBESITY

Relative risk in persons 20–44 years of age:

Diabetes, 3.8

Hypertension, 5.6

Hypercholesterolemia, 2.1

FIGURE 15-3. Obesity is associated with a substantially increased risk for diabetes and cardiovascular disease, even in young persons.

OBESITY AND TYPE 2 DIABETES

80% to 90% of patients with type 2 diabetes are obese

Weight loss (as little as 10–20 pounds) can be adequate treatment

Most people (> 90%) cannot lose weight successfully

Patients with type 2 diabetes are at risk for usual complications, including cardiovascular disease, retinopathy, neuropathy, and nephropathy

FIGURE 15-4. Obesity and type 2 diabetes. Type 2 diabetes typically occurs in obese persons and has a significant component of insulin resistance. Even modest weight loss can lead to normalization of glucose control or to improved control with any given dose of oral medication. However, successful weight loss is unusual.

REGIONAL FAT DEPOSITS

Visceral	Subcutaneous
Mesenteric	Superficial
Omental	Deep
Retroperitoneal	
Perirenal	

FIGURE 15-5. Regional fat deposits. Visceral fat deposits include mesenteric, omental, retroperitoneal, and perirenal deposits. According to location, fat deposits have different metabolic characteristics and thus pose different levels of risk for the complications of obesity. Central fat can be assessed by computed tomography, but a fairly good estimate can also be obtained by determining the waist-to-hip ratio. The abdominal circumference halfway between the lower rib and the iliac crest is compared to the circumference at the level of the greater trochanter [3]. Consideration of the waist-to-hip ratio augments evaluation of the risks of obesity. Data from a study by Goodpaster *et al.* [4] indicate that in men, for any given body mass index, increased waist-to-hip ratio confers additional risk. This increase is also seen in women. (*See* Fig. 15-37 for relative risk.) Recent data from mouse models suggest that the enzyme 11-β hydroxysteroid dehydrogenase may contribute to visceral obesity. This enzyme, which is expressed in fat, activates glucocorticoids. Mice overexpressing this enzyme in adipose tissue develop a syndrome of central obesity that mimics the metabolic syndrome [5].

Role of Molecular Mechanisms

REQUIREMENT FOR STABLE WEIGHT

Calories In	Calories Out
Can only equal what one eats	Basal metabolic rate
	Thermogenesis
	Activity

FIGURE 15-6. Requirement for stable weight. Stable weight requires a match between calories consumed and calories expended. Fat-free mass is a major determinant of resting energy expenditure [6]. Weight gain leads to an increase in both fat and fat-free mass; thus, the basal metabolic rate of obese persons is higher than that of lean persons of the same height [7]. Obesity results from chronic excess of calories ingested over calories expended. Calories expended include the resting metabolic rate, the thermic effects of food and exercise, and adaptive thermogenesis. Body fat is not significantly influenced by resting energy expenditure or the thermic effect of food [8], but changes in energy expenditure resulting from physical activity influence weight and body composition [9].

VIEWS OF ENERGY HOMEOSTASIS

Very old view
   Obesity is the result of excess calories and inactivity; voluntary
   overeating and laziness indicate moral fault
Old view
   Obesity is the result of excess calories, but some lucky people can
   eat more because they have a "faster metabolism"
New view
   Obesity is the result of interactions between factors that regulate
   appetite and total energy expenditure

FIGURE 15-7. Energy homeostasis. For many years, obesity was considered to be the consequence of a moral fault. Eating was considered a process entirely under voluntary control, and decreased energy expenditure was ascribed to inactivity. Over time, various studies revealed that thermogenesis varied among people and that when placed on diets consisting of equal calories, people might gain, maintain, or even lose weight. The discovery of leptin in 1994 revolutionized understanding of the pathophysiologic basis of obesity. It is now clear that multiple factors regulate appetite and total energy expenditure. The demonstration that single gene defects can lead to obesity has also proven that excessive eating is a process that is not always amenable to conscious control.

HYPOTHALAMIC ORGANIZATION

Lateral hypothalamus—eating center (1951)
   Stimulates eating behavior
   Triggers feeding
   Ablative lesions cause aphagia, adipsia, and weight loss
Medial hypothalamus—satiety center (1940)
   Inhibits eating behavior
   Electrical stimulation of ventromedial hypothalamus inhibits eating
   Ablative lesions (surgical and goldthioglucose) cause hyperphagia
   and obesity

FIGURE 15-8. Hypothalamic organization. The role of the hypothalamus in the regulation of eating behavior was initially defined decades ago in studies of electrical stimulation and anatomical lesions. The role of the lateral hypothalamus in mediating eating was first considered in 1951 [10]. Experimental hypothalamic lesions of the ventromedial hypothalamus were reported to produce obesity in 1940 [11].

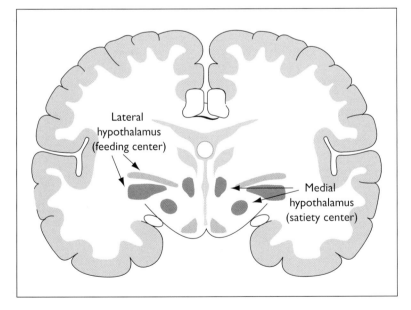

FIGURE 15-9. Hypothalamic areas implicated in eating behavior. The lateral hypothalamus is green (the lighter green area indicates the zona incerta). Melanin-concentrating hormone [12] and orexin [13] localize to this area and stimulate feeding. The medial hypothalamus (ventral medial and dorsal medial) is red, and the paraventricular nucleus is yellow. The arcuate nucleus, in which cell bodies making neuropeptide Y, preproopiomelanocortin (the precursor to melanocyte-stimulating hormone), agouti-related peptide, and cocaine- and amphetamine-regulated transcript [CART] are localized, is pink. Neuropeptide Y and agouti-related peptide stimulate eating, and melanocyte-stimulating hormone and CART inhibit eating.

Monoamines also play a role in appetite regulation. In experimental animals, administration of norepinephrine leads to an acute increase in food intake, and chronic administration leads to weight gain. This effect appears to be dependent on the receptor stimulated because $\alpha 2$ agonists increase food intake while $\alpha 1$ and $\beta 2$ agonists lead to decreased food intake [14–16]. Dopamine plays an important role in regulating food intake; however, effects are dependent on where it is released. Administration of dopamine in the lateral hypothalamus leads to decreased meal size [17] while release in the nucleus accumbens increases food intake [18]. Serotonin also affects food intake; however, the effects are complex and vary depending on the anatomic area of the brain targeted and the receptor activated.

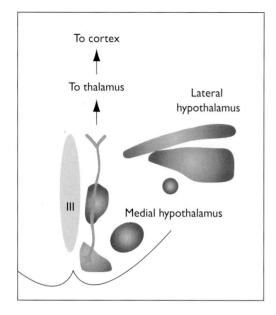

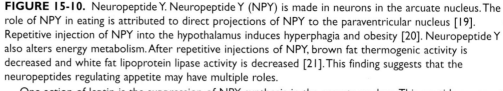

FIGURE 15-10. Neuropeptide Y. Neuropeptide Y (NPY) is made in neurons in the arcuate nucleus. The role of NPY in eating is attributed to direct projections of NPY to the paraventricular nucleus [19]. Repetitive injection of NPY into the hypothalamus induces hyperphagia and obesity [20]. Neuropeptide Y also alters energy metabolism. After repetitive injections of NPY, brown fat thermogenic activity is decreased and white fat lipoprotein lipase activity is decreased [21]. This finding suggests that the neuropeptides regulating appetite may have multiple roles.

One action of leptin is the suppression of NPY synthesis in the arcuate nucleus. This peptide appears to function as an important central regulator in eating behavior. Injection of NPY into rat lateral ventricles leads to a marked increase in eating; NPY-treated animals eat six- to tenfold more than control animals over the ensuing 24-hour period. Repetitive injections over several days cause weight gain. Neuropeptide Y also suppresses energy expenditure through actions on the sympathetic nervous system. Although NPY is diffusely expressed, it is the NPY-synthesizing neurons in the arcuate nucleus that project to paraventricular nucleus, and the dorsal medial hypothalamus that is responsible for mediating eating behavior. In the ob/ob mouse, messenger RNA (mRNA) levels in the arcuate nucleus are two- to threefold higher than mRNA levels in control mice; peptide levels are also increased in the ob/ob mouse. Similar results are seen in the Zucker fatty rat.

Both central intracerebroventricular and peripheral leptin treatment of ob/ob animals reduced NPY messages in the arcuate nucleus, suggesting that NPY is a leptin target. In normal animals, peripheral administration of leptin significantly inhibits the increase in the arcuate NPY mRNA levels seen with starvation. Although NPY may normally mediate eating behavior, NPY knockout mice lacking NPY in all tissues have no demonstrable changes in eating behavior. Crossbreeding of the NPY knockout mice with ob/ob mice revealed that the double-knockout offspring mice had an attenuated obesity phenotype. These data indicate that NPY is an important but not exclusive regulator of eating behavior and energy expenditure.

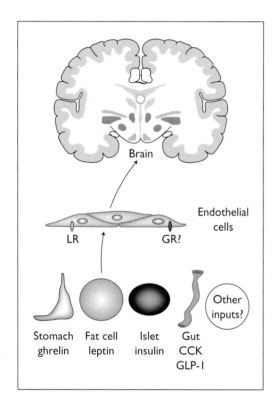

FIGURE 15-11. A number of peripheral factors that contribute to appetite may act on the brain [22]. Ghrelin, which is synthesized in the stomach, has been found to play a role in meal initiation, possibly through actions on target neurons in the hypothalamus [23,24]. Peptide YY is synthesized in the gut and has an orexigenic effect through action in the brain [25]. Anorectic agents may also be produced by the gut. Glucagon-like peptide 1 (GLP-1) is synthesized in the gut and acts to suppress appetite in animals and humans [26]. Cholecystokinin (CCK), which is made in enteroendocrine cells, also acts to inhibit appetite [27]. Finally, insulin, which is made in the pancreas in response to meals, may also act on the brain to regulate food intake and energy expenditure [28]. GR—ghrelin receptor; LR—leptin receptor.

CLINICAL FEATURES OF HUMAN LEPTIN RECEPTOR MUTATION*

Age, y	Sex	Weight, kg	BMI	Genotype	Leptin level, mg/mL
12	Male	37	16	wt/wt	5.6
13	Female	159	71.5	m/m	670
16	Male	87	30	wt/m	212
17	Female	102	34	wt/wt	88
19	Female	166	65.5	m/m	600
19	Female	133	52.5	?	526
22	Female	76	27.5	m/wt	240
24	Female	67.8	26.5	m/wt	294

*Additional features: growth delay; no overnight burst of growth hormone; poor response of growth hormone to stimulation tests; low IgF levels; low TSH; sustained TSH response to thyroid-releasing hormone; hypothalamus-pituitary-adrenal axis grossly normal.

FIGURE 15-18. Human leptin receptor mutation. Leptin-receptor deficiency has been described in a large family [39]. The proband presented with significant obesity and hypogonadotrophic hypogonadism. Affected homozygotes have 100-fold increased leptin levels (body mass index [BMI]) in excess of fat content. Affected heterozygotes had BMIs in the preobese or minimally obese range and leptin levels of approximately 200 mg/mL. TSH—thyroid-stimulating hormone level.

THE STRANGE LINK BETWEEN EATING AND PIGMENTATION

Agouti

Melanocortin-4 receptor

Melanocyte-stimulating hormone

Agouti-related peptide

Melanin-concentrating hormone

FIGURE 15-19. Peptides involved in regulating eating behavior and pigmentation. The intriguing connection between pigmentation and eating was first suggested by the finding that spontaneously mutant yellow mice (Ay), known as agouti mice, were also markedly obese. Agouti (normally expressed in the skin) acts on melanocytes as a paracrine factor to inhibit the conversion of phycomelanin (yellow) to eumelanin (black). Most mice are brown because of variable mixtures of these two pigments. Ay mice express agouti in all tissues and in an unregulated form. These findings suggested that melanocortin receptors have a role in mediating eating behavior.

Agouti protein is expressed in the skin and regulates skin coloration acting through the melanocortin 1 receptor, where it inhibits the action of melanocyte-stimulating hormone; when expressed ubiquitously, it leads to yellow pigmentation (inhibiting melanocortin-1 receptor) and obesity by inhibiting centrally expressed melanocortin-4 receptors. These receptors are expressed in the central nervous system; when activated by melanocyte-stimulating hormone, they mediate inhibition of eating behavior [40]. Melanin-concentrating hormone regulates skin pigmentation in fish, where it is made in the pituitary and released into the circulation and acts on melanophores (cells containing pigment granules) to cause granule aggregation and skin darkening. It has no known role in pigmentation in mammals, but in mammals it is made in the lateral hypothalamus; it stimulates eating behavior through a still-unidentified receptor. A potential endogenous antagonist ligand for the hypothalamic melanocortin receptors is agouti-related protein, a recently cloned homologue of agouti. This protein is expressed in the arcuate nucleus of the hypothalamus, and its messenger RNA is up-regulated in both ob/ob and db/db mice. Agouti-related protein appears to inhibit the melanocortin receptor in a manner similar to that of agouti.

THE AY MOUSE

Heterozygote is obese, macrosomic, insulin-resistant

Heterozygote has mustard yellow color

Syndrome results from ectopic expression of agouti in all organs

   Why is the mouse yellow?

   Why is the mouse obese?

FIGURE 15-20. The Ay mouse, in which normal agouti protein is expressed ectopically, is yellow and obese [41].

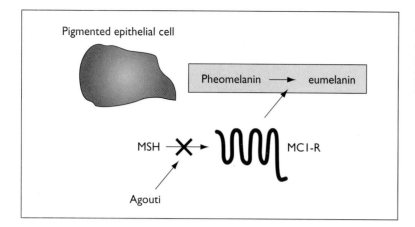

FIGURE 15-21. Agouti protein. Agouti protein is normally expressed in hair follicles in the skin and regulates pigmentation of skin and fur. Agouti protein expressed peripherally inhibits the melanocortin-1 receptor (MC1-R) and prevents the melanocyte-stimulating hormone (MSH)–mediated conversion of yellow pigment to black pigment [42]. If MSH is made in the pituitary, it regulates pigmentation; if it is made in the hypothalamus, it regulates feeding.

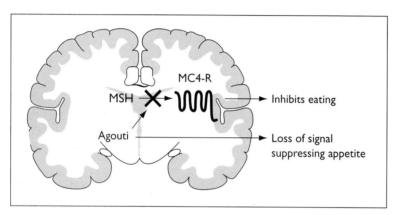

FIGURE 15-22. Agouti protein. Agouti (Ay) protein expressed centrally acts on the melanocortin-4 receptor (MC4-R) [43] and inhibits melanocyte-stimulating hormone (MSH)–mediated inhibition of eating. The obesity syndrome could be mimicked by genetically engineering a mouse that lacked MC4-R [44]; this capability demonstrates the importance of this receptor. In the Ay mouse, agouti is expressed in the brain. Agouti blocks MC4-R, one of two brain melanocortin receptors. The MC4-R cannot respond to α-MSH. The inhibitory effects of α-MSH on feeding are lost; thus, the Ay mouse is obese.

EXPRESSION OF AGOUTI AND AGRP

Agouti is not expressed in brain of normal animals

A related peptide, AgRP, is expressed in the brain

AgRP is found exclusively in arcuate neurons, which are leptin-responsive and co-express neuropeptide Y

FIGURE 15-23. Expression of agouti and agouti-related peptide (AgRP). Because agouti is not normally expressed in the central nervous system, the finding of the agouti effect on centrally expressed melanocortin receptors led to a search for agouti-like peptides in the central nervous system. Agouti-related peptide [45,46] is expressed in the arcuate nucleus and is one of the central nervous system peptides regulating the melanocortin-4 receptor (MC4-R). In addition, attention has focused on α-melanocyte–stimulating hormone (MSH), a product of preproopiomelanocortin in the arcuate, and on the role of α-MSH in the regulation of eating by acting as an agonist on MC4-R.

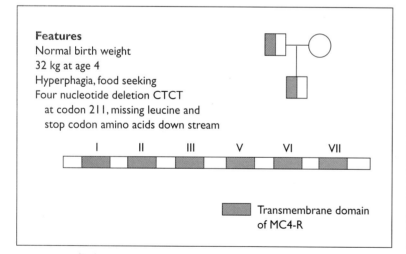

Features
Normal birth weight
32 kg at age 4
Hyperphagia, food seeking
Four nucleotide deletion CTCT
at codon 211, missing leucine and
stop codon amino acids down stream

I   II   III   V   VI   VII

■ Transmembrane domain of MC4-R

FIGURE 15-24. Mutations in melanocortin-4 receptor (MC4-R). A cohort of severely obese children was screened for mutations in MC4-R by using direct nucleotide sequencing [47]. One patient was heterozygous for a 4–base pair deletion at codon 211 of the MC4-R. This mutation resulted in a stop codon in the region encoding for the fifth transmembrane domain. Residues at the fifth and sixth transmembrane domain are important for MC4-R signaling, so this mutation results in a nonfunctional receptor. The proband's mother is normal weight, but the father is obese (body mass index, 41). The same mutation was identified in the father.

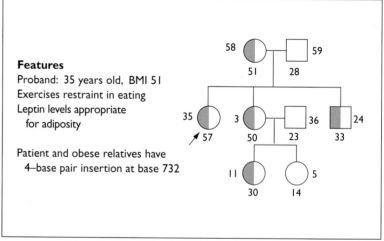

Features
Proband: 35 years old, BMI 51
Exercises restraint in eating
Leptin levels appropriate
    for adiposity

Patient and obese relatives have
    4–base pair insertion at base 732

FIGURE 15-25. Melanocortin-4 receptor (MC4-R) frameshift mutations and dominantly inherited human obesity. A French population was screened by selecting persons with a history of obesity in infancy and highest lifetime body mass index (BMI) at any given age [48]. The entire single exon of MC4-R was evaluated by using five primer pairs. Direct sequencing identified a proband in which a heterozygous frameshift mutation resulted in a nonfunctional truncated receptor. The proband's family was screened, and additional relatives with the mutation were identified. All of these relatives had similar levels of adiposity. Age of individuals is indicated to side of symbol, and BMI is below the symbol.

OBESITY, ADRENAL INSUFFICIENCY, AND RED HAIR PIGMENTATION ASSOCIATED WITH *POMC* MUTATIONS

Patient 1

Obesity of very early onset, red hair, ACTH deficiency; ACTH deficiency led to clinical presentation

Two mutations in exon 3

  Paternal allele

    G→T at nt 7013 leads to premature stop codon 79 (complete absence of ACTH, α-MSH, β-endorphin)

  Maternal allele

    1–base pair deletion nt 7133 leads to a frameshift–disrupting binding motif of ACTH and α-MSH

Patient 2

Obesity of very early onset, red hair, ACTH deficiency; ACTH deficiency led to clinical presentation

Homozygous C→A transversion at nt 3804 leads to out-of-frame start codon

Abolishment of translation of wild-type protein

FIGURE 15-26. *POMC* mutations. Mutations in the *POMC* gene lead to a syndrome of adrenal insufficiency, red hair pigmentation, and obesity. Preproopiomelanocortin (POMC) is the precursor for many peptides, including adrenocorticotropin hormone (ACTH), melanocyte-stimulating hormone (MSH), and β-endorphin. In patient 1, two different POMC mutations led to interference with appropriate synthesis of ACTH and MSH. The adrenal insufficiency results from the absence of ACTH. Red hair results from the absence of MSH regulation of pigmentation in the hair follicle, which would be mediated by the melanocortin-1 receptor. Obesity results from the absence of centrally acting MSH, which would regulate eating through the melanocortin-4 receptor [41]. A syndrome of obesity, adrenal insufficiency, and red hair pigmentation was seen in another patient described by Krude *et al.* [49]. This patient was homozygous for a mutation that abolished POMC translation.

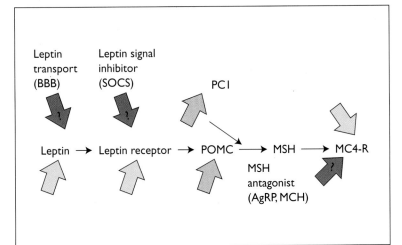

FIGURE 15-27. Summary of mutations in central nervous system pathways that may be associated with obesity in humans. *Blue arrows* point to mutations that have been identified. *Gray arrows* with question marks point to sites where mutations may occur but that have not yet been confirmed. AgRP—agouti-releasing peptide; BBB—blood–brain barrier; MC4-R—melanocortin-4 receptor; MCH—melanin-concentrating hormone; MSH—melanocyte-stimulating hormone; PC1—prohormone convertase-1; POMC—preproopiomelanocortin; SOCS—suppressors of cytokine signaling.

PROHORMONE CONVERTASE 1 GENE AND OBESITY

Extreme childhood obesity

Abnormal glucose homeostasis, hypogonadotropic hypogonadism, hypocortisolism, elevated plasma proinsulin level, low insulin level, elevated POMC level

Compound heterozygote in PC1

  Gly→Arg 483 prevents processing of prepro PC1 and retention in endoplasmic reticulum

  A→C + 4 intron 5-splice site, skipping of exon 5, loss of 26 residues, frameshift, and premature stop codon

Similarity in genetic abnormality and phenotype to fat/fat mouse

FIGURE 15-28. *Prohormone convertase 1* gene and obesity. At least one severely obese patient with a prohormone convertase-1 (PC1) mutation has been described. The patient was a compound heterozygote for the *PC1* gene [50]. This patient's clinical syndrome was very similar to that seen in the fa/fa rat. POMC—preproopiomelanocortin.

PPAR-GAMMA2

358 unrelated German patients

121 were obese (BMI >29)

Examined for mutations at or near serine phosphorylation site at amino acid 114. This site
negatively regulates transcriptional activity of the protein

Mutation identified: proline→glutamine at position 115

  4 of 121 obese patients had this mutation

  0 of 237 non-obese patients had this mutation

Overexpression of the mutant gene in fibroblasts led to synthesis of a phosphorylation defective
protein and accelerated differentiation of cells into adipocytes

FIGURE 15-29. PPAR-gamma2. Peroxisome proliferator-activated receptor (PPAR)-gamma2 is an important regulator of adipocyte differentiation. In a large study of German patients, four obese patients with a missense mutation in PPAR-gamma2 were identified [51]. This mutation resulted in the conversion of proline at position 115 to a glutamine. Overexpression of the mutant gene in mouse fibroblasts revealed that the mutant protein is defective in phosphorylating a serine in position 114. Fibroblasts expressing the mutant gene showed accelerated differentiation into adipocytes. BMI—body mass index.

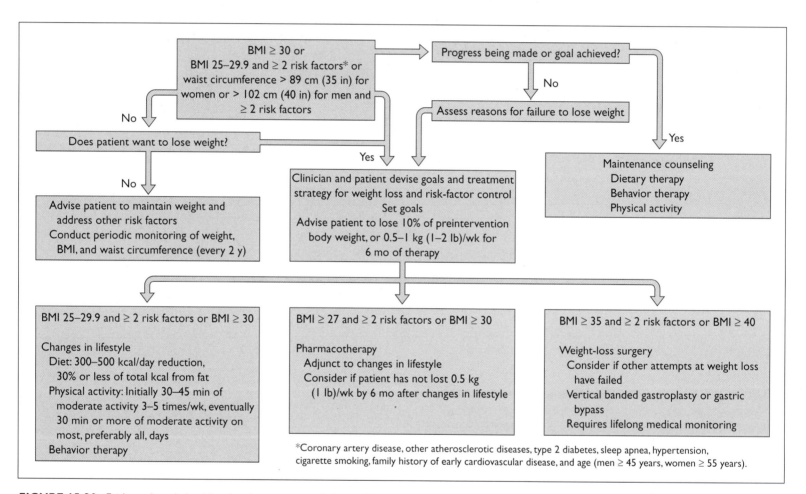

FIGURE 15-30. Evidence-based algorithm for the treatment of obesity. BMI—body mass index. (*Adapted from* [52].)

Treatment of Obesity

NIH ASSESSMENT CONFERENCE: METHODS OF VOLUNTARY WEIGHT LOSS AND CONTROL, BETHESDA, MARYLAND, 1992

40% of women and 24% of men attempt weight loss at any time

Most people can lose 10% of initial weight

One third to one half regain weight within 1 year, and most regain weight within 5 years

For many overweight persons, achieving and maintaining a healthy weight is a lifelong challenge

FIGURE 15-31. Voluntary weight control. The treatment of obesity poses major challenges. A large proportion of the United States population is trying to lose weight at any given time. Although most persons lose a modest amount of weight, weight loss is not usually maintained. NIH—National Institutes of Health.

RATIONALE FOR LONG-TERM USE OF OBESITY MEDICATIONS

Obesity is a chronic disease with morbid consequences

If medications are effective at weight loss, affect morbid consequences, and are safe, they should be used

Precise cut-off point for use of therapy must be determined through clinical trials, as is the case with therapies for other conditions (eg, hypertension, diabetes, hyperlipidemia)

FIGURE 15-32. Long-term use of obesity medications. Obesity is a chronic illness associated with complications. Some chronic illnesses, such as hypertension, may respond to dietary maneuvers (eg, reduction in salt intake). However, patients may be unable to make the necessary changes or the response may be inadequate. Safe medications that help obese individuals achieve sustained weight loss would substantially affect the morbidity and mortality associated with obesity.

RECENT AND FUTURE APPROACHES TO WEIGHT LOSS

Sibutramine—novel serotonin and norepinephrine reuptake inhibitor

Orlistat—inhibitor of intestinal fat absorption

Old standbys—phentermine, diethylpropion, mazindol

β-3 adrenergic agonists

Leptin or leptin analogues/mimics

Centrally acting agents based on new discoveries

  Antagonists of melanin-concentrating hormone, orexin, neuropeptide Y, galanin

  Agonists of melanocortin-4 receptor, corticotropin-releasing hormone receptors

Inhibitors of leptin resistance

FIGURE 15-33. Pharmacologic approaches to weight loss. Many potential medications are available for the treatment of obesity. The odds of successful pharmacologic therapy are increased when drug therapy is combined with a behavior modification program. Commercial programs may be as effective as hospital-based programs. Sibutramine [53] leads to effective weight loss in a subset of motivated patients; its effectiveness appears to be similar to that of phentermine used as a sole agent. The Food and Drug Administration has recently approved orlistat. One-year trials of orlistat with doses of 120 mg three times daily revealed that in the treatment group, weight loss at 1 year was approximately 50% greater than that in the control group (10.3 kg compared with 6.1 kg) [54]. Although the drug was effective in large clinical trials, its effectiveness in patients seen in a standard office practice has not yet been evaluated. Novel therapies, such as β-3 adrenergic agonists, leptin mimetics, or agents based on neuropeptide regulation, are the subject of intense investigation.

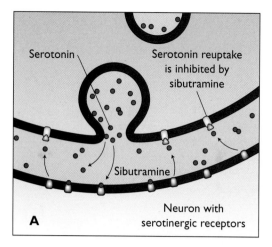

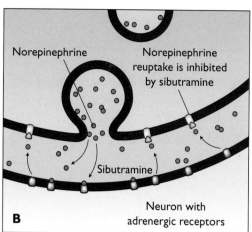

FIGURE 15-34. Mechanisms of action of sibutramine. Sibutramine acts to inhibit reuptake of norepinephrine, serotonin, and dopamine. Treatment is associated with modest degrees of weight loss of about 5% over placebo over a 6-month period. Hypertension is a side effect that may limit the usefulness of sibutramine in obese patients with metabolic syndrome. In the presynaptic neuron, sibutramine and its active metabolites inhibit the reuptake of serotonin (**A**) and norepinephrine (**B**), thereby prolonging the actions of these neurotransmitters at their postsynaptic receptors. (*Adapted from* Yanovski and Yanovski [55].)

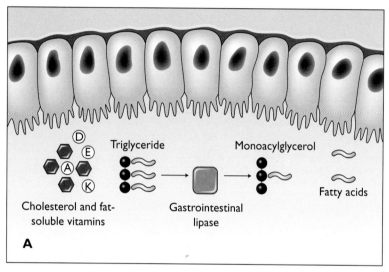

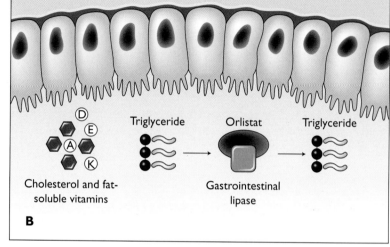

FIGURE 15-35. Inhibition of fat absorption by orlistat. Orlistat acts locally within the bowel to prevent absorption of lipids by inhibiting intestinal lipases. It is associated with local side effects such as loose bowels, diarrhea, and increased flatulence, but has no systemic side effects. **A,** Under normal function, the formation of micelles in the intestinal lumen allows absorption of approximately 90% of dietary triglyceride as monoacylglycerol and fatty acids; cholesterol and fat-soluble vitamins are absorbed with lipids. **B,** With orlistat, approximately one third of dietary triglyceride is excreted unchanged in stool.

Patients taking orlistat should be advised to take a vitamin supplement containing fat-soluble vitamins because absorption of these vitamins is also reduced. Weight-loss effects of orlistat are modest. About 35% of patients will achieve greater than 5% weight loss at 1 year, compared with about 20% of placebo-treated patients. Weight loss of 10% of initial body weight is seen in about 20% of treated patients. (*Adapted from* Yanovski and Yanovski [55].)

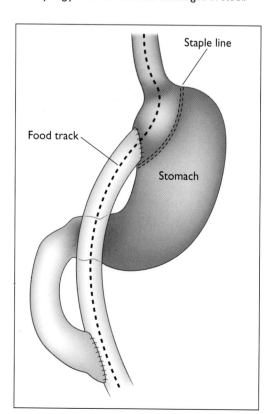

FIGURE 15-36. One of the few effective treatments for morbid obesity is surgical therapy. Although a number of surgical procedures can be performed, the most widely performed surgical procedure is the Roux-en-Y gastric bypass. This achieves permanent (longer than 14 years) and significant weight loss and has a relatively low incidence of side effects. When patients are screened appropriately, 90% of patients will lose 50% or more of excess body weight. Successful surgery is associated with marked improvements in many of the co-morbidities associated with obesity, including glucose homeostasis, blood pressure, and lipid profiles [56].

Relative Risk for Obesity

RELATIVE RISK FOR OBESITY ASSOCIATED WITH BODY MASS INDEX AND FAT DISTRIBUTION IN MEN			
	Waist-to-Hip Ratio		
BMI	**< 0.85**	**0.85–1.0**	**> 1.0**
20 to < 25	Very low	Low	Medium
25 to < 30	Low	Medium	High
30 to < 35	Medium	High	Very high
35 to < 40	High	Very high	Very high
> 40	Very high	Very high	Very high

FIGURE 15-37. Relative risk for obesity with body mass index (BMI) and fat distribution in men. For any particular BMI, the lower the waist-to-hip ratio, ie, the smaller the intra-abdominal deposits, the lower the risk.

References

1. Flegal KM, Carrp MD, Kuczmarski RJ, et al.: Overweight and obesity in the United States: prevalence and trends, 1960–1994. Int J Obesity 1998, 22:39–37.

2. Vanitallie TB: Body weight, morbidity and longevity. In Obesity. Edited by Bjorntorp P, Brodoff BN. Philadelphia: JB Lippincott; 1992.

3. Smith SR: Regional fat distribution. In Nutrition, Genetics and Obesity. Edited by Bray GA, Ryan DH. Baton Rouge, LA: Louisiana State University Press; 1999:433–458.

4. Goodpaster B, Thaete F, Somoneau J, et al.: Subcutaneous abdominal fat and thigh muscle composition predict insulin sensitivity independently of visceral fat. Diabetes 1997, 46:1579–1585.

5. Masuzaki H, Paterson J, Shinyama H, et al.: A transgenic model of visceral obesity and the metabolic syndrome. Science 2001, 294:2071–2072.

6. Ravussin E, Lillioja S, Anderson TE, et al.: Determinants of 24-h energy expenditure in man. J Clin Invest 1986, 778:1568–1578.

7. Prentice AM, Black AE, Coward WA, et al.: High levels of energy expenditure in obese women. Br Med J 1986, 292:983–987.

8. Flatt JP: Importance of nutrient balance in body weight regulation. Diabetes Metab Rev 1988, 4:571–581.

9. Flatt JP, Gupte S: In Nutrition, Genetics and Obesity. Edited by Bray GA, Ryan DH. Baton Rouge, LA: Louisiana State University Press; 1999:73–88.

10. Anand BK, Brobeck JR: Hypothalamic control of food intake in rates and cats. Yale J Biol Med 1951, 24:123.

11. Hetherington A, Ranson SW: Hypothalamic lesions and adiposity in the rat. Anat Rec 1940, 78:149.

12. Qu D, Ludwig DS, Gammeltoft S, et al.: A role for melanin concentrating hormone in the central regulation of feeding behavior. Nature 1996, 380:243–246.

13. Sakurai T, Amemiya A, Ishii M, et al.: Orexins and orexin receptors: a family of hypothalamic neuropeptides and G protein-coupled receptors that regulate feeding behavior. Cell 1998, 92:1–696.

14. Wellman PJ: Norepinephrine and the control of food intake. Nutrition 2000, 16:837–842.

15. Tsujii S, Bray GA: A beta-3 adrenergic agonist (BRL-37,344) decreases food intake. Physiol Behav 1998, 63:723–728.

16. Yamashita J, Onai T, York DA, Bray GA: Relationship between food intake and metabolic rate in rats treated with beta-adrenoceptor agonists. Int J Obes Relat Metab Disord 1994, 18:429–433.

17. Yang ZJ, Meguid MM, Chai JK, et al.: Bilateral hypothalamic dopamine infusion in male Zucker rat suppresses feeding due to reduced meal size. Pharmacol Biochem Behav 1997, 58:631–635.

18. Pothos EN, Creese I, Hoebel BG: Restricted eating with weight loss selectively decreases extracellular dopamine in the nucleus accumbens and alters dopamine response to amphetamine, morphine and food intake. J Neurosci 1995, 15:6640–6650.

19. Turton MD, Oshea D, Bloom SR: Central effects of neuropeptide Y with emphasis on its role in obesity and diabetes. In Neuropeptide Y and Drug Development. Edited by Grundemar L, Bloom SR. San Diego: Academic Press; 1997:15–39.

20. Stanley BG, Kyrkouli SE, Lampert S, et al.: Neuropeptide Y chronically injected into the hypothalamus: a powerful neurochemical inducer of hyperphagia and obesity. Peptides 1986, 7:1189–1192.

21. Billington CJ, Briggs JE, Grace M, et al.: Effects of intracerebroventricular injection of neuropeptide Y on energy metabolism. Am J Physiol 1991, 260(2 Pt 2):R321–R327.

22. Halford JC, Blundell JE: Pharmacology of appetite suppression. Prog Drug Res 2000, 54:25–58.

23. Horvath TL, Diano S, Sotonyi P, et al.: Minireview: ghrelin and the regulation of energy balance—a hypothalamic perspective. Endocrinology 2001, 142:4163-9.

24. Hansen TK, Dall R, Hosoda H, et al.: Weight loss increases circulating levels of ghrelin in human obesity. Clin Endocrinol 2002, 56:203–206.

25. Hagan MM: Peptide YY: a key mediator of orexigenic behavior. Peptides 2002, 23:377–382.

26. Naslund E, Barkeling B, King N, et al.: Energy intake and appetite are suppressed by glucagon-like peptide-1 (GLP-1) in obese men. Int J Obes Relat Metab Disord 1999, 23:304–311.

27. Degen L, Matzinger D, Drewe J, Beglinger C: The effect of cholecystokinin in controlling appetite and food intake in humans. Peptides 2001, 22:1265–1269.

28. Woods SC, Seeley RJ: Adiposity signals and the control of energy homeostasis. Int J Obes Relat Metab Disord 2001, 25(Suppl 5):S35–S38.

29. Zhang Y, Proenca R, Maffei M, et al.: Positional cloning of the mouse obese gene and its human homologue. Nature 1994, 372:425–432.

30. Halaas JL, Gajiwala KS, Maffei M, et al.: Weight-reducing effects of the plasma protein encoded by the obese gene. Science 1995, 269:543–546.

31. Ahima RS, Prabakaran D, Mantzoros C, et al.: Role of leptin in the neuroendocrine response to fasting. *Nature* 1996, 383:250–252.

32. Shimada M, Tritos NA, Lowell BB, et al.: Mice lacking melanin concentrating hormone are hypophagic and lean. *Nature* 1998, 396:670–674.

33. Ericson JC, Clegg KE, Palmiter RD: Sensitivity to leptin and susceptibility to seizures in mice lacking neuropeptide Y. *Nature* 1996, 381:415–418.

34. Erickson JC, Hollopeter G, Palmiter RD: Attenuation of the obesity syndrome of ob/ob mice by the loss of neuropeptide Y. *Science* 1996, 274:1704–1707.

35. Tartaglia LA, Dembski M, Weng X, et al.: Identification and expression cloning of a leptin receptor, OB-R. *Cell* 1995, 83:1263–1271.

36. Elias CF, Saper CB, Maratos-Flier E, et al.: Chemically defined projection linking the mediobasal hypothalamus and the lateral hypothalamic area. *J Comp Neurol* 1998, 402:442–459.

37. Mountjoy KG, Robbinsa LS, Mortrud MT, et al.: The cloning of a family of genes that encode the melanocortin receptors. *Science* 1992, 257:1248–1251.

38. Montague CT, Farooqi IS, Whitehead JP, et al.: Congenital leptin deficiency is associated with severe early-onset obesity in humans. *Nature* 1997, 387:903–908.

39. Clement K, Vaisse C, Lahlou N, et al.: A mutation in the human leptin receptor gene causes obesity and pituitary dysfunction. *Nature* 1998, 392:398–401.

40. Tsujii S, Bray GA: Acetylation alters the feeding response to MSH and beta-endorphin. *Brain Res Bull* 1989, 23:165–169.

41. Yen TT, Gill AM, Frigeri LG, et al.: Obesity, diabetes and neoplasia in the yellow Avy/- mice: ectopic expression of the agouti gene. *FASEB J* 1994, 8:481–488.

42. Blanchard SG, Harris CO, Ittoop OR, et al.: Agouti antagonism of melanocortin binding and action in the B16F10 murine melanoma cell line. *Biochemistry* 1995, 34:10406–10411.

43. Lu D, Willard D, Patel IR, et al.: Agouti protein is an antagonist of the melanocyte-stimulating hormone receptor. *Nature* 1994, 371:799–802.

44. Huszar D, Lynch CA, Fairchild-Huntress V, et al.: Targeted disruption of the melanocortin-4 receptor results in obesity in mice. *Cell* 1997, 88:131–141.

45. Shutter JR, Graham M, Kinsey AC, et al.: Hypothalamic expression of ART, a novel gene related to agouti, is up-regulated in obese and diabetic mutant mice. *Genes Dev* 1997, 11:593–602.

46. Ollmann MM, Wilson BD, Yang YK, et al.: Antagonism of central melanocortin receptors in vitro and in vivo by agouti-related protein. *Science* 1997, 281:135–138.

47. Yeo GS, Farooqi IS, Aminian S, et al.: A frameshift mutation in MC4R associated with dominantly inherited human obesity. *Nat Genet* 1998, 20:111–112.

48. Vaisse C, Clement K, Guy-Grand B, et al.: A frameshift mutation in human MC4R is associated with a dominant form of obesity. *Nat Genet* 1998, 20:113–114.

49. Krude H, Biebermann H, Luck W, et al.: Severe early-onset obesity, adrenal insufficiency and red hair pigmentation caused by POMC mutations in humans. *Nat Genet* 1998, 9:155–157.

50. Jackson RS, Creemers JW, Ohagi S, et al.: Obesity and impaired prohormone processing associated with mutations in the human prohormone convertase 1 gene. *Nat Genet* 1997, 16:303–306.

51. Ristow M, Muller-Wieland D, Pfeiffer A, et al.: Obesity associated with a mutation in a genetic regulator of adipocyte differentiation. *N Engl J Med* 1998, 339:953–959.

52. The practical guide: identification, evaluation, and treatment of overweight and obesity in adults. Bethesda, MD: National Heart, Lung, and Blood Institute, North American Association for the Study of Obesity, 2000. (NIH publication n.00-4048.) Available at http://www.nhlbi.nih.gov/guidelines/obesity/practgde.htm. Accessed May 7, 2002.

53. Bray GA, Blackburn GL, Ferguson JM, et al.: Sibutramine produces dose-related weight loss. *Obes Res* 1999, 7:189–198.

54. Hauptman J, Guerciolini R, Nichols G: Orlistat: a novel treatment for obesity. In *Nutrition, Genetics and Obesity*. Edited by Bray GA, Ryan DH. Baton Rouge, LA: Louisiana State University Press; 1998.

55. Yanovski SZ, Yanovski JA: Obesity. *N Engl J Med* 2002, 346(8):591–602.

56. Mun EC, Blackburn GL, Matthews JB: Current status of medical and surgical therapy for obesity. *Gastroenterology* 2001, 120:669–681.

DIABETES AND PREGNANCY

Lois Jovanovic

16

Hyperglycemia during pregnancy is the most common metabolic problem of pregnancy today [1]. The prevalence of hyperglycemia during pregnancy may be as high as 13% [2] (0.1% of the pregnant population per year have type 1 diabetes, 2% to 3% have type 2 diabetes, and up to 12% of the population have gestational diabetes mellitus [GDM]). Although all types of diabetes increase the risk of complications to the mother and the fetus, it is most important to distinguish among the types, as each has a different impact on the course of pregnancy and the development of the fetus. Pregestational diabetes mellitus (type 1 or type 2) is more serious because it is present before pregnancy; thus its effect begins at fertilization and implantation, and continues throughout pregnancy and thereafter. In particular, organogenesis may be disrupted, leading to a high risk of early abortion [3], severe congenital defects [4–7], and retarded growth [8]. Maternal manifestations are also more serious, especially in the presence of vascular complications such as retinopathy or nephropathy [9]. Gestational diabetes mellitus usually appears in the second half of pregnancy and affects mainly fetal growth rate [10]. The offspring of mothers with GDM have a higher risk of subsequent obesity and slower systemic and psychosocial development, and probably other long-term metabolic effects [11,12].

Historically, few women with pregestational diabetes lived to childbearing age before the advent of insulin therapy. Until insulin became commercially available in 1924, less than 100 pregnancies were reported in diabetic women, and most likely these women had type 2, and not type 1, diabetes. Even with this assumption, these cases of diabetes and pregnancy were associated with a greater than 90% infant mortality rate and a 30% maternal mortality rate [13]. As late as 1980, some physicians were still counseling diabetic women to avoid pregnancy [14]. This philosophy was justified because of the poor obstetric history in 30% to 50% of diabetic women. Infant mortality rates finally began to improve after 1980, when treatment strategies stressed better control of maternal plasma glucose levels, and after self-monitoring of blood glucose and hemoglobin A_{1c} became available to enable better metabolic control in persons with diabetes [15]. As the pathophysiology of pregnancy complicated by diabetes has been elucidated, and as management programs have achieved and maintained near normoglycemia throughout pregnancy complicated by type 1, type 2, and GDM, perinatal mortality rates have become comparable with those of the general population [16]. The Pedersen [17] hypothesis links maternal hyperglycemia-induced fetal hyperinsulinemia to morbidity of the infant. Fetal hyperinsulinemia may cause increased fetal body mass (macrosomia) and, subsequently, a difficult delivery, or cause inhibition of pulmonary maturation of surfactant and, therefore, respiratory distress of the neonate. The fetus may also have decreased serum potassium levels caused by the elevated insulin and glucose levels that may induce fatal cardiac arrhythmias. Neonatal hypoglycemia may cause permanent neurologic damage. The literature since the advent of insulin has documented that programs of near-normal glycemia are associated with improved outcome [18–20]. Therefore, treatment strategies have been developed to minimize the fetal exposure to either sustained or intermittent periods of hyperglycemia [21–23]. The maternal postprandial glucose level has been shown to be the most important variable to affect the subsequent risk of neonatal macrosomia [24–26]. When the postprandial glucose levels are blunted 1 hour after beginning the meal, the risk of macrosomia is minimized [26].

There is an increased prevalence of congenital anomalies and spontaneous abortions in type 1 and type 2 diabetic women who are in poor glycemic control during the period of fetal organogenesis, which is nearly complete by 7 weeks postconception [27]. It also has been reported that some women with gestational diabetes are also at risk for bearing a malformed infant because they most probably had undiagnosed (and thus untreated) type 2 diabetes during the time of organogenesis. Because women may not know they are pregnant during the critical time period for organ formation, prepregnancy counseling and planning is essential for all pregestational diabetic women of childbearing age [20,28].

For the past 30 years, the classification, diagnosis, and treatment of GDM have been based on the recommendations of the International Workshop-Conference on Gestational Diabetes Mellitus [29]. As of 1997, three such international meetings had been held and their recommendations were adopted by major medical institutions in Europe and America (American College of Obstetrics and Gynecology, American Diabetes Association, European Association for the Study of Diabetes, World Health Organization). Despite decades of debate on the optimal screening and diagnostic criteria, there still remains divided opinion as to the best means to diagnose gestational diabetes. At present there is an ongoing multinational trial (Hyperglycemia and Adverse Outcome in Pregnancy [HAPO]) that has as its objective to elucidate the optimal diagnostic criteria for gestational diabetes. The HAPO trial will be completed in 2004, and it is hoped that the results will recommend the best method to diagnose hyperglycemia during pregnancy.

Since 1980, the inception of "tight glycemia control" achieved by "intensive conventional therapy" (including self-monitoring of blood glucose) has become an integral part of the treatment program for pregnancies complicated by hyperglycemia. As early as 1954, Pedersen [13] observed that "the common maternal, fetal, and neonatal complications of a diabetic pregnancy could be diminished by carefully supervised regulation of maternal metabolism." There is now a wealth of literature and experience to justify intensive approaches toward achieving normoglycemia in pregnancy. It is time to invest energy to simplify and disseminate these systems.

Pregestational Diabetes

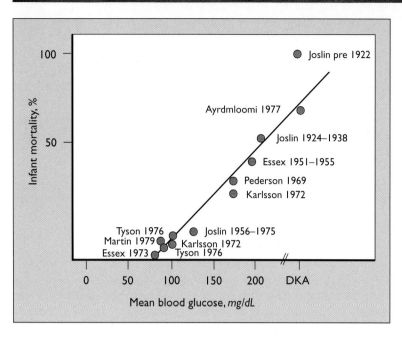

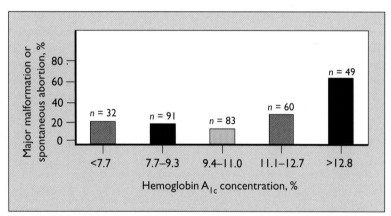

FIGURE 16-1. Literature review of the relationship between mean maternal glucose concentrations and infant mortality. Before the advent of insulin, an infant of a diabetic mother rarely survived. Prior to 1922, the fewer than 100 reported cases of survival are probably the offspring of type 2 and not type 1 diabetic women [13]. A review of the major studies over the years since insulin became commercially available and when intensive glucose control systems were developed reveals that as the mean maternal blood glucose concentrations decrease, the percent infant mortality decreases [30–32]. A linear regression line drawn through the points on this graph indicates that at a mean maternal glucose level of 84 mg/dL, there would be no increased risk of infant mortality over the risk in the general population. The report by Parretti *et al.* [34] on the blood glucose levels in normal, healthy pregnant women shows that the overall daily mean fasting glucose level is 56 mg/dL and the peak postprandial response occurs at 1 hour after the meal. This peak level never exceeds 105.2 mg/dL. The calculated mean glucose concentration in their population was 85 mg/dL, close to the projected mean glucose concentration derived from the literature review [33]. (*Adapted from* Jovanovic and Peterson [33].)

FIGURE 16-2. Combined prevalence of major malformation and spontaneous abortion according to the glycosylated hemoglobin (HbA$_{1c}$) concentration during the first trimester of pregnancy. In the woman with pre-existing diabetes (pregestational diabetes), pregnancy should be deferred until the patient is under good glycemic control and has been thoroughly evaluated for complications of diabetes. Prepregnancy counseling should begin at the onset of puberty, with the need for abstinence or effective contraception clearly explained and understood [20]. HbA$_{1c}$ values provide the best assessment of the degree of chronic glycemic control, reflecting the average blood glucose concentration during the preceding 6 to 8 weeks. As a result, measurement of HbA$_{1c}$ can, in early pregnancy, estimate the level of glycemic control during the period of fetal organogenesis [19,28,30–32]. There are two important consequences in this regard: 1) HbA$_{1c}$ values early in pregnancy are correlated with the rates of spontaneous abortion and major congenital malformations, and 2) normalizing blood glucose concentrations before and early in pregnancy can reduce the risks of spontaneous abortion and congenital malformations nearly to that of the general population [5,28,32]. One report compared 110 women who were already 6 to 30 weeks pregnant at the time of referral with 84 women recruited before conception and then put on a daily glucose-monitoring regimen [28]. The mean blood glucose concentration was between 60 and 140 mg/dL (3.3 and 7.8 mmol/L) in 50% of the latter women. The incidence of anomalies was 1.2% in the women recruited before conception versus 10.9% in those first seen during pregnancy. Very similar findings were noted in another study: 1.4% versus 10.4% incidence of congenital abnormalities [32]. Major congenital malformations (specifically caudal regression, 252 times more common in the infant of the diabetic mother; situs inversus, 84 times common than in the normal population; and renal and cardiac defects, 6 and 4 times more common than in the infant of the diabetic mother compared with the normal population, respectively), which either require surgical correction or significantly affect the health of the child, are more common in infants of mothers with poorly controlled diabetes [27]. There is also a substantial increase in spontaneous abortions in women who enter pregnancy in poor metabolic control as reflected by an elevated HbA$_{1c}$ level [3]. The teratogenicity of glucose appears to be the major factor before the seventh gestational week [27].

This figure depicts the combined prevalence of major malformation and spontaneous abortion according to the HbA$_{1c}$ concentration during the first trimester of pregnancy in 315 women with type 1 diabetes. The risk rises markedly at HbA$_{1c}$ concentrations of about 11%; other studies have found an increase at levels above 9.5% [4,5,28,30–32].

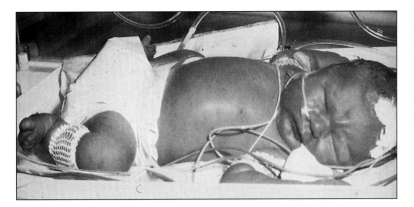

FIGURE 16-3. (See Color Plate) Diabetic fetopathy. The most common and significant neonatal complication clearly associated with diabetes in pregnancy is macrosomia: an oversized baby with a birthweight greater than the 90th percentile for gestation age and sex, or a birthweight greater than 2 SD above the normal mean birthweight. This infant was macrosomic, weighed 4583 g, was delivered a month prematurely, and had all of the signs of an infant of a diabetic mother (hypoglycemia, hypocalcemia, hyperbilirubinemia) and died of respiratory distress 2 days after this photograph was taken.

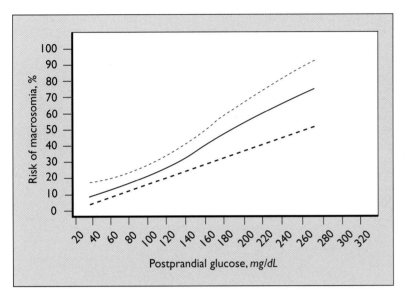

FIGURE 16-4. The relationship between the peak postprandial glucose concentration and risk of macrosomia. Although controversial, the rate of complications in pregnancies complicated by diabetes has been tied to metabolic control of maternal glucose [5,18,19,24–26,28,30–32]. Perhaps the debate remains because many of the reports claim that neonatal complications occur despite excellent metabolic control, but these reports fail to measure postprandial glucose levels [24–26]. Postprandial glucose control has been suggested as key to neonatal outcome for the pregnant woman with either type 1 or gestational diabetes [23,24]. The Diabetes in Early Pregnancy (DIEP) study was a multicenter trial of type 1 diabetic pregnant women who were compared with control women throughout pregnancy. This group studied the relationship of maternal glucose levels and risk of macrosomia [24]. The DIEP study reported that the 1-hour postprandial glucose levels predicted 28.5% of the macrosomic infants born to diabetic mothers. This figure shows that the risk of macrosomia is a continuum. Any postprandial peak increases the risk of macrosomia above that seen in the normal population (10% risk). In addition, when the peak postprandial response is greater than 120 mg/dL, then the risk of macrosomia rises rapidly. (*Adapted from* Jovanovic et al. [24].)

STEPWISE LOGISTIC REGRESSION OF MATERNAL METABOLIC FACTORS AND ESTIMATES OF NEONATAL BODY COMPOSITION*

	r^2	$*\Delta*r^2$
Birthweight		
Insulin sensitivity index†	0.28	—
Maternal weight gain	0.48	0.20
Fat-free mass		
Insulin sensitivity index†	0.33	—
Maternal weight gain	0.53	0.20
Fat mass		
Insulin sensitivity‡	0.15	—
Parity	0.29	0.14
Neonatal sex	0.39	0.10
Insulin sensitivity index†	0.46	0.07

*In 16 neonates of women with normal glucose tolerance (n = 6) or gestational diabetes (n = 10).
†Late pregnancy.
‡Pregravid.

FIGURE 16-5. Stepwise logistic regression of maternal metabolic factors and estimates of neonatal body composition. Catalano et al. [10] evaluated the relationship of various aspects of maternal carbohydrate metabolism and estimates of neonatal body composition. They evaluated 16 infants of women who participated in a long-term study of alterations in glucose metabolism. The results of a stepwise logistic regression of maternal carbohydrate metabolism factors showed that maternal weight gain played the most significant role. (*Adapted from* Catalano et al. [10].)

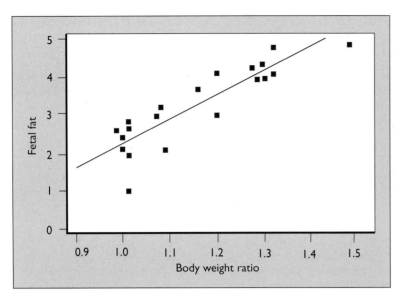

FIGURE 16-6. Relationship between fetal fat and subsequent birthweight. Using MRI, Jovanovic et al. [35] also found that the mother's adiposity was a predictor of birthweight. The relationship of fetal fat, as determined by the mean of two points of maximal thickness of the fetal abdominal wall subcutaneous fat on the MRI taken at 36 weeks of gestation, compared with the infant birthweight ratio was highly significant ($P < 0.001$; $r = 0.88$). (*Adapted from* Jovanovic et al. [35].)

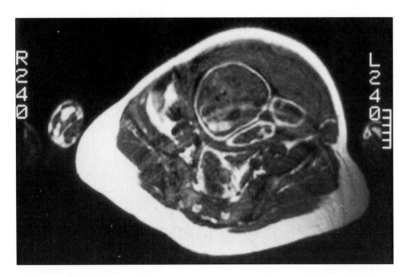

FIGURE 16-7. Magnetic resonance image of the fetus of a diabetic woman in excellent glucose control. This image was taken at the level of the maternal umbilicus at 38 weeks of gestation [35]. The mother had gestational diabetes mellitus and maintained excellent glucose control with preprandial glucose concentrations 70 to 90 mg/dL; all of her blood glucose levels at 1 hour after the meal were less than 120 mg/dL. This infant weighed 3900 g at birth and was normal for percent body fat. (*From* Jovanovic et al. [35]; with permission).

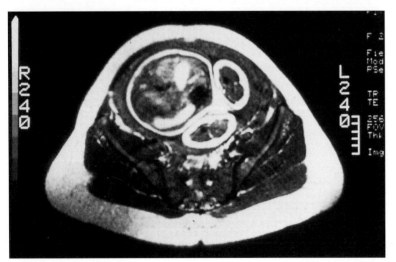

FIGURE 16-8. Magnetic resonance image of the fetus of a diabetic woman in poor glucose control. This image was taken at the level of the maternal umbilicus at 38 weeks of gestational age. As can be seen, this fetus not only has increased subcutaneous fat, but also already has accrual of visceral fat [35]. This mother had no antenatal care and presented to the emergency room with a urinary tract infection. She was found to have severe hyperglycemia. Her glucose concentration on admission was 396 mg/dL, probably indicative that she had undiagnosed type 2 diabetes. This fetus weighed 4340 g at birth, had 50% of its neonatal weight composed of fat, and had all of the signs of an infant of a diabetic mother. (*From* Jovanovic et al. [35]; with permission.)

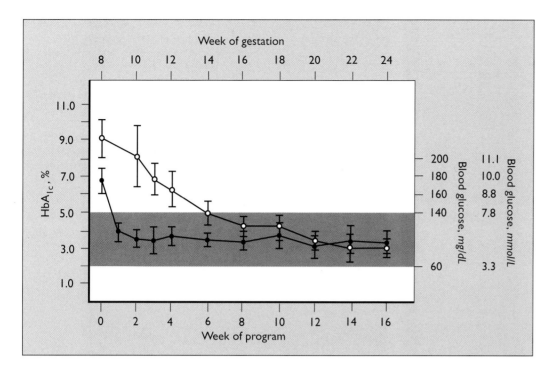

FIGURE 16-9. The time course for normalization of maternal glycosylated hemoglobin level in relationship to the normalization of maternal glucose concentrations. One of the first reports of a significant improvement in the outcome of type I diabetic pregnancies was published by Jovanovic et al. in 1980 [19]. We showed that when maternal blood glucose levels were normalized by the eighth gestational week, the birthweights of the infants were also normalized. This figure shows the time course for the normalization of glycosylated hemoglobin (HbA$_{1c}$) and blood glucose for 10 pregnant women with type I diabetes. The *open circles* represent the mean HbA$_{1c}$ ± SD. The *closed circles* represent mean blood glucose concentrations of ± SD (each time point is based on 8 to 10 glucose determinations obtained from all 10 patients over 2-week intervals). The *shaded area* is the normal range for both HbA$_{1c}$ and blood glucose concentrations in the third trimester. All 10 women had normal infants at term. (*Adapted from* Jovanovic et al. [19].)

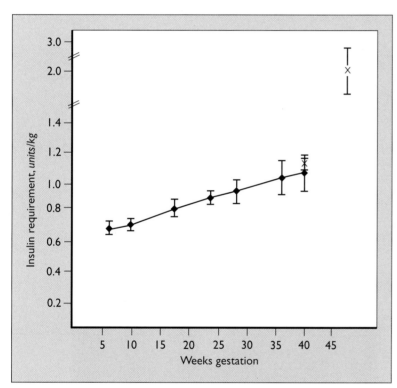

FIGURE 16-10. The insulin requirement throughout pregnancy in type I diabetic women. In a larger study of type I diabetic women who were maintained with normoglycemia from the sixth gestational week onward, we showed that there is a smooth rise in the insulin requirement throughout pregnancy. Fifty-three infants born to 52 type I diabetic women were all normal at birth. The insulin requirement of the woman who delivered twins was double that of the other 51 women. This increased need for insulin was manifested from the sixth gestational week onward. The "×" shows the mean ± SD daily dosage of insulin during weeks 34 to 37 of gestation. (*Adapted from* Jovanovic et al. [18].)

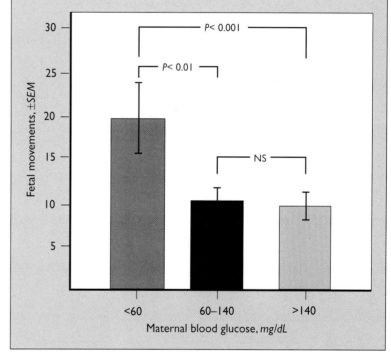

FIGURE 16-11. The relationship between fetal movements and maternal glucose concentrations. In this same population of diabetic women whose glucose control was documented in the study shown in Figure 16-10, the assessment of fetal well-being using the parameter of fetal movements associated with heart rate acceleration is shown here. The *bars* show comparison of fetal movements with accelerations with maternal blood glucose concentrations less than 60 mg/dL, with maternal blood glucose concentrations of 60 to 140 mg/dL, and with maternal blood glucose concentrations greater than 140 mg/dL. It can be seen that the fetuses had significantly more movements with heart rate acceleration when the blood glucose concentrations were low. It appears, therefore, that transient, mild hypoglycemia is well tolerated by the fetus and may in fact be preferred by the fetus. (*Adapted from* Holden et al. [36].)

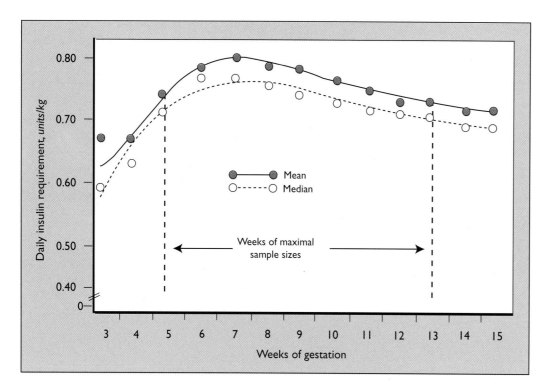

FIGURE 16-12. The declining insulin requirement in the first trimester of type 1 diabetic pregnant women. In the Diabetes in Early Pregnancy Study, the insulin requirement in the first trimester was studied. The daily insulin dosage (expressed as either a weekly mean or median in units per kg from weeks 3 to 8) increased, but there was an insulin dosage decrease in the late first trimester. The *open circles* represent the mean dosage of 346 type 1 diabetic women who had healthy infants. The *closed circles* represent the median dosage of these same patients. (*Adapted from* Jovanovic *et al.* [37].)

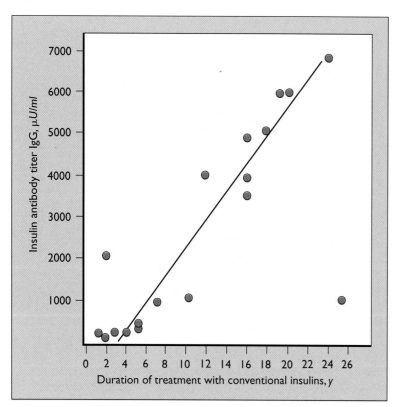

FIGURE 16-13. The relationship between anti-insulin antibody levels and duration of treatment with animal insulin. Although maternal glucose is the most likely causal agent of neonatal macrosomia, some have suggested that neonatal morbidity is secondary to the variability of maternal serum glucose and presence of antibodies to insulin. Placental transfer of insulin bound to immunoglobulin G (IgG) has also been associated with fetal macrosomia in mothers with near-normal glycemic control during gestation. Menon *et al.* [38] reported that antibody-bound insulin transferred to the fetus was proportional to the concentration of antibody-bound insulin measured in the mother. Also, the amount of antibody-bound insulin transferred to the fetus correlated directly with macrosomia in the infant, and was independent of maternal blood glucose levels. In contrast, researchers found that only improved glucose control, as evidenced by lower postprandial glucose excursions, but not lower insulin antibody levels, correlated with lower fetal weight [39]. They showed that insulin antibodies to exogenous insulin do not influence infant birthweight or insulin dosage. They did report, however, that there is a relationship between duration of treatment with conventional insulin and IgG antibody titer as shown here. (*Adapted from* Jovanovic *et al.* [40].)

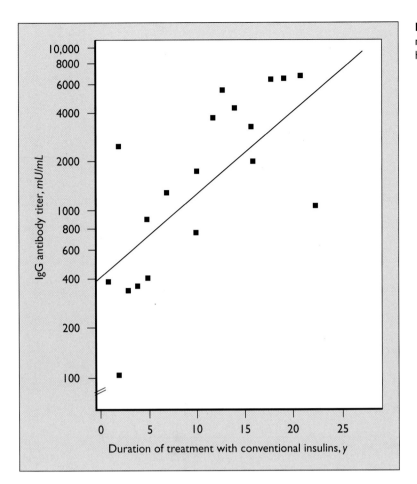

FIGURE 16-14. The relationship between antibody levels and years of treatment with animal insulin. The longer the treatment with animal insulin, the higher the immunoglobulin G (IgG) antibody levels.

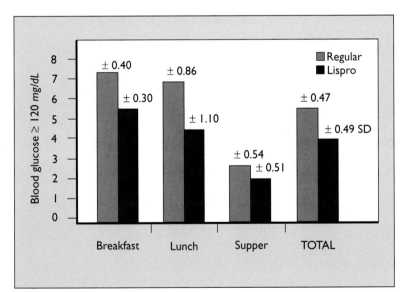

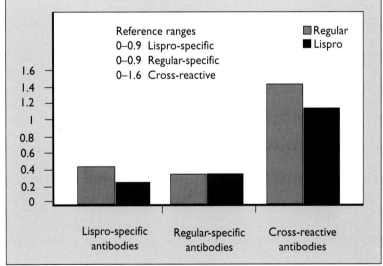

FIGURE 16-15. The postprandial glucose concentrations of diabetic women treated with insulin lispro compared with the postprandial glucose concentrations of diabetic women treated with human insulin during pregnancy. Our group reported that insulin lispro, an analog of human insulin with a peak insulin action achieved within 1 hour after injection, significantly improves the postprandial glucose concentrations in pregnant diabetic patients. We showed that the postprandial glucose level is significantly lower throughout pregnancy in insulin-requiring gestational diabetic women treated with lispro insulin compared with gestational diabetic women treated with human insulin. (*Adapted from* Jovanovic et al. [41].)

FIGURE 16-16. Insulin antibody findings. The antibody levels were no different in the women treated with lispro insulin compared with human insulin. In addition, they were not able to detect lispro in the cord blood of the infants whose mothers were treated with lispro. Because of the importance of blunting the postprandial peak glucose concentration, and the lack of immunogenicity of rapid-acting insulin analogues, the treatment of choice in pregnancy is now to suggest that these insulins be used in pregnancies complicated by diabetes. Large clinical trials in type 1 diabetic women have not yet been published, however. (*Adapted from* Jovanovic et al. [41].)

Insulin dosage regimen for diabetic pregnancy

□ 1. Pregnancy NPH plus regular insulin schedule   Patient weight in kg =

Date &   Nursing will calculate and administer the starting dose of insulin as outlined below: "Big I" = total daily units of insulin.
Time
    Date: Circle One: Gestational weeks = 0–12 | 13–28 | 29–34 | 35–40 |
                          Units of insulin   =   0.7 | 0.8 | 0.9 | 1.0 | OTHER

"BIG I"

Calculate desired units of insulin from above line.
"Big I" = _____ (units X weight KG/24 hours) divide so that 4/9 of "Big I" is NPH given before breakfast, and 1/6
of "Big I" is NPH given before bedtime.
Regular insulin is given before breakfast as 2/9 of "Big I", and before dinner as 1/6 of "Big I". The regular insulin
is titrated based on the blood glucose.

BREAKFAST

Do not
feed the
patient
until the
blood
sugar is
below
120 mg/dL.

0730 Pre-breakfast: NPH = 4/9 "Big I" = _____.
    Check yesterday's pre-dinner BS:
        If yesterday's pre-dinner BS is <60, then decrease today's AM NPH by 2 units.
        If yesterday's pre-dinner BS is 60–90, no change in today's AM NPH.
        If yesterday's pre-dinner BS is >90, then increase today's AM NPH by 2 units.
    Regular = 2/9 Insulin "Big I" = _____ to be adjusted according to the following scale:
        BS <60 = _____ = (2/9 "Big I" dose) - 3% of the "Big I".
        60–90 = _____ = 2/9 "Big I" dose.
        90–120 = _____ = (2/9 "Big I" dose) + 3% of "Big I".
        >121 = _____ = (2/9 "Big I" dose) + 6% of "Big I".
    If today's BS 1 hour after breakfast is <110, then decrease tomorrow's pre-breakfast regular insulin by 2 units.
    If today's BS 1 hour after breakfast is 110–120, no change in tomorrow's pre-breakfast regular insulin.
    If today's BS 1 hour after breakfast is >120, then increase tomorrow's pre-breakfast regular insulin by 2 units.

LUNCH

Do not
feed the
patient
until the
blood
sugar is
below
120 mg/dL.

1130 Pre-lunch: Regular insulin is given based on the following scale:
        BS <90 = 0 insulin.

    91–120 = (1/18 "Big I") = _____.

    121–140 = (1/18 "Big I") + 2 units = _____.

    >141 = (1/18 "Big I") + 4 units = _____.

DINNER

Do not
feed the
patient
until the
blood
sugar is
below
120 mg/dL.

1700 Pre-dinner: Regular insulin is 1/6 "Big I" = _____ and is based on the following scale.
        BS <60 = _____ = (1/6 "Big I" dose) - 3% of "Big I".
        60–90 = _____ = 1/6 "Big I" dose.
        91–120 = _____ = (1/6 "Big I" dose) + 3% of "Big I".
        >121 = _____ = (1/6 "Big I" dose) + 6% of "Big I".
    If today's BS 1 hour after dinner is <110, then decrease tomorrow's dinner regular insulin by 2 units.
    If today's BS 1 hour after dinner is 110–120, no change in tomorrow's dinner regular insulin.
    If today's BS 1 hour after dinner is >120, then increase tomorrow's dinner regular insulin by 2 units.

BEDTIME

2330 Bedtime NPH: Give 1/6 "Big I" = _____.

    If today's pre-breakfast BS is <60, then decrease today's bedtime NPH by 2 units.
    If today's pre-breakfast BS is 60–90, no change in today's bedtime NPH.
    If today's pre-breakfast BS is >90, then check the 3 AM BS and, if it is <70 (regardless of today's pre-breakfast BS),
    decrease today's bedtime NPH by 2 units.
    If today's pre-breakfast BS is >90, and the 3 AM BS >70, increase today's bedtime NPH by 2 units.
    Also, if the 3 AM BS is >90, then call the doctor for 3 AM regular insulin scale equal to the pre-lunch regular insulin scale.

FIGURE 16-17. Insulin dosage regimen for diabetic pregnancy. This treatment algorithm has proven to achieve normal glycemia in pregestational diabetic women. The insulin doses are divided into frequent injections to provide the basal and the meal-related insulin needs. The smooth increase in the total daily insulin requirement throughout pregnancy is calculated based on gestational week and maternal pregnant weight. The insulin requirement at 0 to 12 weeks is 0.7 U/kg/d (with careful monitoring of the blood glucose levels to prevent hypoglycemia from occurring if there is a decline in dosage during weeks 9 to 12). During weeks 13 to 28 of gestation, the dosage is 0.8 U/kg/d; during weeks 29 to 34 the insulin requirement is 0.9 U/kg/d. At term, the insulin requirement is 1.0 U/kg/d [18]. BS—blood sugar. (*Adapted from* Jovanovic and Peterson [22].)

IMPORTANT TESTS FOR MONITORING CONCOMITANT DISEASES AND GLUCOSE DURING PREGNANCIES COMPLICATED BY TYPE I DIABETES

Test	Frequency
Eye examination	Prior to conception and then once each trimester
Fundus photography and/or dilated examination by an ophthalmologist	Prior to conception and once each trimester
Kidney function	Prior to conception and once each trimester
Creatinine clearance with total microalbumin	Prior to conception and once a month
Thyroid function	Premeals and 1-h postmeals
Free T_4 and TS-11	Target: capillary whole blood glucose:
HbA_{1c}	Premeal <90 mg/dL
Self–blood glucose monitoring	Postmeal <120 mg/dL
Blood pressure and weight	Prior to conception and at each visit

FIGURE 16-18. Recommended testing protocol for women with pregestational diabetes. Ideally, a diabetic woman would plan her pregnancy so that there is time to create an individualized algorithm of care. When a diabetic woman presents in her first few weeks of pregnancy, there is no time for individualization, and rather rigid protocols must be instituted urgently to provide optimal control within 24 to 48 hours, and maintain control thereafter [20,28]. The table lists the important tests for monitoring concomitant diseases and the maternal vascular status during pregnancy [23]. HbA_{1c}—hemoglobin A_{1c}; T_4—thyroxine.

A. WHITE CLASSIFICATION OF PREGESTATIONAL DIABETES

Group	Age at Onset, y	Duration of Disease, y	Vascular Complication
B	>20	<10	None
C	<10 and/or 10–19		None
D	<10 and/or >20		Retinopathy-background type
F	All ages	Any duration	Nephropathy
R	All ages	Any duration	Retinopathy-proliferative
H	All ages	Any duration	Cardiac disease
T	All ages	Any duration	After organ transplantation

FIGURE 16-19. Two classifications of pregestational diabetes. Classifications of pregestational diabetes have been formulated to help the physician predict the outcome of pregnancy for both the mother and child [43,44]. **A,** The White [43] classification categorized diabetic women based on the mode of therapy, duration, age at onset of diabetes, and the degree of vascular compromise of each patient at the beginning of the pregnancy. White class A referred to gestational diabetes, but many of these women probably had undiagnosed type 2 diabetes. The White classification also led to confusion, because the "B" determination was given to both the pregnancy-related diabetes (gestational diabetes), which necessitated insulin, and to the pregestational woman with fewer than 10 years of insulin therapy. Treatment for all groups consisted of diet and insulin.
B, Revised classification. As evidence mounts that maternal normoglycemia is beneficial at the time of conception, during fetal organogenesis, and throughout gestation, a newer classification that places more emphasis on maternal plasma glucose concentrations is an acceptable alternative to the White version. This classification is based on vascular status and type of complication, with an emphasis on glycemic control [23]. ASCVD—atherosclerotic cardiovascular disease.

B. CLASSIFICATION OF RISK ASSOCIATED WITH PREGESTATIONAL DIABETES (TYPES 1 AND 2) DURING PREGNANCY BASED ON GLYCEMIC CONTROL, VASCULAR DISEASE, AND TYPE OF DISEASE

Condition			Risk Classification
Optimal glucose control*	No vascular disease		Low
	Vascular disease	Retinopathy	Minimal
		Neuropathy	Minimal
		Nephropathy	Moderate
		ASCVD	
Less than optimal glucose control†	No vascular disease		High
	Vascular disease	Retinopathy	High
		Neuropathy	High
		Nephropathy	High
		ASCVD	High

*Optimal glucose control is defined as fasting blood glucose (BG) concentrations of 55–65 mg/dL, average BG level of 84 mg/dL, and 1-h postprandial BG value of <120 mg/dL [5].
†Less than optimal glucose control status is diagnosed when optimal control fails to occur.

Gestational Diabetes Mellitus

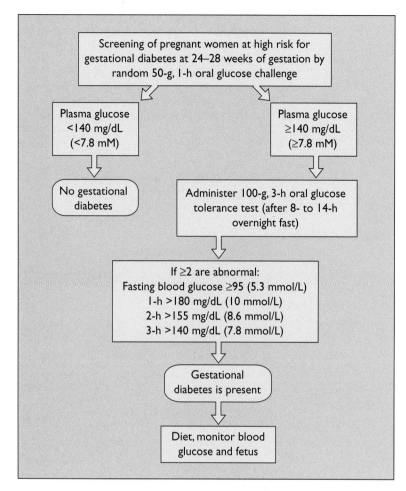

Screening of pregnant women at high risk for gestational diabetes at 24–28 weeks of gestation by random 50-g, 1-h oral glucose challenge

Plasma glucose <140 mg/dL (<7.8 mM)

Plasma glucose ≥140 mg/dL (≥7.8 mM)

No gestational diabetes

Administer 100-g, 3-h oral glucose tolerance test (after 8- to 14-h overnight fast)

If ≥2 are abnormal:
Fasting blood glucose ≥95 (5.3 mmol/L)
1-h >180 mg/dL (10 mmol/L)
2-h >155 mg/dL (8.6 mmol/L)
3-h >140 mg/dL (7.8 mmol/L)

Gestational diabetes is present

Diet, monitor blood glucose and fetus

FIGURE 16-20. Treatment protocol for the screening and diagnosis of gestational diabetes. Gestational diabetes mellitus (GDM) is defined as glucose tolerance of variable severity with onset or first recognition during pregnancy. The prevalence of gestational diabetes is dependent on ethnic background and degree of adiposity, and thus varies from 0.1% to 12% [16]. Most medical centers today use the two-stage diagnostic procedure suggested at the Third International Workshop-Conference on Gestational Diabetes held in Chicago in 1991, namely, glucose challenge screen with confirmation, if necessary, by oral glucose tolerance test. The current position paper, presented in 1997 at the Fourth International Workshop-Conference on Gestational Diabetes Mellitus in Chicago, summarizes the most recent recommendations [29]. The glucose challenge test (GCT) is performed in weeks 24 to 28 of gestation for patients at moderate risk, and in early pregnancy for patients at high risk, regardless of the time of the last meal. The test involves the oral intake of 50 g of glucose within 2 minutes and measurement of plasma glucose level after 1 hour. Patients with a glucose level of more than 140 mg/dL on the GCT (14% to 18% of all pregnant women) must then undergo the oral glucose tolerance test (OGTT) for confirmation of GDM. This subgroup accounts for about 80% of all women with GDM. Some medical centers use a cutoff of 130 mg/dL on the GCT, which identifies over 90% of all affected patients, but it increases the subgroup that requires an OGTT to 20% to 25% of all pregnant women. The OGTT identifies patients with diabetes by glucose loading. Prior to testing, patients ingest a 3-day diet of more than 150 g carbohydrate with regular physical activity followed by a fast of at least 8 hours (but not more than 14 hours). The test is performed in the morning of the fourth day. For diagnosis, the values of two of the four criteria listed in this figure must surpass the predetermined cutoff value, as indicated. According to the most recent recommendations [29], clinicians can use a 75 g or 100 g glucose load and cutoff values equal to both tests. It is important to emphasize that capillary fingerstick glucose values are not accepted for diagnosis. The diagnosis of GDM must be based solely on plasma glucose levels on an OGTT.

DIAGNOSIS OF GESTATIONAL DIABETES MELLITUS BY RISK ASSESSMENT

A. Low risk of developing GDM*
   GCT is not necessary if all of the following criteria are met:
      Absence of diabetes in first-degree relatives
      Age <25 y
      Normal prepregnancy weight
      No history of poor carbohydrate metabolism
      No history of adverse pregnancy outcome

B. Average risk of developing GDM
   GCT should be performed in weeks 24 to 28 of pregnancy. One of the following options may be chosen:
      Two-stage testing
         Stage 1: GCT; if results on GCT are abnormal, go to stage 2
         Stage 2: OGTT; diagnosis is based on values listed in Figure 16-5
      One-stage testing
         OGTT for all suspected cases; diagnosis is based on values listed in Figure 16-20

C. High risk of developing GDM
   Pregnant women who are obese or who have a family history of diabetes mellitus type 2, GDM in a past pregnancy, or known carbohydrate intolerance or high urine glucose level should undergo the GCT and/or OGTT according to the accepted criteria for diagnosis of GDM. Testing should be done as soon as feasible during pregnancy and immediately after the first visit (early first trimester). If GDM is not detected at this stage, the GCT and/or OGTT should be repeated in weeks 24 to 28 or at the first suspicious signs of diabetes.

*Because few women will meet all the criteria for low risk, we recommend that all patients be classified in groups B and C.

FIGURE 16-21. Risk assessment guide for women who need to be screened for gestational diabetes. The risk of gestational diabetes mellitus (GDM) is stratified into low, average, and high [29]. Risk assessment should be undertaken at the first prenatal visit. Women with clinical characteristics consistent with a high risk (obesity, personal history of GDM, glycosuria, or strong family history of diabetes) must be tested as soon as feasible. Women at average risk should be tested in weeks 24 to 28 of gestation, and women at low risk need not be tested at all. However, there are many who favor universal screening for all pregnant women because there is no way to guarantee that a woman with "no risk" does not have GDM [44]. An 8- to 14-h fasting glucose level over 126 mg/dL and/or a casual plasma glucose level over 200 mg/dL are diagnostic of diabetes; thus, no further tests are needed. Evaluation should be done as early during pregnancy as possible. New guidelines may be expected on completion of the 4-year multinational Hyperglycemia and Adverse Pregnancy Outcome (HAPO) study, being conducted under the aegis of the National Institutes of Health in 16 leading medical centers, including two in Israel. The study seeks to set criteria for the 75-g glucose load, which is already accepted in several European countries, to standardize the diagnosis of GDM with the diagnosis of diabetes in the nonpregnant state. GCT—glucose tolerance test; OGTT—oral glucose tolerance test.

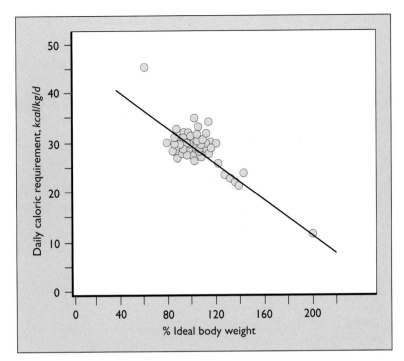

FIGURE 16-22. The caloric needs for a pregnant woman based on her ideal body weight. The main goal of treatment of gestational diabetes mellitus (GDM) is to prevent adverse effects to mother and infant. Normalization of glucose levels is a proven factor to achieve this goal. In addition, postprandial glucose levels are more closely associated with macrosomia than fasting levels. Women with GDM must follow an individually tailored diet prepared by a dietitian who also takes into account the amount, time, and type of insulin injection (if necessary). The diet must satisfy the minimum daily nutritional requirements for all pregnant women. The caloric intake must be compatible with the state of pregnancy and ensure the proper weight gain according to the patient's ideal weight before and during pregnancy. In this figure, the caloric needs of pregnancy are related to maternal body weight. The closed circles show that for a woman who is normal body weight (between 80% and 120% ideal body weight), the caloric requirement is 30 kilocalories per kilogram (present pregnant weight) per day. For overweight women, fewer calories are needed. Most overweight women are 130% above ideal body weight and they require 24 kilocalories per kilogram. Morbidly obese women (greater than 150% above ideal body weight) may require as few as 12 kilocalories per kilogram (present pregnant weight) [46]. (Adapted from Jovanovic [45].)

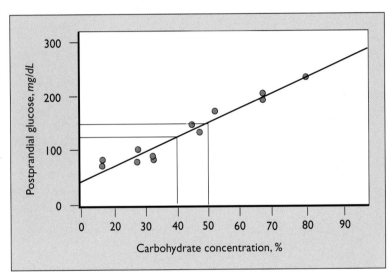

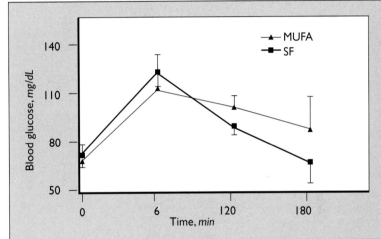

FIGURE 16-23. The relationship between carbohydrate concentration, the meal plan, and the peak postprandial response. The calories are divided into frequent small feedings with the caveat that breakfast needs to be the smallest meal of the day, with less than 33% carbohydrate. This degree of carbohydrate restriction is necessary because the hypercortisolemia seen normally in early waking hours is potentiated in pregnancy. Once the cortisol levels wane, then the other meals can be composed of 40% carbohydrate. This figure shows clearly that when the carbohydrate concentration in lunch and dinner is greater than 40%, then the peak postprandial glucose level is greater than 120 mg/dL, or that level reported to be associated with a rapidly increasing risk of neonatal macrosomia [24]. (Adapted from Peterson and Jovanovic [47].)

FIGURE 16-24. The postprandial glucose concentrations after a saturated fat (SF) meal compared with those concentrations after a monounsaturated fat (MUFA) meal. This figure demonstrates that the addition of SF or MUFA to the meal plan has different effects on the postprandial glucose concentrations. Despite the near-equal peak of the postprandial response at the 1-hour time point with SF compared with MUFA, by the 2- and 3-hour time points, the blood glucose levels are significantly lower with an SF meal. If macrosomia is caused by the total postprandial glucose load, then SF meal plans may actually be a means to minimize the need for insulin therapy in patients with gestational diabetes mellitus. (Adapted from Ilic et al. [48].)

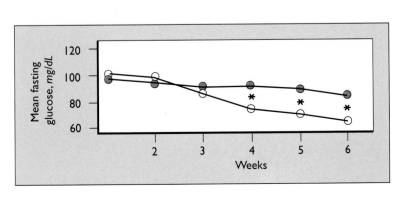

FIGURE 16-25. Weekly fasting glucose concentrations during a cardiovascular training program compared with no exercise program in women with gestational diabetes. An arm exercise has been shown to be a safe and effective mode of therapy for treating these women. Our group documented that women with gestational diabetes can train using arm ergometry, and that a program of this kind of cardiovascular conditioning exercise results in lower levels of glycemia than a program of diet alone. The effects of exercise on fasting glucose concentrations became apparent after 4 weeks of training, as shown in the solid circles. (Adapted from Jovanovic et al. [49].)

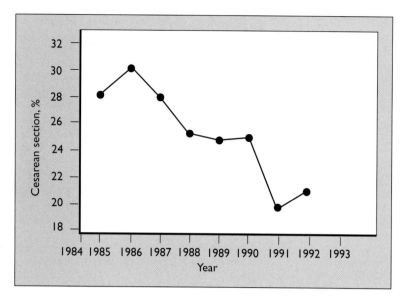

FIGURE 16-26. The fall in cesarean section rate in Santa Barbara County concomitant with the introduction of a program of universal screening and treatment of hyperglycemia in pregnancy. When the glucose level cannot be maintained within recommended limits (90 mg/dL before meals and no higher than 120 mg/dL at 1 hour after meals) by diet and exercise, then insulin treatment is needed. Rapid-acting insulin analogues can improve glycemic levels, and their use is increasing in most leading centers in the United States and Europe. Our experience in Santa Barbara County Health Care Service [44] with a program of universal screening and treatment of postprandial glucose by targeting the blood glucose level to be less than 120 mg/dL (with diet, exercise, and initiation of insulin when blood glucose levels are elevated) has shown that the birthweight is normalized. This degree of intensive care for all gestational diabetic women results in over $2000 saved per pregnancy by avoiding cesarean sections necessitated to deliver macrosomic infants and neonatal intensive care admissions of sick infants. (*Adapted from* Jovanovic and Bevier [44].)

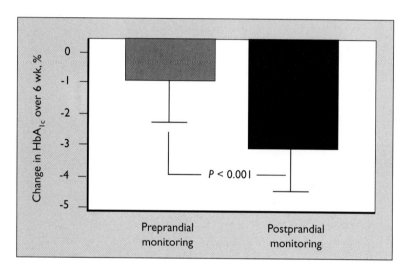

FIGURE 16-27. The glycosylated hemoglobin levels after 6 weeks of monitoring only preprandial glucose concentrations in gestational diabetic women needing insulin therapy compared with the glycosylated hemoglobin levels achieved in a matched population of women who were also monitoring postprandial glucose concentrations. de Veciana *et al.* [26] have also shown that when the insulin-requiring gestational diabetic women measure their preprandial glucose levels alone, the prevalence of macrosomia is 42%. When the postprandial glucose levels are measured and the treatment designed to maintain the levels less than 120 mg/dL, the prevalence of macrosomia was decreased to 12%. With only 6 weeks of treatment designed to blunt the postprandial glucose levels, the glycosylated hemoglobin was significantly lower than in the group of gestational diabetes patients who were only monitoring glucose preprandially.

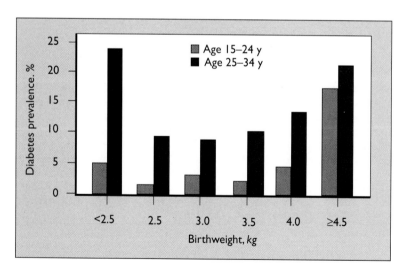

FIGURE 16-28. Relation of birthweight to the risk of subsequent diabetes. Women who have had gestational diabetes mellitus previously should be advised to undergo repeated oral glucose tolerance tests once yearly and maintain a healthy lifestyle with regular exercise and normal body weight for their habitus. They should seek consultation before their next pregnancy [29]. The follow-up of the offspring of diabetic mothers should include careful measurement of growth and development and concern for glucose intolerance during childhood. Children of diabetic mothers are at higher risk of obesity and glucose intolerance. Evidence is accumulating that good metabolic control in the mother during pregnancy can decrease this risk. There appears to be a U-shaped curve that relates birthweight to the risk of subsequent diabetes. Both at the low and high birthweights, it appears that the infants have a lack of pancreatic reserve of insulin and thus as they grow and develop, they cannot increase their insulin secretion sufficiently to maintain glucose homeostasis. (*Adapted from* McCance *et al.* [50].)

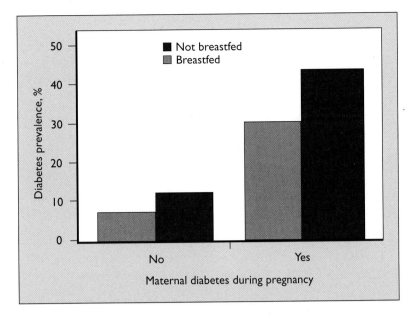

FIGURE 16-29. Predictors of subsequent diabetes in the offspring in Pima Indians. Pettitt and Knowler [12] reported that there is a long-term consequence of the intrauterine environment. When they adjusted for age, sex, birth-weight, presence of diabetes in either parent, and whether or not the child was breast-fed for at least 2 months after birth, the strongest predictors of subsequent diabetes in the child was the presence of maternal diabetes and not being breast-fed. The *dark bars* represent the children who were not breast-fed; the *light bars* represent the children who were breast-fed. Thus it is clear that the intrauterine environment must be normalized and sufficient nutrition must be provided (but not overnutrition). Maintaining the nutritional status of the child after birth is paramount in decreasing the rapidly rising rate of diabetes in the future. (*Adapted from* Pettitt and Knowler [12].)

References

1. American Diabetes Association, Clinical Practice Recommendations 2001: Gestational Diabetes. *Diabetes Care* 2001, 24(Suppl 1):S77–S79.

2. Hod M, Diamant YZ: Diabetes in pregnancy. Norbert Freinkel Memorial Issue. *Isr J Med Sci* 1991, 27:421–532.

3. Mills JL, Simpson JL, Driscoll SG, et al.: Incidence of spontaneous abortion among normal women and insulin dependent diabetic women whose pregnancies were identified within 21 days of conception. *N Engl J Med* 1988, 319:1617.

4. Mills JL, Knopp RH, Simpson JL, et al.: Lack of relation of increased malformation roles in infants of diabetic mothers to glycemic control during organogenesis. *N Engl J Med* 1988, 318:671.

5. Fuhrmann K, Ruher H, Semmler K, et al.: Prevention of congenital malformations in infants of insulin-dependent diabetic mothers. *Diabetes Care* 1983, 6:21–23.

6. Miller E, Hare JW, Clogerty JP, et al.: Elevated maternal hemoglobin A$_{1c}$ in early pregnancy and major congenital anomalies in infants of diabetic mothers. *N Engl J Med* 1981, 304:1331–1335.

7. Cousins L: Etiology and prevention of congenital anomalies among infants of overt diabetic women. *Clin Obstet Gynecol* 1991, 34:484–485.

8. Petersen M, Pedersen SA, Greisen G, et al.: Early growth delay in diabetic pregnancy: relation to psychomotor development at age 4. *Br Med J* 1988, 296:598–601.

9. van Dijk DJ, Axer-Siegel R, Erman A, Hod M: Diabetic vascular complications and pregnancy. *Diabetes Rev* 1995, 3:632–642.

10. Catalano PM, Drago NM, Amini S: Maternal carbohydrate metabolism and its relationship to fetal growth and body composition. *Am J Obstet Gynecol* 1995, 172:1464–1470.

11. Hod M, Diamant YZ: The offspring of a diabetic mother—short- and long-range implications. *Isr J Med Sci* 1992, 28:81–86.

12. Pettitt DJ, Knowler WC: Long-term effects of the intrauterine environment, birth weight, and breast-feeding in Pima Indians. *Diabetes Care* 1998, 21:B138–B141.

13. Pedersen J: Fetal mortality in diabetes in relation to management during the latter part of pregnancy. *Acta Endocrinol* 1954, 15:282–294.

14. Freinkel N: Banting Lecture 1980: Of pregnancy and progeny. *Diabetes* 1980, 29:1023–1035.

15. Jovanovic L, Peterson CM: Moment in history: turning point in blood glucose monitoring of diet and insulin dosing. *Trans Am Soc Artif Intern Organs* 1990, 36:799–804.

16. Buchanan TA, Unterman T, Metzger BE: The medical management of diabetes in pregnancy. *Clin Perinatol* 1985, 12:625–650.

17. Pedersen J, Pedersen LM: Diabetes mellitus and pregnancy: the hyperglycemia, hyperinsulinemia theory and the weight of the newborn baby. In: Rodriguez RR, Vallance-Owen J, eds. *Proceedings of the 7th Congress of the International Diabetes Federation.* Amsterdam: Excerpta Medica; 1971:678–690.

18. Jovanovic L, Druzin M, Peterson CM: The effect of euglycemia on the outcome of pregnancy in insulin-dependent diabetics as compared to normal controls. *Am J Med* 1981, 71:921–927.

19. Jovanovic L, Saxena BB, Dawood MY, et al.: Feasibility of maintaining euglycemia in insulin-dependent diabetic women. *Am J Med* 1980, 68:105–112.

20. Steel JM, Johnstone FD, Hepburn DA, Smith AF: Can prepregnancy care of diabetic women reduce the risk of abnormal babies? *BMJ* 1990, 301:1070–1073.

21. Jovanovic L, Peterson CM: Rationale for prevention and treatment of glucose-mediated macrosomia: A protocol for gestational diabetes. *Endocr Pract* 1996, 2:118–129.

22. Jovanovic L, Peterson CM: The art and science of maintenance of normoglycemia in pregnancies complicated by type 1 diabetes mellitus. *Endocr Pract* 1996, 2:130–142.

23. Jovanovic L: *Medical Management of Pregnancy Complicated by Diabetes.* Alexandria, VA: American Diabetes Association; 1993, revised 1995 and 2000.

24. Jovanovic L, Peterson CM, Reed GF, et al.: Maternal postprandial glucose levels and infant birth weight: the Diabetes in Early Pregnancy Study. The National Institute of Child Health and Human Development—Diabetes in Early Pregnancy Study. *Am J Obstet Gynecol* 1991, 164:103–111.

25. Combs CA, Gunderson E, Kitzmiller JL, et al.: Relationship of fetal macrosomia to maternal postprandial glucose control during pregnancy. *Diabetes Care* 1992, 15:1251–1257.

26. de Veciana M, Major CA, Morgan MA, et al.: Postprandial versus preprandial blood glucose monitoring in women with gestational diabetes mellitus requiring insulin therapy. *N Engl J Med* 1995, 333:1237–1241.

27. Mills JL, Baker L, Goldman A: Malformations in infants of diabetic mothers occur before the seventh gestational week: implications for treatment. *Diabetes* 1979, 23:292–295.

28. Kitzmiller JL, Gavin LA, Gin GD, et al.: Preconception care of diabetes: glycemic control prevents congenital anomalies. JAMA 1991, 265:731–726.

29. Metzger BE, Coustan DR: Proceedings of the Fourth International Workshop-Conference on Gestational Diabetes Mellitus. Diabetes Care 1998, 21(Suppl 2):B1–B167.

30. Ylinen K, Aula P, Stenman UH, et al.: Risk of minor and major fetal malformations in diabetics with high hemoglobin A_{1c} values in early pregnancy. Br Med J 1984, 289:345–349.

31. Hanson U, Persson B, Thunell S: Relationship between haemoglobin A_{1c} in early type 1 (insulin-dependent) diabetic pregnancy and the occurrence of spontaneous abortion and fetal malformation in Sweden. Diabetologia 1990, 33:100–104.

32. Greene MF, Hare JW, Cloherty JP, et al.: First-trimester hemoglobin A_1 and risk for major malformation and spontaneous abortion in diabetic pregnancy. Teratology 1989, 39:225–231.

33. Jovanovic L, Peterson CM: Management of the pregnant diabetic woman. Diabetes Care 1980, 3:63–68.

34. Parretti E, Mecacci F, Papini M, et al.: Third trimester maternal glucose levels from diurnal profiles in non-diabetic pregnancies: correlation with sonographic parameters of fetal growth. Diabetes Care 2001, 24:1319–1323.

35. Jovanovic L, Crues J, Durak E, Peterson CM: Magnetic resonance imaging in pregnancies complicated by gestational diabetes predicts infant birth weight ratio and neonatal morbidity. Am J Perinatol 1993, 10:432–437.

36. Holden KP, Jovanovic L, Druzin ML, Peterson CM: Increased fetal activity with low maternal blood glucose levels in pregnancies complicated by diabetes. Am J Perinat 1984, 1:161–164.

37. Jovanovic L, Knopp RH, Brown A, et al.: Declining insulin requirements in the late first trimester of diabetic pregnancy. Diabetes Care 2001, 24:1130–1136.

38. Menon RK, Cohen RM, Sperling MA, et al.: Transplacental passage of insulin in pregnant women with insulin-dependent diabetes mellitus. Its role in fetal macrosomia. N Engl J Med 1990, 323:309–315.

39. Jovanovic L, Kitzmiller JL, Peterson CM: Randomized trial of human versus animal species insulin in diabetic pregnant women: improved glycemic control, not fewer antibodies to insulin, influences birth weight. Am J Obstet Gynecol 1992, 167:1325–1330.

40. Jovanovic L, Mills JL, Peterson CM: Anti-insulin titers do not influence control or insulin requirements in early pregnancy. Diabetes Care 1984, 7:68–71.

41. Jovanovic L, Ilic S, Pettitt DJ, et al.: The metabolic and immunologic effects of insulin lispro in gestational diabetes. Diabetes Care 1999, 22:1422–1426.

42. Pedersen J: The pregnant diabetic and her newborn: problems and management. Baltimore: Williams & Wilkins; 1967:30–32.

43. White P: Pregnancy and diabetes. In Joslin's Diabetes Mellitus, edn II. Edited by Marble A, White P, Bradley RF, Krall LP. Philadelphia: Lea & Febiger; 1971:50.

44. Jovanovic L, Bevier W: The Santa Barbara County Health Care Services Program: birth weight change concomitant with screening for and treatment of glucose-intolerance of pregnancy: a potential cost-effective intervention. Am J Perinatol 1997, 14:221–228.

45. Jovanovic L: Time to reassess the optimal dietary prescription for women with gestational diabetes [editorial]. Am J Clin Nutr 1999, 70:3–4.

46. Jovanovic L: Nutritional management of the obese gestational diabetic woman [guest editorial]. J Am Coll Nutr 1992, 11:246–250.

47. Peterson CM, Jovanovic L: Percentage of carbohydrate and glycemia response to breakfast, lunch, and dinner in women with gestational diabetes. Diabetes 1991, 40(Suppl 2):172–174.

48. Ilic S, Jovanovic L, Pettitt DJ: Comparison of the effect of saturated and monounsaturated fat on postprandial plasma glucose and insulin concentration in women with gestational diabetes mellitus. Am J Perinatol 2000, 16:489–495.

49. Jovanovic L, Durak EP, Peterson CM: Randomized trial of diet versus diet plus cardiovascular conditioning on glucose levels in gestational diabetes. Am J Obstet Gynecol 1989, 161:415–419.

50. McCance DR, Pettitt DJ, Hanson RL, et al.: Birth weight and non-insulin dependent diabetes: thrifty genotype, thrifty phenotype, or surviving small baby genotype? Br Med J 1994, 308:942–945.

CHILDHOOD DIABETES

17

Francine Ratner Kaufman

Diabetes has a unique impact on children and their families. The daily life of children and youth is affected by the rigors of the diabetes regimen and the need to frequently monitor blood glucose levels, give glucose-lowering agents, and balance the effect of activity and food. Despite this, pediatric patients must still strive to reach the normal developmental milestones of childhood and adolescence, succeed in school, and develop eventual autonomy. To accomplish these tasks, an organized system of diabetes care utilizing a multidisciplinary team versed in pediatric issues must be in place to assure optimal physical and emotional health for the affected child as well as offer support and education for the family, caregivers, and school personnel. In this way, children with type 1 or type 2 diabetes can reach adulthood with as little adverse impact on their well-being as possible.

One of the major risks of type 1 diabetes for children is the development of diabetic ketoacidosis (DKA). Diabetic ketoacidosis remains a major source of morbidity and mortality in pediatric patients due to cerebral edema. The treatment of DKA in patients under 20 years of age involves meticulous rehydration with electrolyte-containing solutions, intravenous insulin administration via a low-dose continuous infusion, avoidance of bolus bicarbonate therapy, and extremely close monitoring of neurologic status. There is increasing evidence that risk factors for cerebral edema include severe dehydration as evidenced by a high initial blood urea nitrogen concentration and failure of the serum sodium level to rise with therapy. In addition to brain swelling, brain infarction can be a consequence of DKA and its treatment, and may lead to persistent neurologic deficit. Since it remains unclear how to avoid the neurologic sequelae of DKA-associated cerebral edema, it becomes imperative to avoid DKA altogether. This can be done by giving patients and families detailed sick day guidelines so that dehydration, acidosis, and severe hyperglycemia can be avoided during intercurrent illness or when diabetes management is appropriate.

Since the completion of the Diabetes Control and Complications Trial, the benefits of following a system of diabetes management that allows for optimal glycemia has become increasingly apparent for infants, children, and youth with type 1 diabetes. The benefit not only appears to be immediate but also long-term, and the management system should be instituted in the prepubertal child as well as in the postpubertal child. Systems of diabetes management that improve glycemic control must be well defined, with age-specific targets, and must be carefully taught to patients and families using algorithms that allow for flexibility of lifestyle. To assure that targets are being met, glucose levels can be assessed with modalities such as continuous glucose monitoring systems that allow for pattern identification. The diabetes regimen can then be altered to optimize glycemic outcome. However, these continuous glucose-monitoring systems, now limited to only intermittent 3-day use, cannot replace home glucose monitoring. The number of blood glucose measurements done at home remains the most modifiable predictor of glycemic control in youth with diabetes. Close multidisciplinary follow-up care with screening for diabetes complications and comorbidities is imperative. Findings such as limited joint mobility, which used to be the most common complication of diabetes in childhood, are decreasing in prevalence, most likely due to improved glycemic outcome. Finally, certain aspects of diabetes care must also be conveyed to school personnel and other caregivers if pediatric subjects are to benefit from an intensive management approach.

The psychologic stress of diabetes, with the fear of immediate and long-term complications, must be addressed by providers of pediatric diabetes care. The child or adolescent with diabetes, as well as other family members including parents and siblings, should be evaluated to assure that there is not a negative effect on family functioning. Quality of life must be an outcome measure. As such, there is evidence that improved diabetes control, with all of its demands, actually improves quality of life. The developmental capabilities of children must be taken into account. As technology advances and more skills and knowledge are required for diabetes management, a limiting factor might be the cognitive and developmental capabilities of some children and their families. Criteria should be established before technologically difficult management tools, such as insulin pumps, are given to a specific patient and family.

As found in the adult population, type 2 diabetes in children and youth is due to the combination of insulin resistance coupled with relative β-cell failure. While there appears to be a host of potential genetic and environmental risk factors for insulin resistance and limited β-cell reserve, perhaps the most significant risk factor is obesity. Obesity in youth has reached epidemic proportions and should be assessed using standard body mass index charts. Few studies have been done to determine the most effective treatment regimens for type 2 diabetes in youth and the role that physical activity and nutrition counseling play in improving glycemic outcome. Since fewer than 10% of youth with type 2 diabetes can be treated with diet and exercise alone, pharmacologic intervention is required for these patients to achieve glycemic targets. In most surveys, practitioners use metformin, insulin, another oral agent, or dual agent therapy. Treatment guidelines have been developed to enable target HbA_{1c} levels to be met and maintained.

While diabetes management remains demanding, children and families can succeed in reaching glycemic targets and in achieving physical and psychologic well-being. The multidisciplinary team, able to appropriately assess and follow the patient, can play a major role in preparing children and youth for as complication-free a future as is possible.

Diabetic Ketoacidosis in the Pediatric Population with Type 1 Diabetes

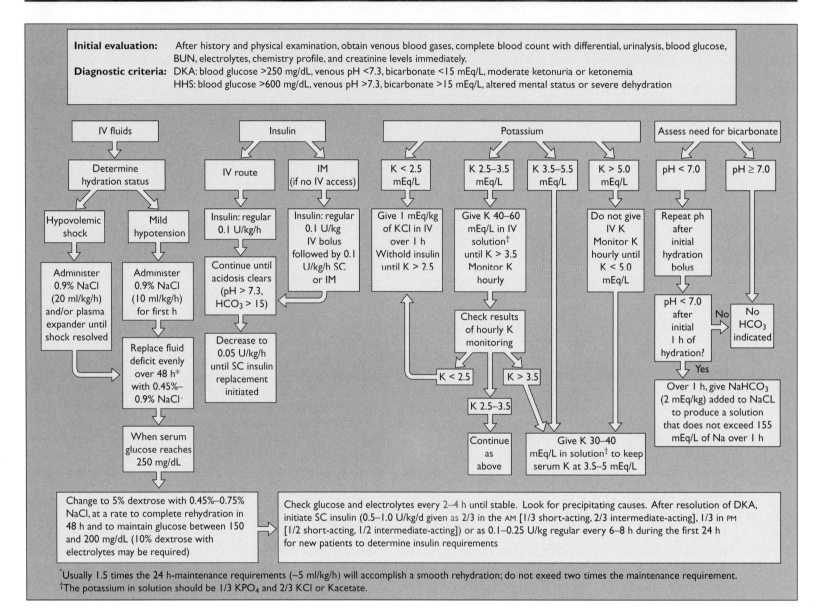

Initial evaluation: After history and physical examination, obtain venous blood gases, complete blood count with differential, urinalysis, blood glucose, BUN, electrolytes, chemistry profile, and creatinine levels immediately.

Diagnostic criteria: DKA: blood glucose >250 mg/dL, venous pH <7.3, bicarbonate <15 mEq/L, moderate ketonuria or ketonemia
HHS: blood glucose >600 mg/dL, venous pH >7.3, bicarbonate >15 mEq/L, altered mental status or severe dehydration

*Usually 1.5 times the 24 h-maintenance requirements (~5 ml/kg/h) will accomplish a smooth rehydration; do not exeed two times the maintenance requirement.
†The potassium in solution should be 1/3 KPO₄ and 2/3 KCl or Kacetate.

FIGURE 17-1. Management of pediatric patients (younger than 20 years) with diabetic ketoacidosis (DKA). The protocol for the management of these patients begins with intravenous (IV) fluid therapy to restore circulation; the rate of fluid administration is dependent on the presence or absence of hypovolemic shock. After fluid resuscitation, IV fluid administration is given at a rate that will complete rehydration in 48 hours. The sodium concentration of the fluid replacement solution is between 0.45% and 0.75%. Insulin infusion is begun after fluid resuscitation at a rate of 0.1 U/kg/h. Insulin can be administered intramus- cularly (IM) if IV access cannot be secured. Potassium is added to the replace- ment fluids at a variable infusion rate depending on the serum potassium level. Bicarbonate is given only for severe acidosis, pH < 7.0, and is administered over 1 hour, not as IV bolus therapy. Glucose is added to the IV solution as the serum glucose level drops. The key to successful management is close monitoring of glucose and electrolytes, and appropriate level of care to detect and treat early neurologic compromise. BUN—blood urea nitrogen; HHS—hyperglycemic hyperosmolar state; SC—subcutaneous. (*Adapted from* [1].)

MULTIVARIATE ANALYSIS OF RISK FACTORS FOR CEREBRAL EDEMA*

Variable†	Relative Risk (95% CI)	P Value
Male sex	0.6 (0.3–1.4)	0.27
Age (per 1-y increase)	0.9 (0.6–1.3)	0.53
Initial serum sodium concentration (per increase of 5.8 mmol/L)	0.7 (0.5–1.02)	0.06
Initial serum glucose concentration (per increase of 244 mg/dL)	1.4 (0.5–3.9)	0.58
Initial serum urea nitrogen concentration (per increase of 9 mg/dL)	1.8 (1.2–2.7)	0.008
Initial serum bicarbonate concentration (per increase of 3.6 mmol/L)	1.2 (0.5–2.6)	0.73
Initial partial pressure of arterial carbon dioxide (per decrease of 7.8 mm Hg)	2.7 (1.4–5.1)	0.002
Rate of increase in serum sodium concentration during therapy (per increase of 5.8 mmol/dL/h)	0.6 (0.4–0.9)	0.01
Rate of decrease in serum glucose concentration during therapy (per decrease of 190 mg/dL/h)	0.8 (0.5–1.4)	0.41
Rate of increase in serum bicarbonate concentration during therapy (per increase of 3 mmol/L/h)	0.8 (0.5–1.1)	0.15
Administration of insulin bolus	0.8 (0.3–2.2)	0.62
Treatment with bicarbonate	4.2 (1.5–12.1)	0.008
Rate of infusion of intravenous fluid (per increase of 5 mL/kg of body weight/h)	1.1 (0.4–3.0)	0.91
Rate of infusion of sodium (per increase of 0.6 mmol/kg/h)	1.2 (0.6–2.7)	0.59
Rate of infusion of insulin (per increase of 0.04 unit/kg/h)	1.2 (0.8–1.8)	0.30

*The cerebral edema group was compared with the matched control group by means of conditional logistic regression.
†The increase or decrease used in the analysis of each continuous variable (except age) represents a change of 1 SD in the variable in the randomly selected control children with diabetic ketoacidosis.

FIGURE 17-2. Multivariate analysis of risk factors for cerebral edema. In a multicenter study, 61 children who developed symptomatic cerebral edema associated with diabetic ketoacidosis (DKA) were compared to 181 randomly selected children with DKA and 174 children with DKA matched according to age, new-onset versus known case, initial pH, and initial serum glucose concentration [2]. Multivariate statistical methods showed that children with DKA-related cerebral edema had lower initial Pco$_2$ values and higher serum urea nitrogen concentrations than the control groups. A lesser rise in serum sodium concentration during treatment was seen in those with cerebral edema, although it is unclear whether this was due to therapy itself or a physiologic response to cerebral injury. The administration of bicarbonate bolus was also associated with the development of cerebral edema, suggesting that bicarbonate therapy, for the most part, is contraindicated in children with DKA. (*Adapted from* Glaser *et al.* [2].)

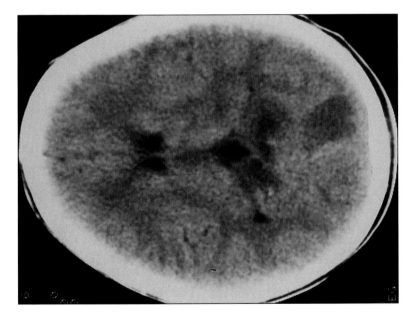

FIGURE 17-3. Magnetic resonance imaging scan of cerebral edema in a 5-year-old boy hospitalized with progressive polyuria and polydipsia. He was found to have a serum glucose level of 1288 mg/dL, sodium 136 mEq/L, potassium 4.0 mEq/L, total CO$_2$ 14 mEq/L, chloride 95 mEq/L, and large ketones. He was started on insulin and fluid therapy and improved over the first 17 hours, at which time he had a generalized convulsion and developed dilated pupils. A CT scan done 6 hours after the neurologic crisis showed infarction in the distribution of the left posterior cerebral artery, including the occipital pole and the undersurface of the temporal lobe. The geniculate nuclei and the posterior part of the left thalamus were also infarcted. At the time of this scan, there was no evidence of cerebral edema. After 2 months, the patient was discharged with a moderate left hemiplegia and was able to do age-appropriate schoolwork. While it is likely that brain edema may have been present initially and before the time of the CT scan, patients with persistent neurologic deficit may also suffer brain infarction during diabetic ketoacidosis-related cerebral edema. The pathophysiology of infarction remains unclear but may be due to a combination of factors including compression of vessels, systemic hypotension and intracranial hypertension, and thrombosis from dehydration, hemoconcentration, and hyperviscosity [3].

Warning signs

Call the health team if:

Vomiting (more than 2 times or longer than 4 h)

Elevated BG level (2 or more readings outside of the target range or >250 mg/dL)

Presence of blood or large urinary ketones

Weakness, dry mouth, or signs of dehydration, excessive thirst

Heavy breathing, shortness of breath

Abdominal pain, diarrhea

Evidence of bacterial infection

Altered level of consciousness or change in mental status

Never stop insulin

Phone numbers: Pediatrician _____

                Diabetes team _____

                Emergency #_____

Log sheet

	1st h	2nd h	3rd h	4th h	5th h	6th h	7th h
Blood sugar							
Ketone level							
Temperature							
Fluid input							
Output urine							
Insulin dose							

Principles for high blood sugar

Give extra rapid-acting (or short-acting) insulin every 2 hours

Add extra insulin for each 50 mg/dL above target (200 mg/dL)

For children <5 years, 0.25 U for each 50 mg/dL

For children ages 5–11 years, 0.5–1.0 U for each 50 mg/dL

For children ages 12–18 years, 1–2 U for each 50 mg/dL

Nonglucose–containing fluids should be given until the blood glucose level reaches 250 mg/dL

Fluids containing sodium and potassium should be used if there is excessive fluid loss

Replacement of fluids is more important than food

Principles for low blood sugar

Glucose-containing fluids should be given in small quantities

Insulin should be decreased by 20%–50%

If persistent hypoglycemia occurs and patients are not able to retain glucose-containing solutions, consider a minidose of glucagon (for children ≤2 years, 20 μg or 2 "units" on the insulin syringe; for children >2 years, 150 μg or 15 "units")

FIGURE 17-4. Sick day management guidelines for the prevention of diabetic ketoacidosis. Early signs of diabetic ketoacidosis (DKA) need to be treated aggressively and the results of treatment carefully monitored to avoid the development of moderate to severe dehydration, hyperglycemia, and acidosis. Precursors to DKA in children and youth with established diabetes include intercurrent illness, infection, incorrect insulin dosage for the glycemic level, inappropriate insulin administration, omission of insulin, psychologic trauma, or surgery [4]. Patients, parents, baby sitters, school personnel, and day care workers need to understand the early signs of DKA and how to access the health care team so that DKA can be reversed. A sick day management guideline can be useful in promoting the early institution of monitoring and treatment to avoid the need for hospitalization and emergency room visits [5,6]. BG—blood glucose.

Importance of Intensive Management

DIABETES CONTROL AND COMPLICATIONS TRIAL RESULTS

	Adults		Adolescents	
	Intensive	**Conventional**	**Intensive**	**Conventional**
Glycemia				
Mean BG mg/dL	155±30	231±55	171±31	260±52
HbA$_{1c}$	7.12±0.03	9.02±0.05	8.06±0.03	9.76±0.12
Risk reduction				
Retinopathy	63%		61%	
Microalbuminuria	54%		35%	
Hypoglycemia				
Episodes/100 patient-years	61.2	18.7	85.7	29.6
Relative risk	3.3		2.8	

FIGURE 17-5. Diabetes Control and Complications Trial (DCCT) results of comparison of adults versus adolescents. The DCCT enrolled adolescent patients; 14% were between the ages of 13 and 17 years at the time of entry into the study [7–9]. Patients under 13 years of age were not enrolled in the study. Compared with adult subjects, the adolescents had higher blood glucose (BG) and HbA$_{1c}$ levels in both the intensive and the conventional groups. Nevertheless, there was still a difference in the mean BG and HbA$_{1c}$ level between the two groups of adolescents. For adolescents, there was a 1.7% + 0.2% decrease in HbA$_{1c}$ in the intensive group compared with the conventional group. The reduction in the development of complications seen in adolescents because of achieving improved glycemia was similar to the reduction appreciated in adults. This reduction was coupled with a greater absolute rate of severe hypoglycemia in adolescents compared with adults. In the follow-up of the DCCT, the Epidemiology of Diabetes Interventions and Complications (EDIC) study [10], 175 of the 195 adolescent subjects were reevaluated with fundus photography and measurement of albumin excretion rate. During 4 years of assessment with the EDIC study, the mean HbA$_{1c}$ levels between the former intensive and the former conventional groups were similar (8.38% vs 8.45%). The prevalence of retinopathy remained reduced in the former intensive therapy group compared to the conventional group (by 74%, P < 0.00, for 3 steps or more worsening of retinopathy and by 78%, P < 0.007, for progression to proliferative or severe nonproliferative retinopathy). The EDIC findings indicate that the benefit of optimal glycemic control for adolescents with type 1 diabetes is not only immediate but also enduring.

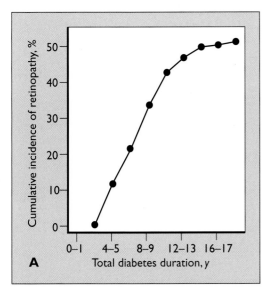 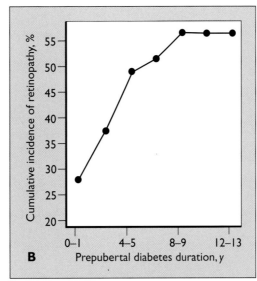

A Total diabetes duration, y
B Prepubertal diabetes duration, y

FIGURE 17-6. Effect of prepubertal diabetes duration on diabetes complications. Controversy exists as to the effect of the duration of diabetes prior to puberty versus the effect of diabetes duration in the postpubertal period. While it is clear that the hormonal changes of puberty, particularly augmentation of the growth hormone-IGF (insulin-like growth factor) axis, may have a permissive role in the damaging effect of diabetes on the microvasculature, the contribution of prepubertal diabetes duration is minimal. To determine the effect of prepubertal diabetes duration on complication rates with regard to retinopathy and albumin excretion rate (AER), 38 prepubertal and 140 pubertal subjects of the same age (10–14 years) and the same diabetes duration (3–12 years) were compared [11]. There were no significant differences between the prepubertal and pubertal groups for retinopathy (27% vs 29%, P = 0.8) and no differences in elevated AER (17% vs 31%, P = 0.1). As shown, longer prepubertal diabetes duration improved the prediction for retinopathy over postpubertal duration alone (P < 0.0005). Since prepubertal diabetes duration significantly is related to the presence of retinopathy in adolescents, it is imperative that patients, parents, and health care providers strive to optimize glycemic control regardless of pubertal status.

GLYCEMIC AND HBA₁c TARGETS FOR PEDIATRIC PATIENTS WITH TYPE I DIABETES

	Age of Patient			
Blood glucose	0–2 y	3–6 y	7–12 y	13 y
Premeal mg/dL	100–180	70–150	70–150	70–150
2–3 h postprandial mg/dL	< 200	< 200	< 180	< 180
Before bed mg/dL	100–200	100–180	90–160	80–150
2–4 AM mg/dL	> 100	> 100	> 90	> 80
HbA₁c, %	< 9.0	< 8.5	< 8.0	< 7.5

FIGURE 17-7. Glycemic and HbA₁c targets for pediatric type I subjects by age. The management goal for infants, children, and adolescents with type I diabetes is to have blood glucose and HbA₁c levels fall within an age-specific target range that takes into account the developmental, cognitive, and communicative abilities and resources of the patient and family [12]. Since it appears that young children are more susceptible to severe hypoglycemia, the target ranges for blood glucose and HbA₁c levels are generally higher. However, as children age, the primary concern shifts from avoidance of excessive hypoglycemia to avoidance of hyperglycemia as a means to decrease long-term diabetes complications.

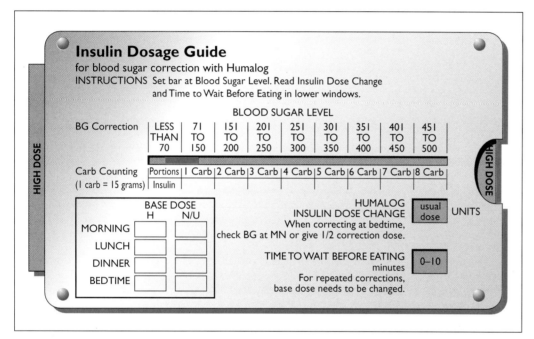

FIGURE 17-8. Insulin dosage guide for correction of blood glucose levels out of the target range. By treating blood glucose (BG) levels that are outside of a predetermined age-specific target range with supplemental oral glucose or extra insulin, children and adolescents can minimize episodes of both hypoglycemia and hyper-glycemia. However, it is challenging to teach insulin dosage adjustment algorithms designed to normalize elevated blood glucose levels and to compensate for alterations in carbohydrate intake. Even with instruction, many families feel uneasy adjusting insulin dosages on their own because of the complexities of these adjustment algorithms, and they often persist in believing that they must have contact with a health care provider to ensure accuracy. A hand-held plastic Insulin Dosage Guide for both rapid- or short-acting insulin in a variety of regimens, including insulin pump therapy, was designed to enable patients to correct abnormal blood glucose levels in a standard consistent fashion and to determine how much insulin to take if they are practicing carbohydrate counting [13]. In 83 patients with issues concerning glycemic control, mean age 11.4 ± 4.3 years and with a mean diabetes duration of 4.4 ± 3.1 years, there was a reduction in HbA₁c levels from 9.5% ± 2.0% at entry to 8.4% + 1.5% at 3 months (P = 0.0002). Improvement was sustained for 12 months (P = 0.0001) while using the Insulin Dosage Guide. Inexpensive, portable, and easy-to-use algorithms for insulin dosage adjustment may improve glycemic control in children and youth and allow for flexibility in lifestyle. H—rapid-acting Humalog or Aspart; MN—midnight; N/U—NPH or Ultralente.

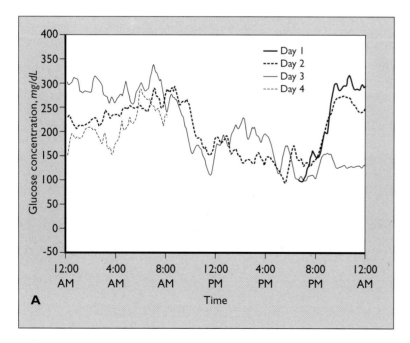

FIGURE 17-9. Continuous glucose monitoring of children with type I diabetes. Continuous subcutaneous glucose monitoring with the MiniMed system (CGMS) (Medtronic MiniMed, Northridge, CA) can be used in pediatric subjects to detect unrecognized nocturnal hypoglycemia and other patterns of abnormal glucose control so that alterations of the diabetes regimen can be made to regulate HbA₁c [14]. **A**, CGMS tracing from a 4-year-old child with a high post-breakfast pattern [15].

(Continued on next page)

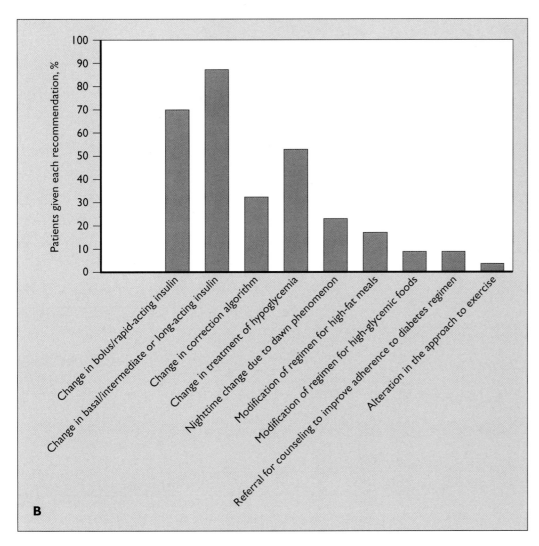

B

FIGURE 17-9. (Continued) B, A recent study involving 47 pediatric patients using CGMS with diabetes management problems showed a variety of abnormal glucose patterns [16]. After these patterns were detected, a mean of 3.3 specific alterations of the diabetes regimen were made. This resulted in an overall significant change in HbA_{1c} from 3 months before using CGMS to 6 months after CGMS was begun (analysis of variance 0,04). Post hoc analysis showed a significant change in HbA_{1c} from 8.6% ± 1.5% at baseline to 8.4% ± 1.3% at 3 months (paired Student's t-test, 0.03). Using continuous glucose monitoring systems will likely help improve glycemic control in pediatric subjects by allowing for pattern detection and alteration of the diabetes regimen. (Panel A adapted from Kaufman et al. [14]; panel B adapted from Kaufman et al. [15].)

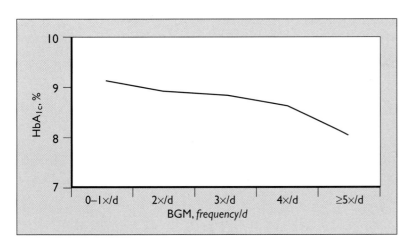

FIGURE 17-10. Predictors of glycemic control and short-term adverse outcomes in youth with type 1 diabetes. Levine et al. [16] examined predictors of glycemic control in 300 youth 7 to 16 years of age with type 1 diabetes who were receiving diabetes specialty care and were followed prospectively for up to 1 year. Incidence rates for adverse outcomes were compared among strata representing tertiles of baseline HbA_{1c}. Blood glucose monitoring (BGM) frequency was the sole modifiable predictor of HbA_{1c} ($P < 0.0001$). Incidence rate of hospitalization was 13/100 person-years, 3 times the general pediatric population. The hospitalization rate was higher in the upper HbA_{1c} tertile ($P = 0.001$). Rate of emergency department use was 29 per 100 person-years and did not differ among tertiles. Incidence of severe hypoglycemia was 62 per100 person-years and high even in those with poorest glycemic control. This study indicates how important it is to encourage blood glucose testing and to strive for reduction in HbA_{1c} levels. (Adapted from Levine et al. [16].)

Diabetes care plan for _____ (name of student) _____ **School** _____ **Effective dates:** _____

To be completed by parents/health care team and reviewed with necessary school staff. Copies should be kept in student's classrooms and school records.

Date of birth: _____ **Grade** _____ **Homeroom teacher:** _____

Contact information _____

Parent/guardian #1: _____ Address: _____

    Telephone-Home: _____ Work: _____ Cell phone: _____

Parent/guardian #2: _____ Address: _____

    Telephone-Home: _____ Work: _____ Cell phone: _____

Student's doctor/health care provider: _____ Telephone: _____

    Nurse educator: _____ Telephone: _____

Other emergency contact: _____ Relationship: _____

    Telephone-Home: _____ Work: _____ Cell phone: _____

Notify parent/guardian in the following situations: _____

Blood glucose monitoring

Target range for blood glucose: _____ mg/dL to _____ mg/dL   Type of blood glucose meter student uses: _____

Usual times to test blood glucose: _____

Times to do extra tests (check all that apply):   _____ Before exercise _____ When student exhibits symptoms of hyperglycemia

         _____ After exercise _____ When student exhibits symptoms of hypoglycemia

         _____ Other (explain): _____

Can student perform own blood glucose tests?   Yes   No   Exceptions: _____

School personnel trained to monitor blood glucose level and dates of training: _____

Insulin

Times, types, and dosages of insulin injections to be given during school:

Time	Type(s)	Dosage
_____	_____	_____
_____	_____	_____
_____	_____	_____

School personnel trained to assist with insulin injection and dates of training: _____

Can student give own injections?   Yes   No

Can student determine correct amount of insulin?   Yes   No

Can student draw correct dose of insulin?   Yes   No

For students with insulin pumps

Type of pump: _____

Insulin/carbohydrate ratio: _____

Correction factor: _____

Is student competent regarding pump?   Yes   No

Can student effectively troubleshoot problems (eg, ketosis, pump malfunction)?   Yes   No

Comments: _____

Meals and snacks eaten at school (The carbohydrate content of the food is important in maintaining a stable blood glucose level.)

	Time	Food content/amount
Breakfast	_____	_____
AM snack	_____	_____
Lunch	_____	_____
PM snack	_____	_____
Dinner	_____	_____

Snack before exercise?   Yes   No

Snack after exercise?   Yes   No

Other times to give snacks and content/amount: _____

A source of glucose, such as _____ should be readily available at all times.

Preferred snack foods: _____

Foods to avoid, if any: _____

Instructions for when food is provided to the class, eg, as part of a class party or food sampling _____

Hypoglycemia (low blood sugar)

Usual symptoms of hypoglycemia: _____

Treatment of hypoglycemia: _____

School personnel trained to administer glucagon and dates of training: _____

Glucagon should be given if the student is unconscious, having a seizure (convulsion), or unable to swallow. If required, glucagon should be administered promptly and then 911 (or other emergency assistance) and parents should be called.

Hyperglycemia (high blood sugar)

Usual symptoms of hyperglycemia: _____

Treatment of hyperglycemia: _____

Circumstances when urine ketones should be tested: _____

Treatment for ketones: _____

Exercise and sports

A snack such as _____ should be readily available at the site of exercise or sports.

Restrictions on activity, if any: _____

Student should not exercise if blood glucose is below _____ mg/dL.

Supplies and personnel

Location of supplies: Blood glucose monitoring equipment: _____ Insulin administration supplies: _____

        Glucagon emergency kit: _____ Ketone testing supplies: _____

        Snack foods: _____

Personnel trained in the symptoms and treatment of low and high blood sugar and dates of training: _____

Signatures

Reviewed by: _____ [student's health provider/date] Acknowledged/received by: _____ [guardian/date] Acknowledged/received by _____ [school representative]

FIGURE 17-11. (Continued on next page)

FIGURE 17-11. *(Continued from opposite page)*
Diabetes in the school and day care center. Approximately 125,000 children of school age in the United States have diabetes. For these young people to be able to attend school or day care, the staff must be knowledgeable about diabetes to be able to provide a safe environment. Parents and the health care team must work in concert to give personnel the information, training, and equipment to allow children with diabetes to participate fully and safely in the school experience and to be in compliance with federal laws that protect these children. The Rehabilitation Act of 1973, the Individuals with Disabilities Education Act of 1991, and the Americans with Disabilities Act of 1992 make it illegal for schools to discriminate against children with special needs. Any school that receives federal funding or is considered open to the public reasonably must accommodate the special needs of children with diabetes with as little disruption to the routine of the school and child as possible, allowing for full participation in all school activities. To ensure this, general guidelines explaining the responsibilities of the parent or guardian, the school or day care provider, the health care team, and the student have been put forth in a Position Statement issued by the American Diabetes Association. Key to the successful implementation of these guidelines is the development of an individualized diabetes care plan that provides specific instructions regarding blood glucose monitoring, insulin administration, recognizing and treating hypoglycemia and hyperglycemia, the meal plan, and testing for ketones. An example of the diabetes care plan is shown to illustrate the complexity of appropriately managing each child with diabetes in the school or day care setting [17]. *(Adapted from* [17].)

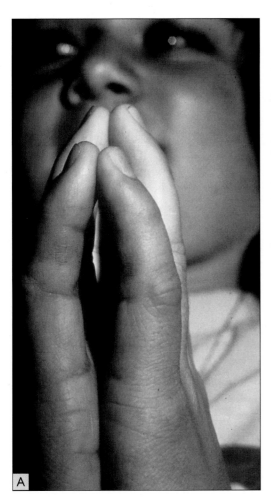

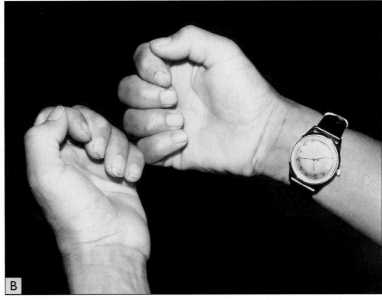

FIGURE 17-12. (See Color Plate) Limited joint mobility: changes in frequency and severity in children with type 1 diabetes between 1976 and 1978 and in 1998. **A, B,** Limited joint mobility (LJM) is the earliest long-term complication of type 1 diabetes in children and youth. It is a risk indicator for microvascular complications and its appearance is primarily affected by long-term metabolic control [18]. Staging for LMJ is as follows: Stage 0: no stiffness or contractures; Stage 1: stiffness of fingers only; Stage 2: stiffness and contractures only of the fifth fingers bilaterally; Stage 3: stiffness and contractures of more than just the fifth fingers bilaterally; Stage 4: stiffness and contractures of the fingers plus the wrists; and Stage 5: spine, neck, and other joints also involved. Limited joint mobility has decreased in prevalence and severity over the last 20 years. In 1998, 312 subjects, 7 to 18 years of age, were examined using the same methods as the 515 subjects in this age group who were examined between 1976 and 1978 [19]. The 1998 cohort was found to have a greater than fourfold reduction in frequency of limited joint mobility (31%) compared to the 1976–1978 cohort (7%). There was a decrease in the proportion of patients with moderate or severe limited joint mobility as well, from 35% to 9%. This decrease in limited joint mobility most likely is the result of improved blood glucose control since the early 1980s [18,19].

COMPONENTS OF THE OUTPATIENT VISIT

Assess

Frequency, causes, and severity of hypoglycemia or hyperglycemia

Results of home glucose monitoring from logbooks and blood glucose meter downloads

Self-adjustments made to diabetes regimen

Integration of home care management behavior, understanding of diabetes management plan and goals

Education assessment and needs

Review of systems for intercurrent problems or diabetes complications

Current medications

Psychosocial issues

Changes in life situations

School performance, after school, weekend, and sports activities

Risk-taking behavior, particularly for adolescents

Physical examination	**Frequency/ recommendations**
Weight, height, BMI	Every 3 mo, assess changes in percentile
Tanner stage	Every 3 mo, note pubertal progression
Blood pressure	Every 3 mo, target < 90th percentile
Eye	Dilated fundoscopic exam every 12 mo after 5 y of diabetes
Thyroid	Every 3 mo, presence of goiter, signs of thyroid dysfunction
Abdomen	Every 3 mo, presence of hepatomegaly, fullness, signs of malabsorption, inflammation
Foot, peripheral pulses	Every 3 mo, inspection; after age 12 y, thorough examination for sensation, pulses, vibration yearly
Skin, joints, injection sites	Every 3 mo, injection sites, joint mobility, lesions associated with diabetes
Neurologic	Every 12 mo, signs of autonomic changes, pain, neuropathy
Laboratory examination	**Frequency**
HbA$_{1c}$	Every 3 mo
Microalbuminuria	Every 12 mo after puberty or after 5 y with diabetes
Urinalysis, creatinine	At presentation and with signs or renal problems
Lipid profile	At diagnosis and every 12 mo
Thyroid function tests	Every 12 mo
Celiac screen	At time of diagnosis, if symptoms, at puberty
Islet antibodies	At diagnosis

FIGURE 17-13. Components of the outpatient visit. Pediatric patients with diabetes should have comprehensive, multidisciplinary outpatient visits at regular intervals [20,21]. The purpose of these visits is to assess health status, to adjust the diabetes regimen as indicated, to promote diabetes knowledge and competency, and to motivate patients and families to improve short-term and long-term outcomes. Diabetes health care providers should insure that the patient receives routine pediatric care to diagnose and treat other medical and psychologic problems and to administer immunizations and anticipatory guidance. At quarterly visits, HbA$_{1c}$ levels should be measured. The results should be available at the time of the clinic visit to allow for a face-to-face discussion if glycemic targets are not met. Thyroid function testing should be done yearly. Thyroid autoantibodies are present in 20% to 30% of pediatric patients with type 1 diabetes; however, overt hypothyroidism occurs in 1% to 5% and compensated hypothyroidism in 5% to 10%. A fasting lipid profile that includes total cholesterol, high-density lipoprotein cholesterol, low-density lipoprotein cholesterol, and triglycerides should be obtained in children and adolescents after glucose control has been established. Microalbumin levels can be measured using a random microalbumin-to-creatinine ratio, timed overnight microalbumin assay-to-albumin excretion rate assessment, or 24-hour timed urinary microalbumin-to-albumin excretion rate measurement. Celiac disease has been reported to occur 10 to 50 times more often in children with diabetes when compared to the general population. Depending on the study, celiac disease may be present in 1% to 10% of children and adolescents with type 1 diabetes. Celiac disease should be considered in children and youth with gastrointestinal symptoms such as diarrhea, pain, flatulence, dyspepsia, or apthous ulcers. Unexplained hypoglycemia, dermatitis herpetiformis, and delayed growth or pubertal development can also be associated with celiac disease. A celiac screen, including anti-endomysial IgA antibody quantitation, should be obtained. At the time of diagnosis, patients should have liver function tests, a serum creatinine test, and urinalysis. Assessment of islet autoimmunity should be made by obtaining specific antibodies to islet antigens. BMI—body mass index.

Adjustment to Childhood Diabetes

PSYCHOSOCIAL ISSUES IN PEDIATRIC DIABETES

Psychosocial Factors Affecting Initial Diabetes Management

Patient's and family's adjustment to losses and uncertainties inherent in diagnosis

Cultural and health beliefs competing with treatment requirements

Emotional reactions to diabetes-specific tasks and complications (fear of injections, BGM, responses to hypo- and hyperglycemia, long-term complications)

Psychiatric and social problems preceding diagnosis

Community and social support surrounding the family

Relationship and communication with health care team

Financial resources for treatment and access to good caretakers

Important Factors in Psychosocial Management

Self-care tasks appropriate to maturity rather than age

Complete supervision in children, discrete supervision in adolescents

Avoidance of extremes of overprotection or total independence

Clear attribution and sharing of responsibilities among family members and patients

Realistic treatment goals according to the patient's acceptance

Empathic understanding of the stresses of living with diabetes

Encouragement of open communication and venting of negative feelings about diabetes

Recognition of diabetes burnout

Problem-solving skills practiced regularly

Help from mental health professionals if necessary

Focus on overall success: age-appropriate developmental skills, adequate social and family relationships, good glycemic control

FIGURE 17-14. Psychosocial issues in pediatric diabetes. The majority of patients diagnosed with diabetes exhibit mild depression, anxiety, and somatic complaints at the time of diagnosis [22]. In most cases, these symptoms are usually self-limited and resolve within 6 to 9 months. However, in a subset of patients, depressive symptoms increase over time and anxiety worsens, more often in girls than boys. Patient adjustment to diabetes at the time of diagnosis predicts later adjustment. The psychosocial factors affecting initial diabetes management are shown. Family characteristics have a major influence on adjustment to diabetes, self-management, and quality of life. Children and adolescents living in families with a high degree of conflict or with parents who are less caring have less optimal metabolic control. To improve psychologic stability and glycemic control, early assessment of family dynamics and, when appropriate, intervention should be done by a multidisciplinary diabetes team equipped to provide social and psychologic support. BGM—blood glucose monitoring.

A. SKILLS, KNOWLEDGE, AND ATTITUDES NEEDED TO USE CSII, BY AGE*

Age, y	Skills	Knowledge/attitude
6–10	Insert pump catheter, wear pump with help	Agree to wear the pump
	Unhook and rehook with help	Know how to protect the pump during activity
	Activate bolus with supervision	
10–12	Protect pump during daily activities without help	Know how to do carbohydrate count
	Unhook and rehook without help	Understand role of exercise
	Activate bolus without assistance	Start to circulate correction dose
12–14	Suspend basal dose	Calculate and deliver bolus dose
	Program basal rates with assistance	Understand need for temporary basal change
	Suspend basal dose	
	Program basal rates with assistance	
15–18	Program change in basal rate	Determine factors that affect basal/bolus, use algorithms
		Understand sick-day protocol

*All patients using CSII must monitor blood glucose 3 to 4 times per day, use insulin algorithms, perform carbohydrate counts, and try the infusion catheter.

FIGURE 17-15. Continuous subcutaneous insulin infusion in pediatrics. Continuous subcutaneous insulin infusion (CSII) has been found to be of benefit to children and youth with diabetes [15,18]. **A,** Criteria for initiating CSII vary at different pediatric centers, but the major criterion for adolescents is the desire to maximize basal/bolus therapy with CSII. Other reasons include frequent hypoglycemia, "dawn" phenomenon, desire for lifestyle flexibility, recurrent diabetic ketoacidosis, and diabetes difficult to control with conventional therapy. To use pump treatment successfully, patients and families must have sufficient knowledge and skills and the appropriate attitudes to manage the technology [23]. In preschool and early school-aged children, the tasks required are done by the parent or guardian. As the child matures, pump management is gradually assumed by the patient, so that by late adolescence, the child can assume responsibility for CSII.

(Continued on next page)

B. CSII THERAPY IN PEDIATRICS

Time	Mean HbA₁c, %	P Value
Pump initiation	8.4±1.8	
3 mo	7.8±1.2	0.006
1 y	8.2±0.9	0.05
2 y	8.1±1.1	0.04

FIGURE 17-15. (Continued) **B,** A decrease in HbA₁c can be expected in pediatric subjects on insulin pump therapy. In a cohort of 83 patients on insulin pump therapy with a mean age of 13.6 ± 3.9 years and a mean diabetes duration of 5.3 ± 3.2 years, a significant drop in HbA₁c after 3 months of pump therapy was sustained for 1 and 2 years [23]. (*Panel A adapted from* Kaufman and Halvorson [15].)

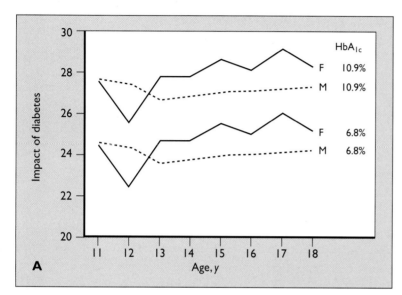

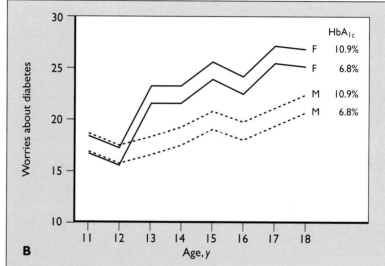

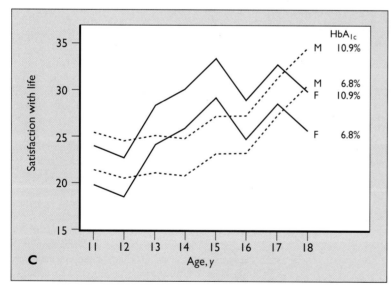

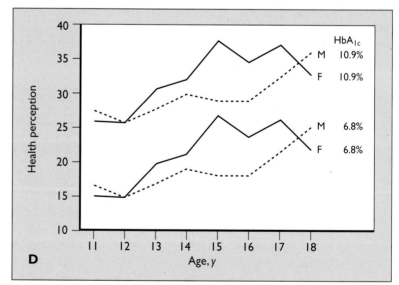

FIGURE 17-16. Metabolic control and quality of life. It is unclear whether the demands of good metabolic control or the consequences of poor control have a greater influence on the quality of life of adolescents with type 1 diabetes. The Diabetes Quality of Life (DQOL) questionnaire was given to 2101 patients, 10–18 years of age, to measure the impact of diabetes, worries about diabetes, satisfaction with life, and health perception [24]. **A–D,** The mean HbA₁c of the group was 8.7%, but those with lower HbA₁c were found to be less impacted by diabetes ($P < 0.0001$) and have fewer worries ($P < 0.05$), greater satisfaction ($P < 0.0001$), and better health perception ($P < 0.0001$). Girls demonstrated increased worries ($P < 0.01$), less satisfaction ($P < 0.01$), and poorer health perception ($P < 0.01$) earlier than boys. Lower HbA₁c was significantly associated with better adolescent-rated quality of life; therefore, improved glycemic control should be encouraged as not only a means to prevent the long-term complications of diabetes, but to lessen the psychologic burden of the disease as well.

Type 2 Diabetes in Children and Youth: a New Epidemic

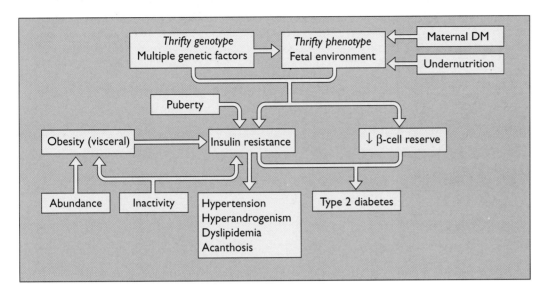

FIGURE 17-17. Associations between insulin resistance and type 2 diabetes in children. Type 2 diabetes in children and adolescents is due to insulin resistance and puts subjects at risk for hyperandrogenism (polycystic ovary syndrome), hypertension, dyslipidemia, and other atherosclerosis risk factors [25,26]. Risk factors for type 2 diabetes include obesity, family history, diabetic gestation, and underweight or overweight for gestational age. Limited β-cell reserve plays a role in progression to frank diabetes. DM—diabetes mellitus. (*Adapted from* Silverstein and Rosenbloom [27].)

TESTING FOR TYPE 2 DIABETES IN CHILDREN

Criteria

Overweight (BMI > 85th percentile for age and sex, weight for height > 85th percentile, or weight > 120% ideal for height)

Plus

Any two of the following risk factors:

Family history of type 2 diabetes in first- or second-degree relative

Race/ethnicity (American Indian, black, Hispanic, Asian/Pacific islander)

Signs of insulin resistance or conditions associated with insulin resistance (acanthosis nigricans, hypertension, dyslipidemia, PCOS)

Age of Initiation

Age 10 years or at onset of puberty if puberty occurs at a younger age

Frequency

Every 2 years

Test

Fasting plasma glucose preferred

FIGURE 17-18. Case finding for type 2 diabetes in children. The American Diabetes Association consensus statement for type 2 diabetes in children and adolescents, which was endorsed by the American Academy of Pediatrics, recommended that overweight children and adolescents with two or more risk factors for type 2 diabetes be tested every 2 years beginning at 10 years of age or at the onset of puberty [26]. BMI—body mass index; PCOS—polycystic ovary syndrome.

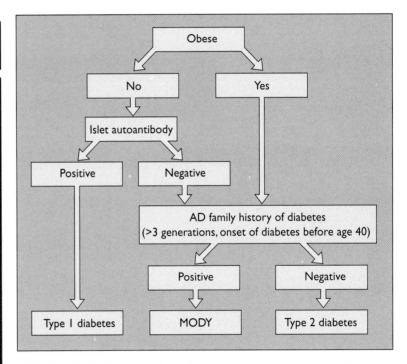

FIGURE 17-19. Research schema for classification of diabetes in children and adolescents to determine the presence of type 2 diabetes. Between 50% to 90% of youth with type 2 diabetes have a body mass index greater than 27 kg/m² or are above the 85th percentile for age. Those children who are obese and have a high fasting C-peptide or insulin level are presumed to have type 2 disease. Autoantibodies should be measured in obese children with low fasting C-peptide or insulin levels. If they are present, the patient likely has type 1 diabetes. If autoantibodies are absent, the patient could have idiopathic diabetes or maturity-onset diabetes of youth (MODY). In nonobese children and adolescents, the presence of autoantibodies indicates type 1 diabetes. Nonobese children with absent antibodies should have C-peptide and insulin levels assessed. If these levels are high, the patient likely has type 2 diabetes; if low, the patient may have idiopathic diabetes or MODY. The final diagnostic classification may require following the patient's clinical course for a few years after diagnosis. AD—autosomal dominant. (*Adapted from* [26].)

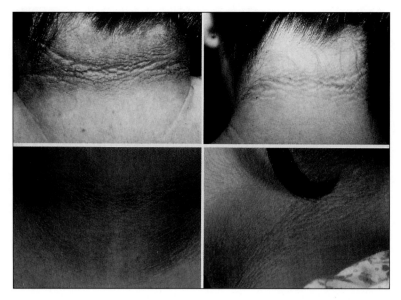

FIGURE 17-20. (See Color Plate) Acanthosis nigricans. Acanthosis nigricans is a marker of insulin resistance frequently associated with type 2 diabetes; 60% to 90% of youth with type 2 diabetes have acanthosis nigricans. The skin is hyperpigmented in intertriginous areas. In a survey by Stuart *et al.* [28] of 1412 students, 7.1% had acanthosis nigricans. The prevalence was highest in black students (13.3%), followed by Hispanics (5.5%) and whites (0.5%). Acanthosis nigricans is highly associated with obesity. The prevalence of diabetes is six times higher in black patients with acanthosis than it is in blacks without this skin lesion. Because acanthosis nigricans is associated with diabetes so highly, it may be used as a screening tool to help identify those at high risk for type 2 diabetes. (*From* Stuart *et al.* [28].)

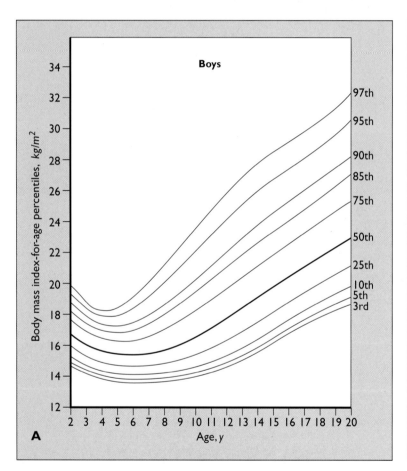

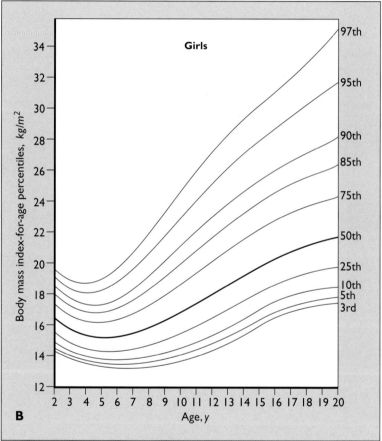

FIGURE 17-21. Body mass index (BMI) growth charts. Children and adolescents should be plotted on BMI-for-age percentile charts. Those with BMI above the 85th percentile are at risk for type 2 diabetes. **A**, BMI chart for boys, 2 to 20 years of age. **B**, BMI chart for girls, 2 to 20 years of age. (*Adapted from* [29].)

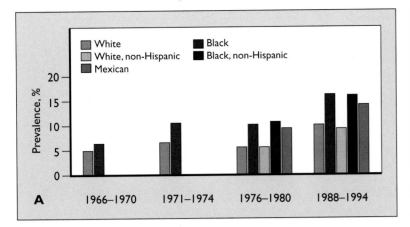

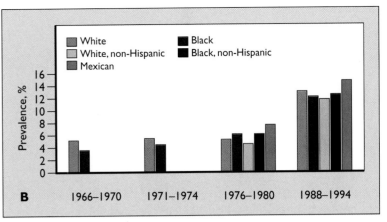

FIGURE 17-22. Prevalence of obesity in adolescents. There has been a marked increase in the prevalence of obesity in girls and boys across all ethnic groups, except white girls, since 1966. The rise in type 2 diabetes in youth mirrors the rise in obesity. **A,** Trends in prevalence of overweight in girls 12 to 17 years of age. **B,** Trends in prevalence of overweight in boys 12 to 17 years of age. Obesity is defined as body mass index at or above the sex- and age-specific 95th percentile. (*Adapted from* [30].)

USE OF METFORMIN IN PEDIATRIC PATIENTS AFTER TYPE 2 DIABETES

	Metformin	Placebo	Difference (Metformin vs Placebo)
Baseline mean FPG (mmol/L)	9.0±2.7	10.7±2.7	
Last double-blind visit mean FPG (mmol/L)	7.0±2.2	11.5±4.5	
Adjusted mean* FPG change from baseline (mmol/L)	-2.4±0.5	1.2±0.5	-3.6±0.8
95% CI	-3.5 to -1.3	0.1 to 2.3	5.1 to -2.0
$P^{\dagger}$			< 0.001‡
Baseline mean HbA_{1c}, %	8.2±1.3	8.9±1.4	
	7.2±1.2	8.9±1.6	
Adjusted mean* HbA_{1c}, %	7.5±0.2	8.6±0.2	-1.2±0.2
95% CI	(7.2–7.8)	(8.3–9.0)	(-1.6–-0.7)
$P^{\S}$			< 0.001

*Mean adjusted for baseline FPG or for baseline HbA_{1c}.

† The P value is based on an ANCOVA, comparing metformin to placebo using baseline FPG as the covariate and treatment as the main effect.

‡Significance level P < 0.03355, where the testwise critical value was adjusted for an 8-week interim analysis of FPG, to preserve an overall α level of ≤0/05 using the O'Brien-Fleming method with an α of 0.025 at the interim analysis.

§P value is based on an ANCOVA, comparing metformin to placebo using baseline HbA_{1c} as the covariate and treatment as the main effect.

FIGURE 17-23. Use of metformin in pediatric patients with type 2 diabetes. Metformin is the first oral agent to be proven safe and effective for the treatment of type 2 diabetes in pediatric subjects. It is the first oral hypoglycemic agent to gain Food and Drug Association approval for type treatment of type 2 diabetes in children. A multicenter study evaluated 82 patients with doses of metformin up to 1000 mg twice daily [31]. Subjects were between 10 and 16 years of age and were treated for up to 16 weeks in a randomized double-blind placebo-controlled trial. Entry criteria were a fasting plasma glucose (FPG) of 126 or higher and 240 mg/dL or lower and HbA_{1c} of 7.0% or greater and C-peptide of 0.5 nmol/L or greater. Subjects had a body mass index above the 50th percentile for age. Metformin showed a beneficial effect when compared to placebo. Improvement in fasting plasma glucose occurred in both sexes and all race groups. Metformin did not have a negative impact on body weight or lipid profile, and the adverse events were similar to those seen in adults. (*Adapted from* Jones et al. [31].)

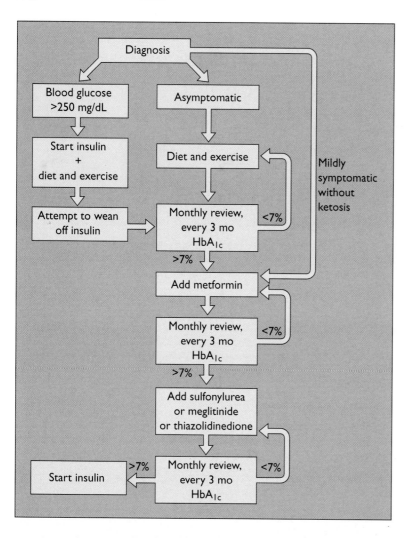

FIGURE 17-24. Treatment of type 2 diabetes in children. The treatment of type 2 diabetes in pediatric patients must include diabetes education for both the family and patient, with emphasis on the importance of regular exercise and appropriate nutrition. Glycemic targets should be established. Maintaining HbA_{1c} below 7.0% and fasting plasma glucose levels as near to 126 mg/dL as possible is difficult in adolescents [27,31]. (*Adapted from* Silverstein and Rosenbloom [27].)

References

1. American Diabetes Association: Hyperglycemic crises in patients with diabetes mellitus. *Diabetes Care* 2001, 24:1992.

2. Glaser N, Barnett P, McCaslin I, *et al.*: Risk factors for cerebral edema in children with diabetic ketoacidosis. *N Engl J Med* 2001, 344:264–269.

3. Roe TF, Crawford TO, Huff KR, *et al.*: Brain infarction in children with diabetic ketoacidosis. *J Diabetes Complications* 1996, 2:100–108.

4. The International Society for Pediatric and Adolescent Diabetes (ISPAD) Consensus Guidelines for the Management of Type 1 Diabetes Mellitus in Children and Adolescents, 2000, Medical Forum International, The Netherlands.

5. Kaufman FR, Halvorson M: The treatment and prevention of diabetic ketoacidosis in children and adolescents with type 1 diabetes mellitus. *Pediatric Annals* 1999, 28:9.

6. Karvonen M, Viik-Kajander M, Moltchanova E, *et al.*: Incidence of child-hood type 1 diabetes worldwide. *Diabetes Care* 2000, 23:1516–1526.

7. Diabetes Control and Complications Trial Research Group: Effect of intensive diabetes treatment in the development and progression of long-term complications in adolescents with insulin-dependent diabetes. *J Pediatr* 1994, 125:177–188.

8. Kaufman FR: Diabetes in children and adolescents: prevention and treatment of diabetes and its complications. *Med Clin North Am* 1998, 82:721–738.

9. White NH, Cleary PA, Dahms W, *et al.*: Beneficial effects of intensive therapy of diabetes during adolescence: outcomes after the conclusion of the Diabetes Control and Complications Trial (DCCT). *J Pediatr* 2001, 139:804–812.

10. Donaghue KC, Fung ATW, Hing S, *et al.*: The effect of prepubertal diabetes duration on diabetes: microvascular complication in early and late adolescence. *Diabetes Care* 1997, 20:77–80.

11. Buckingham BA, Bluck B, Wilson DM: Intensive diabetes management in pediatric patients. *Curr Diabetes Rep* 2001, 1:111–118.

12. Kaufman FR, Halvorson M, Carpenter S: Use of a plastic insulin dosage guide to correct blood glucose levels out of the target range and for carbohydrate counting in subjects with type 1 diabetes. *Diabetes Care* 1999, 22:1252–1257.

13. Chase HP, Kim LM, Owen SL, *et al.*: Continuous subcutaneous glucose monitoring in children with type 1 diabetes. *Pediatrics* 2002, 107:222–226.

14. Kaufman FR, Halvorson M, Carpenter S, *et al.*: Insulin pump therapy in young children with diabetes. *Diabetes Spectrum* 2001, 14:84–89.

15. Kaufman FR, Gibson LC, Halvorson M, *et al.*: A pilot study of the continuous glucose monitoring system. *Diabetes Care* 2001, 24:2030–2034.

16. Levine BS, Anderson BJ, Butler DA, *et al.*: Predictors of glycemic control and short-term adverse outcomes in youth with type 1 diabetes. *J Pediatr* 2001, 139:197–203.

17. Care of children with diabetes in the school and day care setting. American Diabetes Association. *Diabetes Care* 1999, 22:163–166.

18. Brink SJ: Limited Joint Mobility. In *Pediatric and Adolescent Diabetes Mellitus*. Edited by Brink SJ. Chicago: Year Book Medical Publishers; 1987:305–312.

19. Infante JR, Rosenbloom AL, Silverstein JH, *et al.*: Changes in frequency and severity of limited joint mobility in children with type 1 diabetes mellitus between 1976–1978 and 1998. *J Pediatr* 2001, 138:33–37.

20. The American Diabetes Association Clinical Practice Recommendations for 2001. *Diabetes Care* 24:S1–S126.

21. Kaufman FR, Halvorson M: New trends in managing type 1 diabetes. *Contemp Pediatr* 1999, 16:112–123.

22. Schiffrin A: Psychosocial issues in pediatric diabetes. *Curr Diabetes Rep* 2001, 1:33–40.

23. Kaufman FR, Halvorson M, Miller D, *et al.*: Insulin pump therapy in type 1 pediatric patients: now and into the year 2000. *Diabetes Metab Res Rev* 1999, 15:338–352.

24. Hoey H, Aanstoot HJ, Chiarelli F, *et al.*: Good metabolic control is associated with better quality of life in 2,101 adolescents with type 1 diabetes. *Diabetes Care* 2001, 24:1923–1928.

25. Silverstein JH, Rosenbloom AL: Type 2 diabetes in children. *Curr Diabetes Rep* 2001, 1:19–27.

26. Type 2 diabetes in children and adolescents. American Diabetes Association. *Diabetes Care* 2000, 23:381–389.

27. Silverstein JH, Rosenbloom AL: Treatment of type 2 diabetes mellitus in children and adolescents. *J Pediatr Endocrinol Metab* 2000, 13:1402–1409.

28. Stuart CA, Pate CJ, Peters EJ: Prevalence of acanthosis nigricans in an unselected population. *Am J Med* 1989, 87:269–272.

29. CDC Body mass index-for-age percentiles. Available at: http://www.cdc.gov/nchs/about/major/nhanes/growthcharts/set1. Accessed April 23, 2001.

30. CDC/National Center for Health Statistics. Prevalence of overweight among children and adolescents. Available at: http://www.cdc.gov/nchs/products/pubs/pubd/hestats/overwght99.htm. Accessed April 23, 2002.

31. Jones KL, Arslanian S, Peterokova VA, *et al.*: Effect of metformin in pediatric patients with type 2 diabetes. *Diabetes Care* 2002, 25:89–94.

Index

Color Plates

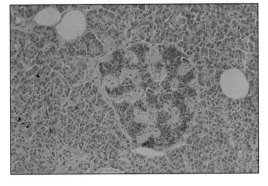

FIGURE 1-20. Page 11

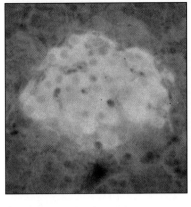

FIGURE 3-2A. Page 28

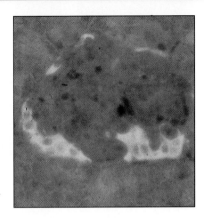

FIGURE 3-2B. Page 28

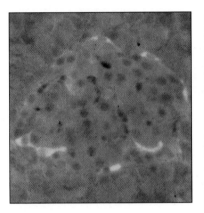

FIGURE 3-2C. Page 28

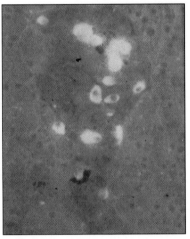

FIGURE 3-2D. Page 28

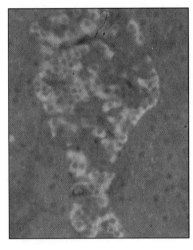

FIGURE 3-2E. Page 28

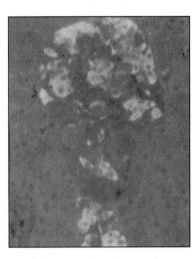

FIGURE 3-2F. Page 28

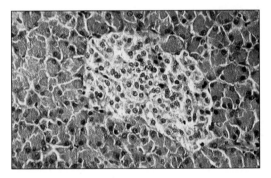

FIGURE 3-4A. Page 30

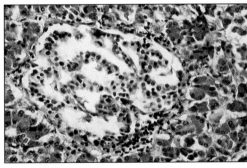

FIGURE 3-4B. Page 30

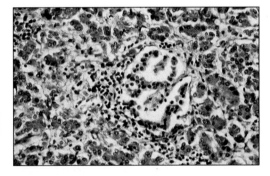

FIGURE 3-4C. Page 30

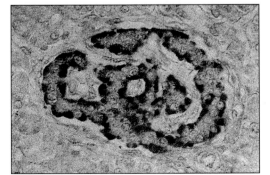

FIGURE 4-11C. Page 48

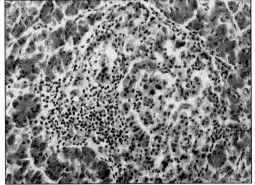

FIGURE 4-11D. Page 49

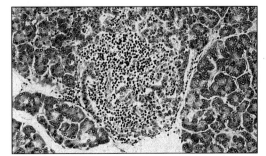

FIGURE 4-12. Page 49

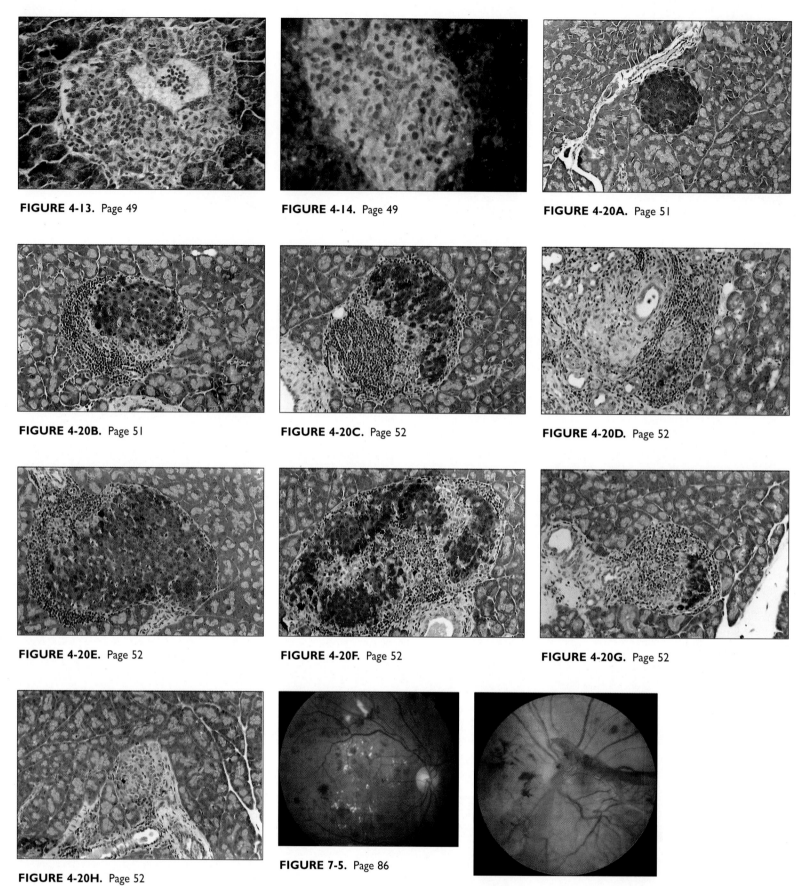

FIGURE 4-13. Page 49

FIGURE 4-14. Page 49

FIGURE 4-20A. Page 51

FIGURE 4-20B. Page 51

FIGURE 4-20C. Page 52

FIGURE 4-20D. Page 52

FIGURE 4-20E. Page 52

FIGURE 4-20F. Page 52

FIGURE 4-20G. Page 52

FIGURE 4-20H. Page 52

FIGURE 7-5. Page 86

FIGURE 7-6. Page 87

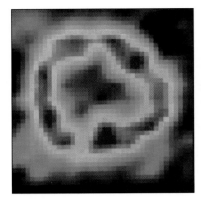

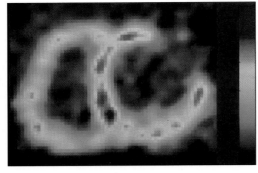

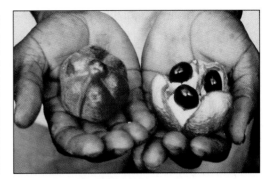

FIGURE 8-9A. Page 100

FIGURE 8-9B. Page 100

FIGURE 9-6. Page 116

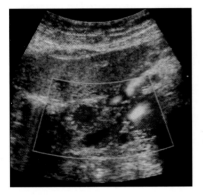

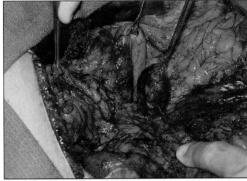

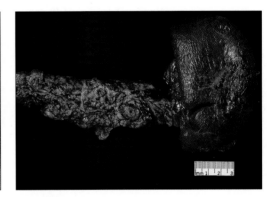

FIGURE 9-14. Page 118

FIGURE 9-18. Page 119

FIGURE 9-19. Page 120

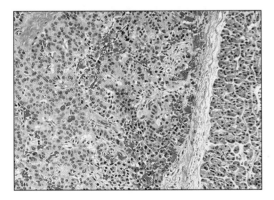

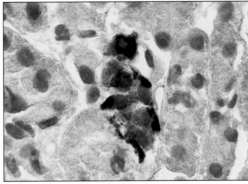

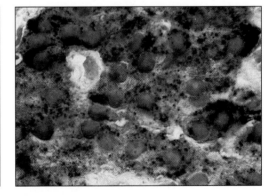

FIGURE 9-20. Page 120

FIGURE 9-21A. Page 120

FIGURE 9-21B. Page 120

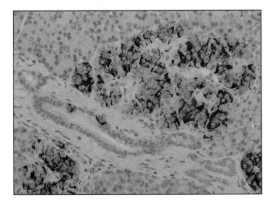

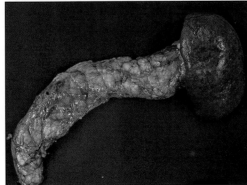

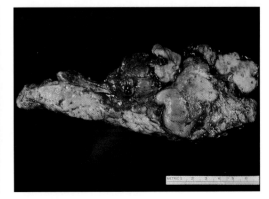

FIGURE 9-22. Page 121

FIGURE 9-23. Page 121

FIGURE 9-24. Page 121

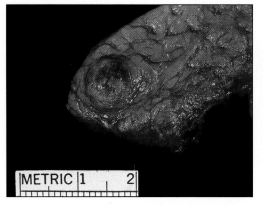

FIGURE 9-25. Page 121

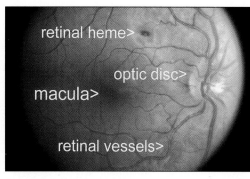

retinal heme>

optic disc>

macula>

retinal vessels>

FIGURE 11-7A. Page 142

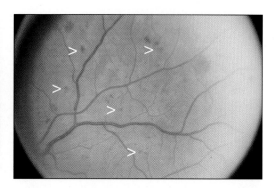

FIGURE 11-7B. Page 142

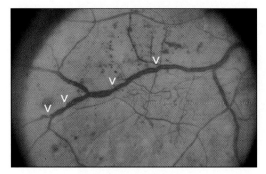

FIGURE 11-7C. Page 143

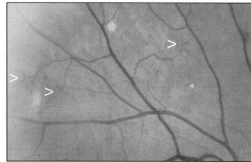

FIGURE 11-7D. Page 143

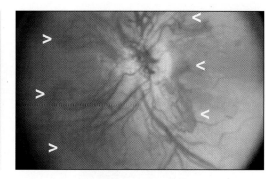

FIGURE 11-9A. Page 144

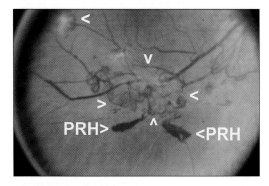

PRH>   <PRH

FIGURE 11-9B. Page 144

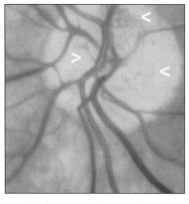

FIGURE 11-9C. Page 144

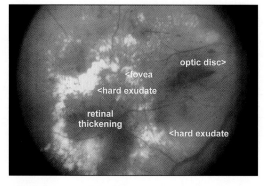

optic disc>

<fovea

<hard exudate

retinal
thickening

<hard exudate

FIGURE 11-10B. Page 144

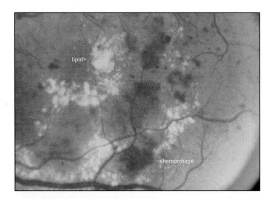

lipid>

<hemorrhage

FIGURE 11-12B. Page 145

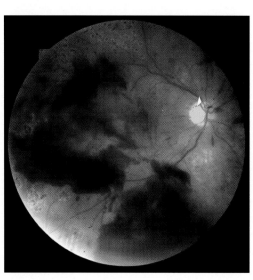

FIGURE 11-12C. Page 146

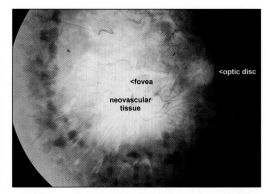

<optic disc

<fovea

neovascular
tissue

FIGURE 11-12D. Page 146

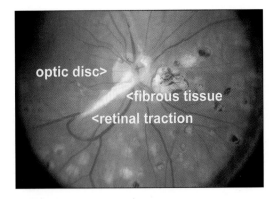

FIGURE 11-13A. Page 146

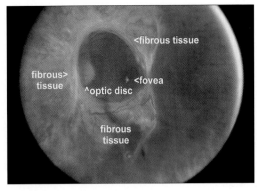

FIGURE 11-13B. Page 146

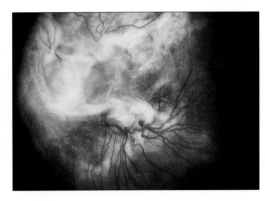

FIGURE 11-13C. Page 147

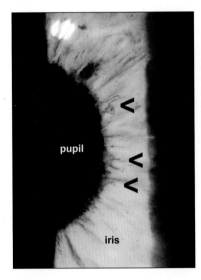

FIGURE 11-14A. Page 147

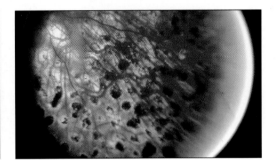

FIGURE 11-15A. Page 148

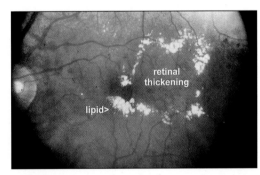

FIGURE 11-15B. Page 148

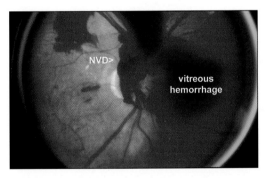

FIGURE 11-15C. Page 148

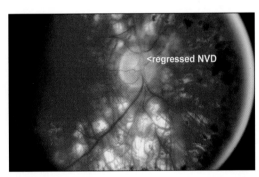

FIGURE 11-15D. Page 148

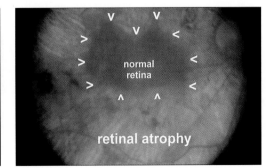

FIGURE 11-16A. Page 149

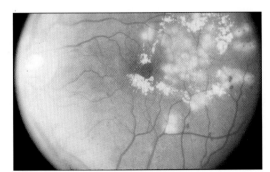

FIGURE 11-16C. Page 149

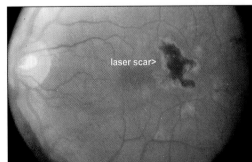

FIGURE 11-16D. Page 149

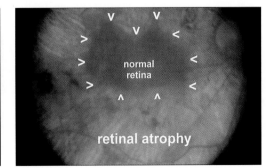

FIGURE 11-18A. Page 150

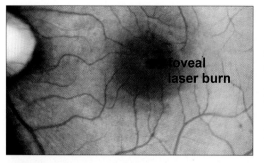

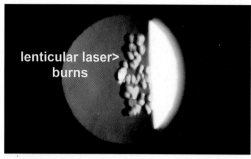

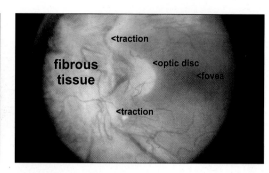

FIGURE 11-18C. Page 151

FIGURE 11-18D. Page 151

FIGURE 11-19B. Page 151

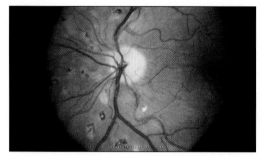

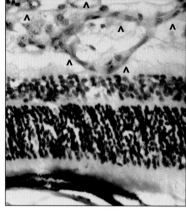

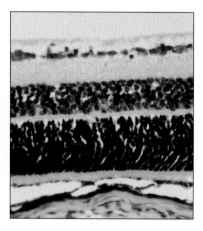

FIGURE 11-19C. Page 151

FIGURE 11-23A. Page 153

FIGURE 11-23B. Page 153

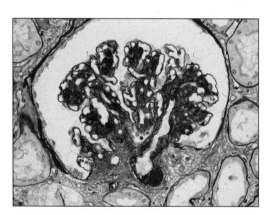

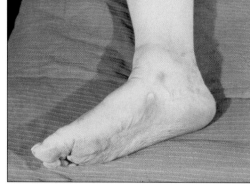

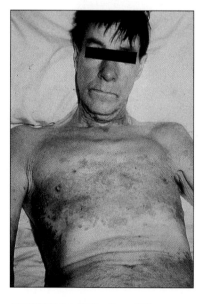

FIGURE 12-6A. Page 159

FIGURE 13-21. Page 178

FIGURE 14-10A. Page 189

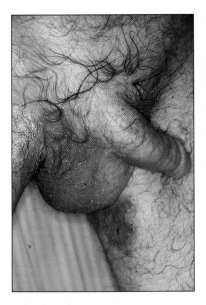

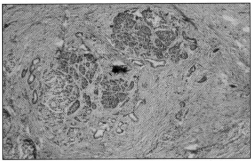

FIGURE 14-16. Page 192

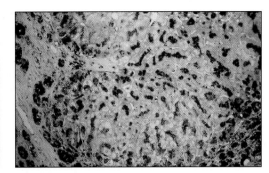

FIGURE 14-17A. Page 192

FIGURE 14-10B. Page 189

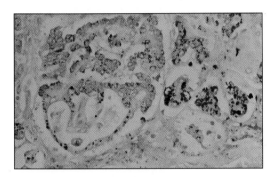

FIGURE 14-17B. Page 192

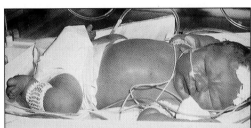

FIGURE 16-3. Page 213

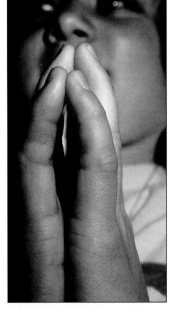

FIGURE 17-12A. Page 233

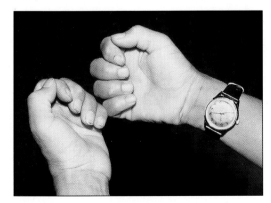

FIGURE 17-12B. Page 233

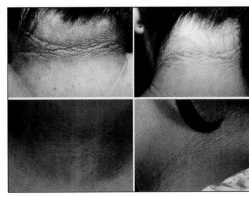

FIGURE 17-20. Page 238